T0276060

Treating Comorbid Opioid
Use Disorder in Chronic Pain

Annette M. Matthews • Jonathan C. Fellers
Editors

Treating Comorbid Opioid Use Disorder in Chronic Pain

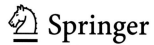 Springer

Editors
Annette M. Matthews, M.D.
Department of Psychiatry
Oregon Health and Science University
Portland, OR, USA

Department of Medical Informatics
    and Clinical Epidemiology
Oregon Health and Science University
Portland, OR, USA

Portland VA Medical Center
Portland, OR, USA

Jonathan C. Fellers, M.D.
Department of Psychiatry
Maine Medical Center
Portland, ME, USA

ISBN 978-3-319-29861-0   ISBN 978-3-319-29863-4   (eBook)
DOI 10.1007/978-3-319-29863-4

Library of Congress Control Number: 2016938003

This Springer imprint is published by Springer Nature
The registered company is Springer International Publishing AG Switzerland

Preface

Chronic noncancer pain affects more than 100 million Americans and can be caused by many conditions including osteoarthritis, low back pain, musculoskeletal pain, injury-related pathology, and diabetic neuropathy. It is estimated that the 1-month prevalence of moderate to severe noncancer pain is 19 %. Opioids can be an effective way to treat this pain, but not without risk. The goal of the book, *Treating Comorbid Opioid Use Disorder in Chronic Pain*, is to address how to approach and treat the chronic pain patient struggling with problematic opioid use.

Chronic pain serves as a conduit for problematic opioid use and addiction. Brain regions including the nucleus accumbens, the amygdala, and the hypothalamus are involved in both the mechanisms of pain and opioid dependence. The problematic use of opioids in this population can present as a range of issues including recreational use, physical dependence, pseudoaddiction, opioid-induced hyperalgesia, engagement in illicit activity, cross-addiction to street heroin, diversion, overdose, and theft. In some cases there is escalating use that may result in drug seeking from other healthcare providers or transitioning to the use of heroin or other drugs purchased on the street, to satisfy cravings. Recognizing these problematic patterns of use and developing ways to address them are important for the clinician prescribing for chronic pain.

Associated with addressing problematic use of opioids are a number of ethical, legal, and policy considerations. In the 1990s and 2000s, there was pressure on physicians by the Board of Medical Examiners and healthcare systems to aggressively treat pain with opioids and other treatments, and prescribers were sued for undertreatment. The pendulum has now swung, and prescribers' licensure can be at risk now for overprescribing. Physicians and others may, however, still find themselves trapped between legal and regulatory issues and the ethics of withholding treatment to someone in pain. Strategies for documentation and for detection of diversion can help mitigate the risk of legal issues or ethical boundary crossings.

To compound this, the healthcare system often struggles in addressing the needs of patients with chronic pain experiencing problematic opioid use. While the patient may start their pain care in primary care, he may intersect with numerous other treatment settings including the emergency room, the mental health clinic, the substance abuse clinic, and the chronic pain clinic, if it exists. As problematic use arises and is detected, it can become less clear who and where in the healthcare system the patient's pain needs are to be met. It also can become very clear that not everyone agrees on how to treat pain, or even knows how to address pain, particularly in those with problematic use of opioids.

We would like to thank Springer for offering us the opportunity to compile this volume and also our families who understood and supported the time needed to produce such a work. We are also deeply indebted to the authors of this volume, without which, it would not exist. We hope this book will provide useful information for practitioners navigating the care of the chronic pain patient who also has an opioid use disorder or other mental health problems.

Portland, OR, USA   Annette M. Matthews
Portland, ME, USA   Jonathan C. Fellers

Contents

Part II   Ethical, Legal, Regulatory, and Policy Issues

Part III   Best Practices and Practice Models

Contributors

Monica L. Broderick, M.D. Department of Psychiatry, Kings County Hospital Center/SUNY Downstate Medical Center, Brooklyn, NY, USA

Jonathan R. Buchholz, M.D. VA Puget Sound Health Care System (S-116 ATC), Seattle, WA, USA

Department of Psychiatry & Behavioral Sciences, University of Washington, Seattle, WA, USA

H. Westley Clark, M.D., J.D., M.P.H. Public Health Program, Santa Clara University, Santa Clara, CA, USA

Sandra D. Comer Division on Substance Abuse, New York Psychiatric Institute and Columbia University Medical Center, New York, NY, USA

Teni Davoudian, Ph.D. VA Portland Health Care System, Portland, OR, USA

Michael I. Demidenko, B.S. Center to Improve Veteran Involvement in Care, VA Portland Health Care System, Portland, OR, USA

Andrea R. Diulio, Ph.D. Mental Health and Clinical Neurosciences, VA Portland Health Care System, Portland, OR, USA

Andrew J. Engel, M.D. Affordable Pain Management, Chicago, IL, USA

Jonathan C. Fellers, M.D. Department of Psychiatry, Maine Medical Center, Portland, ME, USA

Marian Fireman, M.D. Department of Psychiatry, Oregon Health and Science University, Portland, OR, USA

Jeffrey Freeman, M.D. Faculty of Medicine, University of Ottawa, Ottawa, ON, Canada

Stuart Gitlow, M.D., M.P.H., M.B.A. Annenberg Physician Training Program in Addictive Disease, Woonsocket, RI, USA

Stacey Gramann, D.O., M.P.H. Mental Health Division, Portland VA Medical Center, Portland, OR, USA

Jermaine D. Jones, Ph.D. Division on Substance Abuse, New York Psychiatric Institute and Columbia University Medical Center, Portland, OR, USA

Monique M. Jones, M.D. Department of Psychiatry, Oregon Health and Science University, Portland, OR, USA

Jyothsna Karlapalem, M.B.B.S. Department of Psychiatry, SUNY Downstate Medical Center, Brooklyn, NY, USA

Kenneth L. Kirsh, Ph.D. Clinical Research and Advocacy, San Diego, CA, USA

Clinical Affairs, Millennium Health, San Diego, CA, USA

Travis I. Lovejoy, Ph.D., M.P.H. Center to Improve Veteran Involvement in Care, VA Portland Health Care System, Portland, OR, USA

Annette M. Matthews, M.D. Department of Psychiatry, Oregon Health and Science University, Portland, OR, USA

Department of Medical Informatics and Clinical Epidemiology, Oregon Health and Science University, Portland, OR, USA

Portland VA Medical Center, Portland, OR, USA

Sean W. Moore, M.D. C.M., F.R.C.P.C., F.A.C.E.P. University of Ottawa, Ottawa, ON, Canada

Northern Ontario School of Medicine, Emergency Department, Lake of the Woods District Hospital, Kenora, ON, Canada

Laura C. Moss, M.D. Hazelden Springbrook, Part of the Hazelden Betty Ford Foundation, Newberg, OR, USA

Steven D. Passik, Ph.D. Clinical Research and Advocacy, San Diego, CA, USA

Veronica L. Rodriguez, Ph.D. Mental Health and Clinical Neurosciences Division, VA Portland Health Care System, Portland, OR, USA

Andrew J. Saxon, M.D. VA Puget Sound Health Care System (S-116 ATC), Seattle, WA, USA

Department of Psychiatry & Behavioral Sciences, University of Washington, Seattle, WA, USA

Katherine A. Tacker, M.D. Department of Psychiatry, Oregon Health and Science University, Portland, OR, USA

Alicia Trigeiro, M.S. Millennium Health, San Diego, CA, USA

Mary Elizabeth Turner, M.D., J.D. Oregon Health and Science University, Portland, OR, USA

Lori A. Urban, Psy.D., A.B.P.P. Department of Anesthesiology, Pain Management, University of Virginia School of Medicine, Charlottesville, VA, USA

Michael J. Yao, M.D., M.P.H. Mental Health and Neurosciences Division, Portland VA Health Care System, Portland, OR, USA

Part I
Diagnosis and Treatment

Chapter 1
Theories of Pain and Addiction: Type of Pain, Pathways to Opiate Addiction

Jonathan C. Fellers

1.1 Introduction

Unlike other sensations that primarily inform about the environment, pain engages us at an emotional level and plays a protective role for survival. It sends a signal that nature assures we cannot ignore. Through the unpleasant experience of pain, we focus attention on the affected area and marshal our resources to prevent further injury. Take, for example, Descartes' figure of a boy with his foot too close to a fire (Fig. 1.1). First, pain leads the boy to reflexively withdraw his foot from the flame, thereby preventing further burns. Second, pain teaches the boy that this situation should be avoided in the future. And third, pain in his foot limits his activity on the affected foot, thereby enabling healing to occur.

Perhaps because the experience of pain is so unpleasant and engrossing, man has from time eternal sought to understand and master it. Therefore, it is not surprising that medication for pain was one of the first, if not the first, treatments to be developed. The ancient Sumerians began cultivating and extracting opium in the third millennium BC [1]. They called opium "Gil" which means "joy," and the opium poppy was known as "Hul Gil" or the "Joy Plant." Opium was initially reserved for religious and medicinal purposes, though over time access for recreational use grew.

By the seventeenth and eighteenth centuries, addiction to opium was already problematic in Western cultures [2]. The clear link between opioids and addiction led the United States to adopt the Harrison Narcotics Act in 1914. In addition to introducing controls on the production, distribution, and prescription of opioids, the law prevented physicians from prescribing opioids for the treatment of addiction.

J.C. Fellers, M.D. (✉)
Department of Psychiatry, Maine Medical Center,
216 Vaughan Street, Portland 04102, ME, USA
e-mail: jfellers@mmc.org

© Springer International Publishing Switzerland 2016
A.M. Matthews, J.C. Fellers (eds.), *Treating Comorbid Opioid Use Disorder in Chronic Pain*, DOI 10.1007/978-3-319-29863-4_1

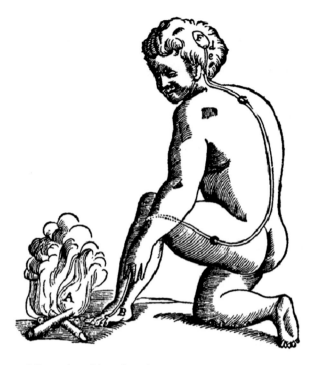

Fig. 1.1 Descartes' illustration of the pain pathway

The recognition of the abuse liability of opioids, many considered to be of "high potential for abuse," continues to this day in the form of the Controlled Substances Act of 1970.

1.2 Theories of Pain

Our understanding of pain has evolved over time. Descartes' [3] initial idea that painful stimuli pulled a thread that then open a valve in the brain has matured as scientific understanding and experimentation have revealed the secrets of our anatomy. Many theories have been developed, but they all fail to fully capture the symptom [4]. Pain is, after all, a subjective experience.

The *Specificity Theory* was first formulated during the nineteenth century. It theorizes that pain is an independent sense, with its own unique receptors, pathways, and "brain center" for perception. Moritz Schiff advanced this theory in 1858 when he was able to show that pain and touch travelled to the spinal cord through separate pathways.

Pain is detected through a variety of receptors on primary afferent neurons. A subgroup called nociceptors specifically detects painful stimuli through free nerve endings [5]. Myelinated nociceptors detect mechanical injury and transmit sharp and stinging sensations quickly. Their axons make up the neospinothalamic tract. Tissue damage from chemical, mechanical, or thermal injury activates non-myelinated nociceptors that transmit dull and aching sensations slowly. These axons form the paleospinothalamic tract.

The neospinothalamic tract transmits peripheral pain to the thalamus and on to the primary somatosensory cortex. There, location and intensity of pain is determined. The paleospinothalamic tract, the more primitive of the two systems, projects to the reticular formation and thalamus and then on to the limbic system, the frontal cortex, and then diffusely throughout the cortex. These structures manage arousal and the emotional components of suffering and pain.

Sinclair and Weddell proposed the *Pattern Theory* in 1955. It proposes that the perception of pain depends upon the temporal and spatial pattern of stimulation. Pain will only be experienced if the summary of stimulation of the individual fibers occurs in the correct combination. This model is able to explain how, based on the intensity of the stimulus, touch can be pleasant as with a caress, or painful like with a hard hit.

In 1965, Melzack and Wall put forth *Gate Control Theory* [6]. They postulated that a "gate" in the dorsal horn of the spinal cord controls the flow of pain signals from the periphery to the central nervous system. Based on the position of the gate, pain signals are either passed or blocked. In the open position, pain sensations are able to pass through the gate and reach the brain where pain is perceived. If the gate is closed, pain signals cannot pass through the gate and therefore no pain signal is sent to brain. In their model, an inhibitory interneuron allows feedback inhibition and augmentation on the projection neuron (Fig. 1.2). The Gate Control Theory is able to explain why after stubbing our toe, we rub it to relieve pain. This is also the basis for transcutaneous electrical nerve stimulation (TENS) pain relief.

They also envisioned a mechanism by which central feedback in the form of "top-down" processing could exert control over the gate. Therefore, the model provides an explanation for how a soldier who is wounded is able to feel no pain while he is focused on something else, like survival.

The most complete theory to date is the *Biopsychosocial Model* [7]. It proposes that pain is more than a biological phenomenon, as it also engages psychological and social factors. The mind–body connection between pain and psychological factors has been appreciated for many years in the field of psychosomatic medicine.

Emotional distress may predispose to and perpetuate pain. Anxiety, depression, and anger are among the negative affect states involved in pain perception. Not only can affective states modulate pain, but also the converse is true: opioid medications can lessen psychiatric symptoms [8]. Prior to modern antidepressants, opiates were commonly used to treat depression. There is also suggestive evidence that other disorders, including PTSD, may respond to opioid medications [9].

Cognitive factors such as pain appraisal and beliefs are also important in pain. Symptom amplification [10], pain catastrophizing, fear and avoidance, negative affectivity, anxiety sensitivity, and illness/injury sensitivity are all associated with increased pain perception. Perceived control, self-efficacy, hope, and optimism are all related to improved pain tolerance.

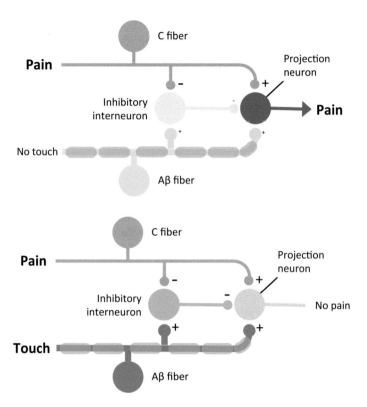

Fig. 1.2 Gate Control Theory. In the *top* figure, an afferent thin C fiber carries a pain signal from the periphery to the "gate" in the dorsal horn of the spinal cord. The thin fiber inhibits an inhibitory interneuron within the *substantia gelatinosa*, thereby "cutting the break-cable" and facilitating pain transmission centrally. However, as shown in the *bottom* figure, when both a thin C fiber (pain) and thick Aβ fiber (touch) are co-activated, the thick fiber enhances the inhibitory contribution of the interneuron, closing the gate and preventing pain transmission

Ultimately, pain is a uniquely individual experience, and multiple psychological and social factors interact with the biological to produce each person's constellation of symptoms and functioning.

1.3 Development of Addiction

Healthcare providers may introduce patients to the effects of opioids when prescribing for painful medical conditions. This differs from how the initial exposure of many other potentially addictive drugs occurs. It has been recognized for some time that the risk for addiction with opioids is significant. Dr. Foster Kennedy suggested, "morphinism is a disease, in the majority of cases, initiated, sustained and left uncured by members of the medical profession" [11].

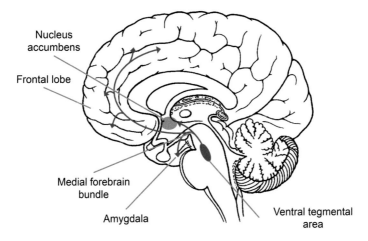

Fig. 1.3 Mesocorticolimbic dopamine system. Dopaminergic cell bodies in the ventral tegmental area project through the medial forebrain bundle to the nucleus accumbens, within the ventral striatum. Projections also pass to the amygdala and the frontal cortex

1.3.1 Positive Reinforcement

In order to appreciate how addiction to opioids develops, it is first useful to review our current understanding of reward processing. Through evolution, our brains have developed an intrinsic reward system. This system is critical for learning and motivating behavior; it assures we repeat activities necessary for survival by associating those activities with pleasure. The anatomic basis for the reward system was first discovered via brain stimulation experiments. Low-voltage stimulation of electrodes placed along the medial forebrain bundle from its origins in the brain stem all the way to the lateral and posterior hypothalamus in rats produces pleasure and is highly reinforcing [12]. Similar studies with intracranial self-stimulation in man reveal that stimulation of these same areas is powerfully reinforcing [13].

Three of these areas (ventral tegmental area, medial forebrain bundle, nucleus accumbens) constitute a major part of the mesocorticolimbic dopamine pathway (Fig. 1.3). Dopaminergic cells located in the ventral tegmental area project rostral through the medial forebrain bundle to the nucleus accumbens, where they release dopamine. Brain stimulation reward activates this pathway, increasing dopamine in the nucleus accumbens as a consequence. Dopamine elevations here convey "incentive salience," rather than pleasure. It is the "do it again" message that makes stimulation so reinforcing.

The mesocorticolimbic dopamine system is highly implicated in the rewarding aspects of drugs of abuse [14, 15]. Drugs of abuse enhance dopamine release within the nucleus accumbens, which has been postulated as the final common pathway for addiction [16]. This is the positive reinforcement aspect of addiction.

Opioid drugs with abuse potential are agonists at the μ opioid receptor. This receptor is found in the brain, spinal cord, and intestinal tract. Acute activation of μ

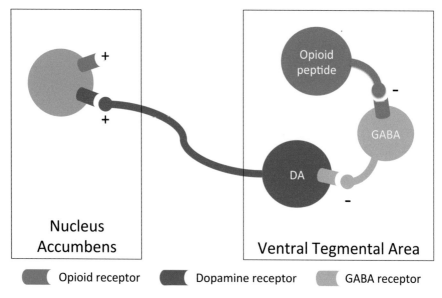

Fig. 1.4 Opioid actions on the mesocorticolimbic dopamine system. Opioids disinhibit ventral tegmental dopamine neurons, thereby facilitating dopamine release in the nucleus accumbens. Opioids also directly stimulate the nucleus accumbens at opioid receptors

receptors leads to analgesia, mood changes including euphoria, sedation, meiosis, respiratory depression, and decreased gastrointestinal motility [17]. Some opioids are better able to induce euphoria than others [18].

Opioid actions on the mesocorticolimbic dopamine system make them liable for abuse [19]. Opioids act indirectly on this system by inhibiting GABA-ergic neurons within the ventral tegmental area. Through disinhibition of the dopaminergic neurons, dopamine release in the nucleus accumbens is facilitated. Opioids also act directly in the nucleus accumbens activating opioid receptors (Fig. 1.4).

1.3.2 Negative Reinforcement

Though activation of brain reward centers by addictive drugs is important for the development of addiction, it alone is not sufficient. Chronic drug use leads to neuroplastic changes in order to maintain homeostasis [20]. Overtime, the recruitment of anti-reward systems leads to the development of a withdrawal state when drug use stops. The unpleasant state can contribute to the development of addiction by negatively reinforcing continued drug use [21].

Chronic opioid use leads to tolerance via up-regulation of compensatory mechanisms. One important system with implications for addiction is the locus coeruleus noradrenergic system (Fig. 1.5). Among other functions, this system is important for arousal and psychological stress.

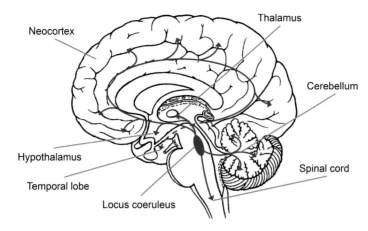

Fig. 1.5 Locus coeruleus noradrenergic system. Noradrenergic neurons in the locus coeruleus project to the thalamus, hypothalamus, cortex, temporal lobe, cerebellum, and spinal cord

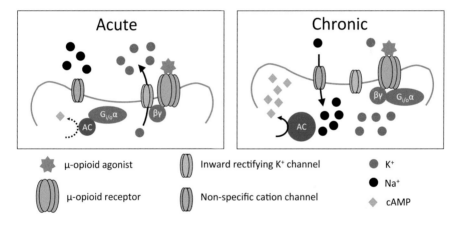

Fig. 1.6 Opioid inhibition of the locus coeruleus. On the *left*, acute opioid use leads to activation of the G-protein-coupled receptor, thereby leading to K^+ efflux, reducing membrane potential, and inhibiting firing. On the *right*, chronic opioid exposure leads to up-regulation of adenylate cyclase, which restores a closed K^+ channel, ultimately leading to normalized firing

With acute opioid use, firing of noradrenergic neurons within the locus coeruleus is suppressed. With continued use, however, compensatory processes are induced to maintain homeostasis. As a result, normal firing returns to the locus coeruleus (Fig. 1.6) [22].

As a consequence of this tolerance, when opioid use is abruptly discontinued, the now unopposed compensatory mechanisms lead to hyperactivity in the locus coeruleus. As a result, the noradrenergic system is activated, leading to the characteristic discomfort of opioid withdrawal. Opioid withdrawal acts as negative reinforcer, thereby contributing to continued opioid use.

1.3.3   Special Considerations in Pain

Even though opioids are reinforcing and with chronic use tolerance and withdrawal will develop, the progression to opioid use disorder is not assured. There has been some suggestion that using opioids in the context of pain is protective against addiction, as the pain provides a natural counterbalance to opioid-induced reward and tolerance during treatment. Good evidence supports that the risk for developing addiction during opioid treatment for acute and cancer pain is minimal [23]. It has been much more difficult to quantify the risk of addiction during treatment of chronic non-cancer pain.

One good study interrogated a large claims database for the development of opioid use disorders after receiving a diagnosis of chronic pain [24]. Those who received opioids for treatment of chronic pain were three times as likely to develop addiction compared to those who were not prescribed opioids. As opioid dose was increased, the risk for addiction also increased; opioid dose is therefore an important factor in abuse liability. The chronicity of treatment also was related to risk; the duration of treatment had a larger effect than the dose in determining risk.

Several recent reviews have examined the risk of developing addiction during opioid treatment for chronic pain [25–28]. A consistent finding has been the paucity of adequate quality studies that can be used to answer this question. A low overall incidence of addiction is reported (0.5–3.3 %), though the range is unacceptably high (0–45 %).

These review findings should be taken with caution. The studies that are available are very heterogeneous. The available studies show little consistency in defining the outcome of addiction. Part of the problem stems from discriminating addiction from pseudoaddiction, a term coined to describe the behavioral manifestations of undertreated pain that mimics diagnostic criteria for addiction [29][30]. Studies often do not identify the opioid used or the dose in morphine-equivalents, therefore a dose-response for addiction risk is not possible. Despite this shortcoming, there is increasing evidence that high doses of opioids incur greater risk [31] [32]. There are also few longer duration studies. Risk for addiction could be related to duration of exposure. Since by definition, chronic pain treatment has no end-date, it represents a higher risk situation.

The generalizability is also questionable, as many of the reported studies carefully selected patients and excluded those with addiction histories and followed patients at a higher level than is possible in most care settings.

1.4   Conclusion

Theories of pain have evolved as our understanding of the biological underpinnings, psychological factors, and social context of this complex experience has grown. The gate control theory and biopsychosocial model remain important in helping us conceptualize this multifaceted yet individualized experience.

Opioids are able to activate the brain's innate reward system, like other drugs of abuse. Through both indirect and direct actions, opioids lead to increased dopamine within the nucleus accumbens, which explains why they are so reinforcing. With chronic use, physical dependence develops and leads to negative reinforcement for continued use. Despite the risk of addiction, opioids remain important medications for pain management. An understanding of the risk/benefit ratio is very important when deciding whether to prescribe opioids. In the case of chronic pain, it is crucial to know that the risk for addiction increases with dose and duration of treatment.

References

1. Brownstein MJ. A brief history of opiates, opioid peptides, and opioid receptors. Proc Natl Acad Sci U S A. 1993;90(12):5391–3.
2. Kramer JC. Opium rampant: medical use, misuse and abuse in Britain and the West in the 17th and 18th centuries. Br J Addict Alcohol Other Drugs. 1979;74(4):377–89.
3. Descartes, R. (1644). L'homme. Paris.
4. Moayedi M, Davis KD. Theories of pain: from specificity to gate control. J Neurophysiol. 2013;109(1):5–12.
5. Lynn, B. (1984). Cutaneous nociceptors. In W. Winlow, & A. V. Holden, The neurobiology of pain: Symposium of the Northern Neurobiology Group, held at Leeds on 18 April 1983 (p. 106). Manchester: Manchester University Press.
6. Melzack R, Wall PD. Pain mechanisms: a new theory. Science. 1965;50(3699):971–9.
7. Gatchel RJ, Peng YB, Peters ML, Fuchs PN, Turk DC. The biopsychosocial approach to chronic pain: scientific advances and future directions. Psychol Bull. 2007;133(4):581–624.
8. Tenore PL. Psychotherapeutic benefits of opioid agonist therapy. J Addict Dis. 2008;27(3):49–65.
9. Seal KH, Shi Y, Cohen G, Cohen BE, Maguen S, Krebs EE, et al. Association of mental health disorders with prescription opioids and high-risk opioid use in US veterans of Iraq and Afghanistan. JAMA. 2012;307(23):2489.
10. Barsky AJ, Goodson JD, Lane RS, Cleary PD. The amplification of somatic symptoms. Psychosom Med. 1988;50(5):510–9.
11. Kennedy F. The effects of narcotic drug addiction. NY Med J. 1914;22:20–2.
12. Olds J, Milner P. Positive reinforcement produced by electrical stimulation of septal area and other regions of rat brain. J Comp Physiol Psychol. 1954;47(6):419–27.
13. Moan CE, Heath RG. Septal stimulation for the initiation of heterosexual behavior in a homosexual male. J Behav Ther Exp Psychiatry. 1972;3(1):25–30.
14. Koob GF. Neural mechanisms of drug reinforcement. Ann N Y Acad Sci. 1992;654:171–91.
15. Wise RA. Neurobiology of addiction. Curr Opin Neurobiol. 1996;6:243–51.
16. Nestler EJ. Is there a common molecular pathway for addiction? Nat Neurosci. 2005;8(11): 1445–9.
17. Koneru A, Satyanarayana S, Rizwan S. Endogenous opioids: their physiological role and receptors. Global J Pharmacol. 2009;3(3):149–53.
18. Wightman R, Perrone J, Portelli I, Nelson L. Likeability and abuse liability of commonly prescribed opioids. J Med Toxicol. 2012;8(4):335–40.
19. Kosten TR, George TP. The neurobiology of opioid dependence: implications for treatment. Sci Pract Perspect. 2002;1(11):13–20.
20. Volkow ND, Wang GJ, Fowler JS, Tomasi D, Telang F. Addiction: beyond dopamine reward circuitry. Proc Natl Acad Sci U S A. 2011;108(37):15037–42.
21. Koob GF, Buck CL, Cohen A, Edwards S, Park PE, Schlosburg JE, et al. Addiction as a stress surfeit disorder. Neuropharmacology. 2014;76(Part B):370–82.

22. Nestler EJ, Alreja M, Aghajanian GK. Molecular control of locus coeruleus neurotransmission. Biol Psychiatry. 1999;46(9):1131–9.
23. Ballantyne JC, LaForge KS. Opioid dependence and addiction during opioid treatment of chronic pain. Pain. 2007;129(3):235–55.
24. Edlund MJ, Martin BC, Russo JE, DeVries A, Braden JB, Sullivan MD. The role of opioid prescription in incident opioid abuse and dependence among individuals with chronic noncancer pain: the role of opioid prescription. Clin J Pain. 2014;30(7):557–64.
25. Chou R, Turner JA, Devine EB, Hansen RN, Sullivan SD, Blazina I, et al. The effectiveness and risks of long-term opioid therapy for chronic pain: a systematic review for a National Institutes of Health Pathways to Prevention Workshop. Ann Intern Med. 2015; 162(4):276–86.
26. Fishbain DA, Cole B, Lewis J, Rosomoff HL, Rosomoff RS. What percentage of chronic nonmalignant pain patients exposed to chronic opioid analgesic therapy develop abuse/ addiction and/or aberrant drug-related behaviors? A structured evidence-based review. Pain Med. 2008;9(4):444–59.
27. Juurlink DN, Dhalla IA. Dependence and addiction during chronic opioid therapy. J Med Toxicol. 2012;8(4):393–9.
28. Minozzi S, Amato S, Davoli M. Development of dependence following treatment with opioid analgesics for pain relief: a systematic review. Addiction. 2013;108(4):688–98.
29. Weissman DE, Haddox JD. Opioid pseudoaddiction - an iatrogenic syndrome. Pain. 1989;36(3):363–6.
30. Lusher J, Elander J, Bevan D. Analgesic addiction and pseudoaddiction in painful chronic illness. Clin J Pain. 2006;22(3):316–24.
31. Shurman J, Koob GF, Gutstein HB. Opioids, pain, the brain, and hyperkatifeia: a framework for the rational use of opioids for pain. Pain Med. 2010;11(7):1092–8.
32. Miller LL, Altarifi AA, Negus SS. Effects of repeated morphine on intracranial self-stimulation in male rats in the absence or presence of a noxious pain stimulus. Exp Clin Psychopharmacol. 2015;23(5):405–14.

Chapter 2
The Epidemiology of Pain and Opioid Abuse

Jermaine D. Jones and Sandra D. Comer

2.1 The Epidemiology of Pain and Opioid Abuse

The medicinal and psychoactive effects of the opium poppy (*Papaver somniferum*) have been known for thousands of years [1]. Several major alkaloids in opium that have been isolated, including morphine (8.0–17.0%) and codeine (0.7–5.0%), are used therapeutically as analgesics, antitussives, and antidiarrheal agents [2, 3]. Our knowledge of the structure of natural *opiates* (morphine, codeine, and thebaine) led to the development of synthetic and semi-synthetic *opioids* (e.g., hydrocodone, oxycodone, hydromorphone, and fentanyl) with varying analgesic potencies and durations of action [4]. The therapeutic diversity of opioid analgesics has made them one of the clinician's most valuable tools to treat moderate-to-severe acute and *chronic pain*. Chronic pain has been defined by the American Society of Interventional Pain Physicians (ASIPP) as, "pain that persists 6 months after an injury and beyond the usual course of an acute disease or a reasonable time for a comparable injury to heal" [5, 6].

Unfortunately, the immense medical utility of opioids is tempered by their potential to be abused. In addition to analgesia, many opioid drugs produce robust euphoric effects. Both properties of opioids are commonly attributed to their actions upon the mu (μ) subtype of opioid receptors ([7, 8, 9]). The intensely pleasurable subjective effects produced by opioids can encourage nonmedical use leading to addiction. Several different types of investigations, from global and national epidemiological studies [10, 11, 12] to controlled laboratory research [13–16], have confirmed the potential for these drugs to be used for nonmedical purposes. As such, the abuse liability of this drug class creates a dilemma as chronic pain and opioid abuse are two major public health concerns. Recent market research indicates that

J.D. Jones, Ph.D. (✉) • S.D. Comer
Division on Substance Abuse, New York Psychiatric Institute and Columbia University
Medical Center, New York, NY, USA
e-mail: JonesJe@NYSPI.Columbia.edu; ComerSa@NYSPI.Columbia.edu

© Springer International Publishing Switzerland 2016
A.M. Matthews, J.C. Fellers (eds.), *Treating Comorbid Opioid Use Disorder in Chronic Pain*, DOI 10.1007/978-3-319-29863-4_2

more than 1.5 billion people worldwide suffer from chronic pain [17]. In the US, it has been conservatively estimated that there are over 100 million chronic pain sufferers, with annual direct (e.g., medical expenditures) and indirect (e.g., loss of productivity) costs of over US$560 billion [18].

The epidemiology and cost of prescription opioid abuse is just as striking. According to the World Health Organization (WHO), the annual global prevalence of opioid abuse was estimated at between 28 and 38 million users [World Drug Report, 2014, heroin (diacetylmorphine) and prescription opioids were not distinguished]. Figures from the US National Survey on Drug Use and Health (NSDUH) place the number of current (within the past month) nonmedical users of opioid analgesics at 4.5 million [19]. Meanwhile, the annual societal costs (direct + indirect) of prescription opioid abuse have been estimated at US$57 billion [20]. Greater than the economic burden of opioid abuse is the mortality and morbidity resulting from fatal and non-fatal overdoses. The number of unintentional overdose deaths from prescription opioids in the United States has more than quadrupled in the first decade of the twenty-first century [19].

Healthcare clinicians are therefore tasked with balancing adequate pain management using opioids with the risk of patients developing abusive patterns of use. In spite of this concern, the use of long-term opioid therapy has increased dramatically over the past two decades [6, 21, 22]. Nowhere has this increase been more dramatic than in the United States where the total number of opioid pain reliever prescriptions has risen from around 76 million in 1991 to nearly 207 million in 2013 [23]. The United States is easily the largest global consumer of opioid analgesics. Though Americans constitute only 4.6 % of the world's population, we consume 80 % of the global opioid analgesic supply [24–27].

Increased availability of opioid analgesics combined with other factors such as greater social acceptability of using these medications and aggressive marketing by pharmaceutical companies are believed to have led to a substantial rise in the incidence of prescription opioid abuse ([6, 28]; Fig. 2.1). In the last few years, policymakers have become increasingly interested in provisions for better pain management, while at the same time reducing opioid analgesic diversion and abuse [29].

Because of the risk of *iatrogenic* abuse (attributable due to medical treatment) as a result of exposure to opioids for pain management, there has been substantial interest in their comorbidity. However, determining the frequency of abusive patterns of opioid use among chronic pain patients has proven difficult. Variability in defining "opioid abuse" operationally has led to substantial inconsistency across estimates of their co-occurrence. Terminologies such as "abuse," "aberrant use," "misuse," "addiction," "pseudo-addiction," and "nonmedical use" have all been employed in attempts to define the same disease state. The *abstracting* (filtering and selecting the relevant aspects of a concept of interest for research purposes) of criteria defining the problematic use of opioids has also been variable and imprecise, encompassing many combinations of behaviors such as:

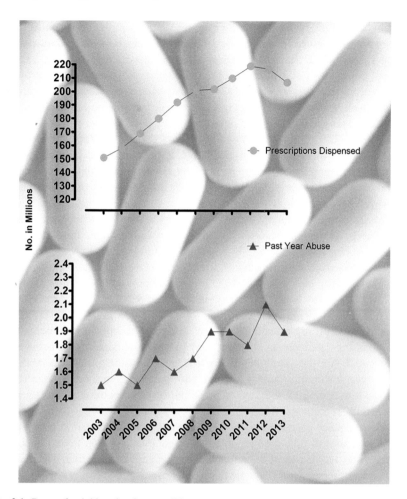

Fig. 2.1 Rates of opioid analgesic prescribing and abuse

- Intravenous and intranasal use
- Using more than prescribed
- Unsanctioned dose escalations
- Obtaining opioids from friends or family
- "Doctor shopping" (obtaining opioids from several medical sources)
- Purchasing opioid medications off the street

An additional challenge is that there are no commonly accepted study design metrics to determine rates of opioid analgesic abuse among chronic pain patients. The methodologies used to quantify the co-epidemiology of pain and opioid abuse have ranged vastly. Internet analyses have been used to capture target keywords from search engines and drug forums to evaluate the frequency of opioid use for nonmedical purposes [30]. Online surveys have also proven to be a rapid method of providing insight into individuals who use prescription opioids non-medically [31, 32]. Structured examinations of clinical notes and chart reviews of pain patients' medical records have also been used to assess abusive patterns of use [33–41]. Similarly, forensic studies utilizing data from prescription monitoring programs [42] and urine toxicology testing [43–49] have been used as ways of gathering information on aberrant opioid use. On a larger scale, population-based assessments have obtained these data using self-report surveys [50–53]. Other population-based data have come from clinical reports of emergency department visits [54] and treatment center admissions [55–59]. In addition to data from events involving healthcare utilization (see also [60]), events involving interaction with law enforcement [61] and adverse events reporting [62-64] have also been used to examine the rates of comorbid pain and opioid abuse.

All of these methods have inherent limitations, examining diverse populations using different endpoints. Accordingly, rates of problematic opioid use among pain patients have ranged broadly (>1–81 %) across studies [65]. Review articles, which combine data across multiple studies, are therefore more likely to provide valid estimates. Portenoy [66] was one of the first to perform an evidence-based, *structured review* (employing an explicit description of what types of studies to be included, to limit selection bias) on this topic. This investigation described and assessed "aberrant drug-related behaviors," which were operationalized as those indicative of the development of "addiction" [67, 68]. He concluded that the literature indicated that the psychological, social, and physiological vulnerability to addiction was uncommon among chronic pain patients, and therefore the risk of abuse was low. However, no rates of comorbidity were reported due to a lack of studies and other technical issues.

There have since been a number of reviews that have attempted to pool data on the risk and rates of opioid abuse among chronic pain patients. Wasan et al. [69] reviewed nine articles they determined were related to iatrogenic addiction in patients treated for acute or subacute pain. They concluded that they could not adequately answer the study question, and that the risk and prevalence of addiction among patients treated with opioids could not be determined. Bartleson [70] also performed a structured review of 11 reports addressing addiction as a result of opioid treatment. They concluded that opioid therapy is associated with a low risk of abuse or drug addiction, as only two of the studies reviewed indicated the development of abuse/addiction to have been a problem. A *narrative review* (an unstructured, unsystematic critical analysis that describes and discusses the state of a topic from a theoretical and contextual point of view) by Aronoff [71] came to a similar conclusion. Another narrative review by provided one of the first detailed rates of comorbidity [72]. Following their review of 25 studies, they concluded that the prevalence of "addiction" among chronic non-malignant pain patients (patients prescribed opioids for cancer pain are typically distinguished and excluded from this research) varied from 0 up to 50 %. In yet another narrative synthesis, Martell et al. [73] placed estimates of current substance use disorders and aberrant medication-taking behaviors at 5–43 %.

It is commonly believed that these wide-ranging estimates are the result of the limited scientific rigor of these previous reviews (mostly attributable to the lack of primary data on the topic), along with inconsistent operationalization of abuse and addiction [33, 74]. More recent reviews have addressed both these limitations. Integrative literature reviews provide the most scientifically rigorous assessments of the current state of knowledge on a topic [75, 76]. An *integrative review* not only summarizes, but also critiques and synthesizes the representative literature an integrated way. Fishbain et al. [77] performed one of the first integrative reviews of research studies aimed at determining the rates of opioid "abuse/addiction and/or aberrant drug-related behaviors" among patients exposed to chronic opioid therapy. An initial literature searches yielded 79 papers on the topic. Study characteristics were extracted and independently evaluated by two raters according to 12 quality criteria, and a quality score was calculated. Studies were not utilized in the final assessment unless their quality score (from both raters) was greater than 65 %. Sixty seven reports were included in the final analysis. They found that the rate of opioid abuse/addiction among patients with pain (e.g., drug problems, drug seeking, psychological dependence, craving, etc.) was slightly higher than the general population (3.27 % versus 1.7 % among Americans aged 12 or older; [12]). In comparison to rates of abuse/addiction, their estimates of the rate of aberrant drug-related behavior (e.g., aggressively requesting medications, unsanctioned dose escalations, etc.) and inconsistent urine toxicology findings (e.g., the presence of opioid medications that are not prescribed) were higher at 11.5 % and 20.4 %, respectively.

Although the data provided by Fishbain et al. [77] are compelling and informative, recent attempts at standardizing terminology concerning opioid misuse and abuse have greatly aided comparisons across studies. A multidisciplinary group of academic, industry, clinical, public health, and regulatory experts in pain and addiction was convened by the Analgesic, Anesthetic, and Addiction Clinical Trials, Translations, Innovations, Opportunities, and Networks (ACTTION; http://www. acttion.org). This panel reviewed existing definitions of misuse, abuse, and related events from consensus efforts, review articles, and major institutions and agencies. Their goal was to develop mutually exclusive and exhaustive consensus definitions of opioid analgesic misuse, abuse, and related events (MARES) to inform clinical trials, post-marketing research, and clinical care [78].

This consensus statement has provided a much better framework for evaluating problematic opioid use in chronic pain patients. Accordingly, Vowles et al. [65] conducted a comprehensive and elegant integrated review aimed at defining rates of problematic opioid use among chronic pain patients. The clinical and scientific literature related to this topic was searched using Science Direct, Google Scholar, PubMed, and PsychINFO/PsycArticles databases. Each potential study identified in the literature search was read in full by two study team members to determine eligibility. In total, data from 38 studies were included (shown below in Fig. 2.2).

The following data were extracted from studies that met inclusion criteria:

- Participant demographics
- Pain details (i.e., sample size, gender, age, pain duration)

Table 2

Characteristics of included studies.

First author (year)	Sample size (country)	Design	Setting	Method of assessment	Rate (%) of problematic use, %			Quality
					Misuse	Abuse	Addiction	
Adams et al.[1],*	4278 (USA)†	Prospective	Not specified	Q	—	—	4.9	7
Banta-Greenet al.[5]	704 (USA)	Retrospective	Primary care	SI	—	8	13	8
Brown et al.[8],*	561 (USA/Puerto Rico)	Prospective	Primary care	CJ, Q, UDS	2-6	—	—	6
Butler et al.[11]	95 (USA)	Prospective	Pain clinic	CJ, Q, UDS	46.3	—	—	5
Butler et al.[10]	226 (USA)	Prospective	Pain clinic	CJ, Q, UDS	34.2	—	—	3
Chelminski et al.[12]	63 (USA)	Prospective	Primary care	CJ, UDS	32	—	—	2
Compton et al.[14]	135 (USA)	Prospective	Pain clinic	CJ, UDS	28	—	—	5
Couto et al.[15],*	938,586 (USA)	Cross-sectional	Toxicology laboratory database	UDS	75	—	—	U
Cowan and Wilson-Barnett[16],*	104 (UK)	Retrospective	Pain clinic	SI	—	—	2.8	7
Edlund et al.[18],*	9279 (USA)	Cross-sectional	Community database	Q	3.3	—	0.7	5
Edlund et al.[17],*	46,256 (USA)	Cross-sectional	Not specified	INSUR CL	3.2	—	—	5
Fleming et al.[20],*	801 (USA)	Cross-sectional	Primary care	SI	—	—	3.8	8
Fleming et al.[21],*	904 (USA)	Cross-sectional	Primary care	SI	—	—	3.4	6
Højsted et al.[23],*	207 (Denmark)	Cross-sectional	Pain clinic	CJ	—	—	14.4-19.3	7
Ives et al.[25],*	196 (USA)	Prospective	Pain clinic	CJ, UDS	32	—	—	4
Jamison et al.[26]	455 (USA)	Prospective	Pain clinic	CJ, SI, UDS	24.0-37.1	—	34.1	4
Jamison et al.[27]‡	110 (USA)	Cross-sectional	Pain clinic	Q	46.4	—	—	1
Katz et al.[29],*	122 (USA)	Retrospective	Pain clinic	CJ, UDS	43	—	—	4
Manchikanti et al.[36]	100 (USA)	Retrospective	Pain clinic	CJ	24	—	—	6
Manchikanti et al.[35],*	500 (USA)	Retrospective	Pain clinic	CJ	9.4	—	8.4	4
Manchikanti et al.[34],*	200 (USA)	Cross-sectional	Pain clinic	UDS	3-12	—	—	1
Manchikanti et al.[33],*	500 (USA)	Prospective	Pain clinic	CJ	9	—	—	5
Manchikanti et al.[30],*	500 (USA)	Prospective	Pain clinic	UDS	9	—	—	3
Meltzer et al.[40]	238 (USA)	Cross-sectional	Primary care	SI	11	—	—	4
Meltzer et al.[39]	264 (USA)	Cross-sectional	Primary care	CR	—	—	23	8
Morasco et al.[42]	127 (USA)	Cross-sectional	Primary care	Q	78	—	—	1
Naliboff et al.[43]	135 (USA)	Prospective	Pain clinic	CJ, UDS	27	—	—	5
Passik et al.[45]	1160 (USA)	Retrospective	Clinical database	CJ	—	—	6-11	7
Portenoy et al.[46]	219 (USA)	Prospective	Clinical trial registry	Q	2.6	—	—	3
Reid et al.[47]	98 (USA)	Retrospective	Primary care	CJ	24-31	—	—	7
Schneider et al.[49]	184 (USA)	Retrospective	Pain clinic	CJ, UDS	—	—	15.7	7
Sekhon et al.[50]	797 (USA)	Retrospective	Primary care	CJ	22.9	—	—	5
Skurtveit et al.[52],*	17,252 (Norway)	Prospective	Prescription database	CJ	0.08-0.3	—	—	3
Vaglienti et al.[57],*	184 (USA)	Retrospective	Pain clinic	CJ, UDS	25.5	—	—	5
Wasan et al.[59]	455 (USA)	Cross-sectional	Pain clinic	CJ, Q, UDS	34.1	—	—	7
Webster and Webster[61]	183 (USA)	Prospective	Pain clinic	Q	56.3	—	—	6
Wilsey et al.[62]	113 (USA)	Cross-sectional	Emergency department	Q	81	—	—	2
Wu et al.[65]	136 (USA)	Prospective	Pain clinic	CJ, UDS	27.9	—	—	3

* The primary study aim was assessment of prevalence of opioid misuse, abuse, or addiction.
† Adams et al.[1]—only data from the group taking hydrocodone used.
‡ Jamison et al.[27]—only baseline data used (ie, patients who screened as "high risk" on questionnaire).
Method of assessment: CJ, clinical judgment (including chart review); INSUR CL, Insurance Claims Database; Q, questionnaire.
SI, structured interview; UDS, urine drug screen; USI, unstructured interview.
Quality: possible range 0 to 8; higher scores indicate higher quality (quality criteria adopted from Chou et al.[13]).

Fig. 2.2 Rates of problematic opioid use behaviors among pain patients determined by systematic review and synthesis

- Primary objective (e.g., assessment of prevalence, medication safety/efficacy)
- Design (i.e., cross-sectional, prospective, retrospective)
- Setting details
- Methods of assessing problematic opioid use (i.e., structured/unstructured clinical interview)

Fig. 2.3 ACTTION committee consensus definitions of problematic opioid use behaviors

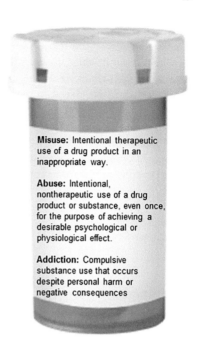

> **Misuse:** Intentional therapeutic use of a drug product in an inappropriate way.
>
> **Abuse:** Intentional, nontherapeutic use of a drug product or substance, even once, for the purpose of achieving a desirable psychological or physiological effect.
>
> **Addiction:** Compulsive substance use that occurs despite personal harm or negative consequences

Problematic opioid use behaviors from the selected articles were then coded using the terms defined in the ACTTION statement (Fig. 2.3): misuse, abuse, and addiction [78]. Average prevalence rates were calculated and weighted by sample size and study quality. Their investigation found that rates of opioid analgesic misuse averaged between 21 and 29 %, while rates of addiction averaged between 8 and 12 %. Abuse was reported in only a single study.

In conclusion, determining the rate of comorbid opioid abuse and misuse among patients with pain has proven to be challenging. However, it is clear that particularly in the U.S., there should be increased scrutiny regarding who is a suitable candidate for opioid treatment, and what are suitable precautions [79]. Greater prescribing of opioids in clinical practice also increases the likelihood that they will be diverted to the illegal market. Furthermore, anecdotal reports and news media suggest that individuals who begin abusing prescription opioids may transition to using heroin. Although causality cannot be determined, increases in the numbers of new heroin users (between 2002 and 2011) parallel rises in prescribing and abuse of prescription opioids [80].

The increased focus on how opioid prescribing contributes to the growing "opioid abuse epidemic" has allowed the field to identify patients who are most at-risk of misusing and abusing prescribed opioids. More specifically, patients with a personal or family history of substance abuse and psychosocial comorbidity may need more carefully structured and monitored opioid treatment [81]. Better understanding of all the psychological, social, and genetics risk factor should help circumvent the development of addiction [82–84]. These issues are discussed in greater detail in a later chapter of this text, so we will not elaborate upon them here.

Much of our thinking on drug abuse is derived from our knowledge and experience with illicit drugs. In contrast, assessment of abusive patterns of prescription opioid use must be placed in the context of a population with germane medical needs and adjusted accordingly. It is a concern that misunderstanding of these behaviors and labeling of patients as "addicts" could lead to unnecessary withholding of medications and undertreatment of pain [85]. Clear and empirical definitions of aberrant opioid analgesic use behaviors will hopefully lead to increased reliability and validity across studies and more scientific consensus to better inform clinical care.

Acknowledgment Financial support for the preparation of this chapter was provided by the NIDA grants: DA030446 to JDJ, DA016759 to SDC.

References

1. Kapoor LD. Opium poppy—botany, chemistry, and pharmacology. Binghamton: Haworth Press; 1995. p. 1–17.
2. Bernard MC. Experimental researches on opium and its alkaloids. Boston Med Surg J. 1865;72:349–57.
3. Schiff PL. Opium and its alkaloids. Am J Pharmaceutical Ed. 2002;66:186–94.
4. Brownstein MJ. Review A, brief history of opiates, opioid peptides, and opioid receptors. Proc Natl Acad Sci USA. 1993;90:5391–93.
5. Manchikanti L, Abdi S, Atluri S, Balog CC, Benyamin RM, Boswell MV, Brown KR, Bruel BM, Bryce DA, Burks PA, Burton AW, Calodney AK, Caraway DL, Cash KA, Christo PJ, Damron KS, Datta S, Deer TR, Diwan S, Eriator I, Falco FJ, Fellows B, Geffert S, Gharibo CG, Glaser SE, Grider JS, Hameed H, Hameed M, Hansen H, Harned ME, Hayek SM, Helm S 2nd, Hirsch JA, Janata JW, Kaye AD, Kaye AM, Kloth DS, Koyyalagunta D, Lee M, Malla Y, Manchikanti KN, McManus CD, Pampati V, Parr AT, Pasupuleti R, Patel VB, Sehgal N, Silverman SM, Singh V, Smith HS, Snook LT, Solanki DR, Tracy DH, Vallejo R, Wargo BW. American Society of Interventional Pain Physicians (ASIPP) guidelines for responsible opioid prescribing in chronic non-cancer pain: Part 2—guidance. Pain Physician. 2012;15(3 Suppl):S67–116.
6. Manchikanti L, Helm 2nd S, Fellows B, Janata JW, Pampati V, Grider JS, Boswell MV. Opioid epidemic in the United States. Pain Physician. 2012;15(3 Suppl):ES9–38.
7. Bertalmio AJ, Woods JH. Reinforcing effect of alfentanil is mediated by mu opioid receptors: apparent pA2 analysis. J Pharmacol Exp Ther. 1980;251:455–60.
8. Matthes HW, Maldonado R, Simonin F, Valverde O, Slowe S, Kitchen I, Befort K, Dierich A, Le Meur M, Dollé P, Tzavara E, Hanoune J, Roques BP, Kieffer BL. Loss of morphine-induced analgesia, reward effect and withdrawal symptoms in mice lacking the mu-opioid-receptor gene. Nature. 1996;383(6603):819–23.
9. Negus SS, Henriksen SJ, Mattox A, Pasternak GW, Portoghese PS, Takemori AE, Weinger MB, Koob GF. Effect of antagonists selective for mu,delta and kappa opioid receptors on the reinforcing effects of heroin in rats. J Pharmacol Exp Ther. 1993;265:1245–52.
10. United Nations Office on Drugs and Crime, World Drug Report 2014 (United Nations publication, Sales No. E.14.XI.

11. European Monitoring Centre for Drugs Addiction (EMCDA), 2014: European Drug Report 2014: Trends and developments. http://www.emcdda.europa.eu/publications/edr/trends-developments/2014. Accessed April 16, 2015.
12. Substance Abuse and Mental Health Services Administration. Results from the 2013 National survey on drug use and health: summary of national findings, NSDUH Series H-48, HHS Publication No. (SMA) 14-4863. Rockville: Substance Abuse and Mental Health Services Administration; 2014.
13. Comer SD, Sullivan MA, Whittington RA, Vosburg SK, Kowalczyk WJ. Abuse liability of prescription opioids compared to heroin in morphine-maintained heroin abusers. Neuropsychopharmacology. 2008;33:1179–91.
14. Comer SD, Zacny JP, Dworkin RH, Turk DC, Bigelow GE, Foltin RW, Jasinski DR, Sellers EM, Adams EH, Balster R, Burke LB, Cerny I, Colucci RD, Cone E, Cowan P, Farrar JT, Haddox JD, Haythornthwaite JA, Hertz S, Jay GW, Johanson CE, Junor R, Katz NP, Klein M, Kopecky EA, Leiderman DB, McDermott MP, O'Brien C, O'Connor AB, Palmer PP, Raja SN, Rappaport BA, Rauschkolb C, Rowbotham MC, Sampaio C, Setnik B, Sokolowska M, Stauffer JW, Walsh SL. Core outcome measures for opioid abuse liability laboratory assessment studies in humans: IMMPACT recommendations. Pain 2012;153(12): 2315–24.
15. Jones JD, Sullivan MA, Vosburg SK, Manubay JM, Mogali S, Metz V, Comer SD. Abuse potential of intranasal buprenorphine versus buprenorphine/naloxone in buprenorphine-maintained heroin users. Addict Biol. 2014;20(4):784–98. doi:10.1111/adb.12163.
16. O'Connor AB, Turk DC, Dworkin RH, Katz NP, Colucci R, Haythornthwaite JA, Klein M, O'Brien C, Posner K, Rappaport BA, Reisfield G, Adams EH, Balster RL, Bigelow GE, Burke LB, Comer SD, Cone E, Cowan P, Denisco RA, Farrar JT, Foltin RW, Haddox JD, Hertz S, Jay GW, Junor R, Kopecky EA, Leiderman DB, McDermott MP, Palmer PP, Raja SN, Rauschkolb C, Rowbotham MC, Sampaio C, Setnik B, Smith SM, Sokolowska M, Stauffer JW, Walsh SL, Zacny JP. Abuse liability measures for use in analgesic clinical trials in patients with pain: IMMPACT recommendations. Pain 2013;154(11): 2324-34.
17. Global Industry Analysts, Inc. Report, January 10, 2011. http://www.prweb.com/pdfdownload/8052240.pdf.
18. Institute of Medicine. Report from the Committee on Advancing Pain Research, Care, and Education: relieving pain in America, a blueprint for transforming prevention, care, education and research. Washington, DC: The National Academies Press; 2011.
19. Pradip et al. Associations of nonmedical pain reliever use and initiation of heroin use in the U.S. center for behavioral health statistics and quality data review. SAMHSA (2013) http://www.samhsa.gov/data/2k13/DataReview/DR006/nonmedical-pain-reliever-use-2013.htm
20. Meyer R, Patel AM, Rattana SK, Quock TP, Mody SH. Prescription opioid abuse: a literature review of the clinical and economic burden in the United States. Popul Health Manag. 2014;17(6):372–87.
21. Boudreau D, Von Korff M, Rutter CM, et al. Trends in long-term opioid therapy for chronic non-cancer pain. Pharmacoepidemiol Drug Saf. 2009;18(12):1166–75.
22. Caudill-Slosberg MA, Schwartz LM, Woloshin S. Office visits and analgesic prescriptions for musculoskeletal pain in US: 1980 vs 2000. Pain. 2004;109(3):514–19.
23. IMS Health, Vector One: National, years 1991-1996, Data Extracted 2011. IMS Health, National Prescription Audit, years 1997-2013, Data Extracted 2014.
24. Califano JA. High society: how substance abuse ravages America and what to do about it. New York: Perseus; 2007.
25. Chou R, Huffman L. Use of chronic opioid therapy in chronic non-cancer pain: evidence review. Glenview: American Pain Society; 2009.
26. Kuehn BM. Opioid prescriptions soar: increase in legitimate use as well as abuse. JAMA. 2007;297:249–51.
27. Pain and Policy Studies Group. International Narcotics Control Board opioid consumption data. http://www.painpolicy.wisc.edu/opioid-consumption-data. Accessed April 13, 2015.

28. Volkow, ND. Director, National Institute on Drug Abuse, National Institutes of Health, U.S. Department of Health and Human Services, before the Subcommittee on Criminal Justice, Drug Policy, and Human Resources Committee, July 26, 2006.
29. U.S. Department of Health and Human Services. Addressing prescription drug abuse in the United States: current activities and future opportunities. 2013. http://www.cdc.gov/HomeandRecreationalSafety/pdf/HHS_Prescription_Drug_Abuse_Report_09.2013.pdf Accessed April 12, 2015
30. Krüger R, Meißner W, Zimmer A. Misuse of opioid analgesics. An Internet analysis. Schmerz. 2014;28(5):473–82.
31. Katz N, Fernandez K, Chang A, Benoit C, Butler SF. Internet-based survey of nonmedical prescription opioid use in the United States. Clin J Pain. 2008;24(6):528–35.
32. Vietri J, Joshi AV, Barsdorf AI, Mardekian J. Prescription opioid abuse and tampering in the United States: results of a self-report survey. Pain Med. 2014;15(12):2064–74.
33. Boscarino JA, Rukstalis MR, Hoffman SN, Han JJ, Erlich PM, Ross S, Gerhard GS, Stewart WF. Prevalence of prescription opioid-use disorder among chronic pain patients: comparison of the DSM-5 vs. DSM-4 diagnostic criteria. J Addict Dis. 2011;30(3):185–94.
34. Cheatle MD, O'Brien CP, Mathai K, Hansen M, Grasso M, Yi P. Aberrant behaviors in a primary care-based cohort of patients with chronic pain identified as misusing prescription opioids. J Opioid Manag. 2013;9(5):315–24.
35. Cowan DT, Wilson-Barnett J, Griffiths P, Allan LG. A survey of chronic noncancer pain patients prescribed opioid analgesics. Pain Med. 2003;4:340–51.
36. Ives TJ, Chelminski PR, Hammett-Stabler CA, Malone RM, Perhac JS, Potisek NM, Shilliday BB, DeWalt DA, Pignone MP. Predictors of opioid misuse in patients with chronic pain: a prospective cohort study. BMC Health Serv Res. 2006;6:46–56.
37. Macey TA, Morasco BJ, Duckart JP, Dobscha SK. Patterns and correlates of prescription opioid use in OEF/OIF veterans with chronic noncancer pain. Pain Med. 2011;12(10):1502–9.
38. Morasco BJ, Dobscha SK. Prescription medication misuse and substance use disorder in VA primary care patients with chronic pain. Gen Hosp Psychiatry. 2008;30:93–9.
39. Palmer R, Carrell D, Cronkite D, Saunders K, Gross D, Masters E, Hylan T, VonKroff M The prevalence and characteristics of patients with indicators of opioid abuse within an integrated group practice. Presented at the American Pain Society 33rd Annual Scientific Meeting; April 30-May 3, 2014. Tampa, FL. http://www.fda.gov/downloads/Drugs/NewsEvents/UCM397249.pdf.
40. Passik SD, Messina J, Golsorkhi A, Xie F. Aberrant drug-related behavior observed during clinical studies involving patients taking chronic opioid therapy for persistent pain and fentanyl buccal tablet for breakthrough pain. J Pain Symptom Manage. 2011;41:116–25.
41. Proctor SL, Estroff TW, Empting LD, Shearer-Williams S, Hoffmann NG. Prevalence of substance use and psychiatric disorders in a highly select chronic pain population. J Addict Med. 2013;7(1):17–24.
42. Sowa EM, Fellers JC, Raisinghani RS, Santa Cruz MR, Hidalgo PC, Lee MS, Martinez LA, Keller AE, Clayton AH. Prevalence of substance misuse in new patients in an outpatient psychiatry clinic using a prescription monitoring program. Prim Care Companion CNS Disord. 2014;16(1).
43. Belgrade MJ, Ismail M, Yoon M, Panopoulos G. Non-compliant drug screens during opioid maintenance analgesia for chronic non-malignant pain. Am Pain Society Meeting, 2001. San Diego A# 787, p. 42.
44. Couto JE, Romney MC, Leider HL, Sharma S, Goldfarb NI. High rates of inappropriate drug use in the chronic pain population. Popul Health Manag. 2009;12:185–90.
45. Fleming MF, Balousek SL, Klessig CL, Mundt MP, Brown DD. Substance use disorders in a primary care sample receiving daily opioid therapy. J Pain. 2007;8:573–82.
46. Manchikanti L, Manchukonda R, Pampati V, et al. Does random urine drug testing reduce illicit drug use in chronic pain patients receiving opioids? Pain Physician. 2006;9:123–9.
47. Manchikanti L, Manchukonda R, Pampati V, Damron KS. Evaluation of abuse of prescription and illicit drugs in chronic pain patients receiving short-acting (hydrocodone) or long-acting (methadone) opioids. Pain Physician. 2005;8:257–61.

48. Michna EJ, Ross EL, Janfaza D, et al. Urine toxicology screening among chronic pain patients on opioid therapy: frequency and predictability of abnormal findings. Clin J Pain. 2007;23:173–9.
49. Vaglienti RM, Huber SJ, Noel KR, Johnstone RE. Misuse of prescribed controlled substances defined by urinalysis. W V Med J. 2003;99:67–70.
50. Edlund MJ, Sullivan M, Steffick D, Harris KM, Wells KB. Do users of regularly prescribed opioids have higher rates of substance use problems than nonusers? Pain Med. 2007;8:647–56.
51. Hudson TJ, Edlund MJ, Steffick DE, Tripathi SP, Sullivan MD. Epidemiology of regular prescribed opioid use: results from a national, population-based survey. J Pain Symptom Manage. 2008;36(3):280–8.
52. Meyer C, Rumpf H, Hapke U, Dilling H, John U. Lebenszeitpraˉvalenz psychicher störungen in der erwachsenen allgemeinbevölkerung [Lifetime prevalence of mental disorders in general adult populations. Results of TACOS study]. Nervenarzt. 2000;71:535–42.
53. Regier D, Farmer M, Rae D, Locke Z, Keith S, Judd L, Goodwin F. Comorbidity of mental disorders with alcohol and other drug abuse. JAMA. 1990;19:2511–8.
54. Wilsey BL, Fishman SM, Tsodikov A, Ogden C, Symreng I, Ernst A. Psychological comorbidities predicting prescription opioid abuse among patients in chronic pain presenting to the emergency department. Pain Med. 2008;9(8):1107–17.
55. Butler SF, Budman SH, Licari A, et al. National Addictions Vigilance Intervention and Prevention Program (NAVIPPRO): a real-time, product-specific, public health surveillance system for monitoring prescription drug abuse. Pharmacoepidemiol Drug Saf. 2008;17:1142–54.
56. Butler SF, Budman SH, Fanciullo GJ, Jamison RN. Cross validation of the Current Opioid Misuse Measure (COMM) to monitor chronic pain patients on opioid therapy. Clin J Pain. 2010;26:770–6.
57. Cicero TJ, Surratt H, Inciardi JA, et al. Relationship between therapeutic use and abuse of opioid analgesics in rural, suburban, and urban locations in the United States. Pharmacoepidemiol Drug Saf. 2007;16:827–40.
58. Cicero TJ, Lynskey M, Todorov A, Inciardi JA, Surratt HL. Co-morbid pain and psychopathology in males and females admitted to treatment for opioid analgesic abuse. Pain. 2008;139(1):127–35.
59. Katz N, Panas L, Kim M, et al. Usefulness of prescription monitoring programs for surveillance—analysis of schedule II opioid prescription data in Massachusetts, 1996–2006. Pharmacoepidemiol and Drug Saf. 2010;19:115–23.
60. Banta-Green CJ, Merrill JO, Doyle SR, Boudreau DM, Calsyn DA. Measurement of opioid problems among chronic pain patients in a general medical population. Drug Alcohol Depend. 2009;104(1-2):43–9.
61. Office of National Drug Control Policy. Arrestee Drug Abuse Monitoring Program II, 2013 Annual Report; https://www.whitehouse.gov/sites/default/files/ondcp/policy-andresearch/adam_ii_2013_annual_report.pdf
62. Hughes AA, Bogdan GM, Dart RC. Active surveillance of abused and misused prescription opioids using poison center data: a pilot study and descriptive comparison. Clin Toxicol. 2007;45:144–51.
63. U.S. Department of Justice, Drug Enforcement Administration, Office of Diversion Control. National Forensic Laboratory Information System (NFLIS). 2013 Annual Report. https://www.nflis.deadiversion.usdoj.gov/DesktopModules/ReportDownloads/Reports/NFLIS2013AR.pdf. Accessed April 12, 2015
64. Woody GE, Senay EC, Geller A, Adams EH, Inciardi JA, Schnoll S, Muñoz A, Cicero TJ.An independent assessment of MEDWatch reporting for abuse/dependence and withdrawal from Ultram (tramadol hydrochloride). Drug Alcohol Depend. 2003;72(2):163–8.
65. Vowles KE, McEntee ML, Julnes PS, Frohe T, Ney JP, van der Goes DN. Rates of opioid misuse, abuse, and addiction in chronic pain: a systematic review and data synthesis. Pain. 2015;156(4):569–76.

66. Portenoy R. Opioid therapy for chronic nonmalignant pain: a review of the critical issues. J Pain Symptom Manage. 1996;11:203–17.
67. Jaffee J. Opiates: clinical aspects. In: Lowenson J, Ruiz P, Mullman R, editors. Substance abuse, a comprehensive text. Baltimore: Williams & Wilkins; 1992. p. 186–94.
68. Lowinson JH, Ruiz P, Milman RB. Substance abuse: a comprehensive textbook. Baltimore: Williams & Wilkins; 1992.
69. Wasan A, Correll D, Kissin I, O'Shea S, Jamison R. Iatrogenic addiction in patients treated for acute or subacute pain: a systematic review. J Opioid Manage. 2006;2:16–22.
70. Bartleson JD. Evidence for and against the use of opioid analgesics for chronic nonmalignant low back pain: A review. Pain Med. 2002;3:260–71.
71. Aronoff G. Opioids in chronic pain management: is there a significant risk of addiction? Curr Rev Pain. 2000;4:112–21.
72. Højsted J, Sjøgren P. Addiction to opioids in chronic pain patients: a literature review. Eur J Pain. 2007;11(5):490–518.
73. Martell B, O'Connor P, Kerns R, Becker W, Morales K, Kosten T, Fiellin D. Opioid treatment for chronic back pain: prevalence, efficacy, and association with addiction. Ann Intern Med. 2007;146:187–92.
74. Sullivan M. Clarifying opioid misuse and abuse. Pain. 2013;154:2239–40.
75. Cooper HM. Synthesizing research: a guide for literature reviews. 3rd ed. Newbury Park: Sage; 2001.
76. Hemingway P, Brereton N. What is a systematic review? Evidenced-based medicine. http://www.medicine.ox.ac.uk/bandolier/painres/download/whatis/syst-review.pdf. Accessed April 15, 2015
77. Fishbain DA, Cole B, Lewis J, Rosomoff HL, Rosomoff RS. What percentage of chronic nonmalignant pain patients exposed to chronic opioid analgesic therapy develop abuse/addiction and/or aberrant drug-related behaviors? A structured evidence-based review. Pain Med. 2008;9(4):444–59.
78. Smith SM, Dart RC, Katz NP, Paillard F, Adams EH, Comer SD, Degroot A, Edwards RR, Haddox JD, Jaffe JH, Jones CM, Kleber HD, Kopecky EA, Markman JD, Montoya ID, O'Brien C, Roland CL, Stanton M, Strain EC, Vorsanger G, Wasan AD, Weiss RD, Turk DC, Dworkin RH. Classification and definition of misuse, abuse, and related events in clinical trials: ACTTION systematic review and recommendations. Pain. 2013; 154: 2287–96.
79. Kotecha MK, Sites BD. Pain policy and abuse of prescription opioids in the USA: a cautionary tale for Europe. Anethesia. 2013;68:1207–19.
80. Muhuri PK, Gfroerer JC, Davies MC. Associations of nonmedical pain reliever use and initiation of heroin use in the United States. CBHDQ Data Review. Rockville, MD: Substance Abuse and Mental Health Services Administration. http://www.samhsa.gov/data/2k13/DataReview/DR006/nonmedical-pain-reliever-use-2013.pdf. Accessed April 27, 2014.
81. Ballantyne JC. Opioid analgesia: perspectives on right use and utility. Pain Physician. 2007;10:479–91.
82. Gordon A, Cone EJ, DePriest AZ, Axford-Gatley RA, Passik SD. Prescribing opioids for chronic noncancer pain in primary care: risk assessment. Postgrad Med. 2014;126(5):159–66.
83. Huffman KL, Shella ER, Sweis G, Griffith SD, Scheman J, Covington EC. Nonopioid substance use disorders and opioid dose predict therapeutic opioid addiction. J Pain. 2015;16(2):126–34.
84. Sehgal N, Manchikanti L, Smith HS. Prescription opioid abuse in chronic pain: a review of opioid abuse predictors and strategies to curb opioid abuse. Pain Physician. 2012;15(3 Suppl):ES67–92.
85. American Academy of Pain Medicine. Use of opioids for the treatment of chronic pain: A statement from the American Academy of Pain Medicine. 2013. http://www.painmed.org/files/use-of-opioids-for-the-treatment-of-chronic-pain.pdf. Accessed April 15, 2015.

Chapter 3
Alternative Treatments

Lori A. Urban

While pharmacologic approaches to the treatment of acute and chronic pain have been utilized for years, alternative/nonpharmacologic approaches have increasingly become acceptable methods of management, especially within a chronic framework. Chronic pain typically requires the coordinated efforts from a variety of professionals due to the complexity of the physical, psychosocial, and spiritual aspects that this pain presents [1]. It is also best conceptualized utilizing a biopsychosocial model, which was introduced several years ago by Engel [2], and is now well-utilized in health psychology and among many physicians. This model purposes an integrative theoretical perspective that incorporates addressing biological, psychological, interpersonal, and social functioning. It has challenged the previous reductionist biomedical model and has helped account for illnesses as human experiences rather than as mind-body dualism. Similarly, the diathesis-stress model of chronic pain [3] integrates cognitive, affective, behavioral, and family/social domains and suggests that they contribute to the perpetuation of the experience of pain and possible future psychopathology. In many models such as the diathesis-stress model, the *context* of the medical condition, illness, or pain is a significant component in understanding both conceptualization and intervention. This concept has guided many healthcare providers from the use of a biomedical model to a biopsychosocial model of understanding chronic illness and pain and the use of alternative methods of managing and treating chronic pain.

The nonpharmacologic approaches may be organized into psychological, physical rehabilitative, and surgical and are often an excellent supplement or adjunct to traditional medication. The numerous benefits and advantages may include improved patient empowerment, decreased anxiety and depression, cost effectiveness, strengthened coping skills, and overall improved quality of life. Of the many

L.A. Urban, Psy.D., A.B.P.P. (✉)
Department of Anesthesiology, Pain Management, University of Virginia School of Medicine, 545 Ray C. Hunt Drive, Suite 316, Charlottesville, VA 22908, USA
e-mail: lau9c@virginia.edu

© Springer International Publishing Switzerland 2016
A.M. Matthews, J.C. Fellers (eds.), *Treating Comorbid Opioid Use Disorder in Chronic Pain*, DOI 10.1007/978-3-319-29863-4_3

approaches that are used with treating chronic pain, a few specific psychological interventions and acupuncture will be addressed here in more detail. These alternative means of managing chronic pain are varied and include CBT, acceptance and commitment therapy, biofeedback, hypnosis, and acupuncture.

3.1   Cognitive–Behavioral Therapy

Interventions based on behavioral and cognitive–behavioral therapy (CBT) have significant empirical support [4] for many different disorders. Within the general body of research, the techniques defined as CBT interventions have included the following: relaxation training, communication strategies, sleep and activity interventions, problem solving, cognitive reframing/restructuring, operant techniques, and imagery. Although CBT for chronic pain has been described as the "gold standard" of psychological treatment [5], the mechanism by which it works has not been fully established, and there is not a standard protocol, varying in both session number and techniques. The emphasis on treating cognitive and affective domains and influences on pain was likely started with the introduction of the gate control theory of pain [6], with subsequent importance found for both social and environmental variables as well. Another significant contribution to the field was by Turk et al. [7], arguing the importance of and influence of cognition on chronic pain.

Behavior therapy and CBT have similar theoretical foundations that engage patients in making lifestyle changes that improve their functional status with management of pain [8]. CBT has become one of the primary psychological treatment modalities for chronic pain, and traditional methods of change include reducing pain and emotional distress and increasing healthy behaviors (physical and role function). This occurs through changing maladaptive thought patterns and behaviors and increasing self-efficacy. Homework assignments are an important method used in CBT and may involve practicing relaxation, working toward goals, or completing a thought log/diary. Guided workbooks are available for individuals, which include activity sheets and assistance in practicing or completing assigned homework tasks. One of these, Managing Pain Before It Manages You [9], includes several topics that impact individuals with chronic pain, such as education on pain and mind–body interactions, relaxation techniques, assertive communication, and even nutrition. Workbooks such as this can often be used within a therapy setting as an aid to increase follow-through and as a reminder of tasks after therapy is completed.

The empirical support for CBT used with chronic pain reveals statistically significant effects. These appear to be small for pain and disability, but moderate on mood and catastrophizing [10]. Pain catastrophizing, or the magnification of the possibility of pain and inability to cope with it, has been associated with greater levels of dysfunction, both physically and psychologically. Other outcome measures have included pain intensity, emotional functioning, physical functioning, global improvement, healthcare utilization, healthcare visits, pain medications, and employment status (or school, if pediatric). CBT interventions were found to be efficacious in these areas when used with individuals with chronic low back pain [11], and studies have also supported the use of CBT with chronic orofacial pain and headaches. The numerous reviews of these studies have supported the efficacy of CBT in treating chronic pain with small to medium effects overall.

CBT can also be expanded and tailored to treat special populations experiencing chronic pain, including children and adolescents, older adults, individuals with neurological conditions, low-literacy, and individuals in rural areas [5]. Within the pediatric population, research on cognitive–behavioral family interventions [12] reveals improvements in predicting and terminating pain episodes (reducing frequency) with use of several interventions, including education, operant behavior techniques, and cognitive procedures (thought stopping, distraction, and imagination). Other empirically supported interventions identified through a systematic review of treatments for recurrent abdominal pain in children and adolescents include self-monitoring, relaxation training, coping skills, and positive imagery [13].

3.2   Acceptance and Commitment Therapy

Acceptance and commitment therapy (ACT) [14] is a process-oriented and mindfulness-based approach that emphasizes observation without judgment, and commitment and behavior change (acceptance versus control). It targets maladaptive response-focused strategies and rejects the causal nature between cognitions, behaviors, and emotions. Application to chronic pain is based on the premise that the struggle with pain causes suffering, rather than the actual pain itself. ACT, therefore, aims to improve psychological flexibility when thoughts, feelings, and behaviors are presented that are associated with pain [15] and to engage in activities that are consistent with valued goals. The more an individual is fused (believes) with pain-related thoughts and feelings and acts accordingly, the more suffering or struggle will ensue. The acceptance ("letting go") may play a key role in decreasing the impact of pain flares, increasing treatment gains, and may predict future functioning. The process may also involve a decrease in physical exertion and muscle tension which subsequently results in interrupting the pain cycle. This mindfulness-based approach counters experiential avoidance and teaches individuals to respond reflectively rather than reflexively. The six important elements used in ACT include acceptance, defusion, contact with the present moment, self as context, values, and committed action.

ACT has had a small, but growing body of empirical support over the last couple of decades that suggests effectiveness with several disorders, including anxiety, depression, pain, trichotillomania, substance abuse, psychosis, and epilepsy and diabetes management. These studies, specifically using ACT in the context of chronic pain, have revealed improvement in pain disability, life satisfaction, fear of movement, depression, psychological inflexibility, medical visits, work status, physical performance, pain-related anxiety, school attendance, catastrophizing, and pain [16]. Although most of the studies use pain intensity as one of the primary outcome measures, reduction in this area is not a primary focus of acceptance-based interventions, and in fact, most controlled studies find that mindfulness-based interventions have a small effect on pain intensity overall. Preliminary trials of an outpatient group-based intervention [17] and of manual-based self-help interventions with some therapist support [18, 19] revealed efficacy of ACT with chronic pain. This includes improvements in acceptance, satisfaction with life, and level of function. Powers et al.'s [20] meta-analytic review found that ACT outperformed several control conditions, but there was no distinct advantage of use over other established treatments, such as CBT, interpersonal therapy, and cognitive therapy. These results have been supported by other meta-analyses [21] as well. A review of articles and research also reveals a need for more well-controlled studies with larger sample sizes, as the methodological rigor appears less stringent than studies related to CBT interventions. Future studies likely need to be time-limited within standard, outpatient clinical settings facilitated by a single discipline.

3.3   Biofeedback

Biofeedback is a form of applied psychophysiology that relies on the premise of early stress research by Selye [22] and involves the relationship between physiological and cognitive processes. An individual is taught to increase awareness of unhealthy mental patterns and improve health by changing physiological functioning. The physiological feedback/input may be presented in the form of peripheral blood flow, heart rate variability, blood pressure, muscle or sweat gland activity, or brain electrical activity. The two most common forms are electromyography (EMG) and skin temperature (indirect measure of peripheral blood volume). The feedback is provided through visual or auditory cues via the connection to electrical sensors which are then relayed on a monitor. Patient education is a vital component of this intervention and involves seven levels of information, including the following: signal presentation; explanation of the signal; explanation of the signal in relation to physiology; explanation of the signal in relation to symptoms; therapist suggestions; information to the therapist; and informing patients that they are successful [23]. The decision of which type of biofeedback to use is the result of empirically based data and the desired outcomes.

Disorders that are most likely to improve with use of biofeedback interventions include tension-type headache, migraine headache, nocturnal enuresis, fecal incontinence, urinary incontinence, pelvic floor disorders, essential hypertension, and phantom limb pain. Other disorders that have empirical support with biofeedback, specifically associated with pain, include irritable bowel syndrome, temporomandibular disorders and bruxism, Raynaud's phenomenon, fibromyalgia, and chronic pain in general [24]. Biofeedback can assist with altering abnormal patterns of muscle tension or managing anxiety that has contributed to recurrent or chronic pain. A recent review of mind–body therapies with chronic pain revealed improvement with chronic low back pain and migraine headache pain in at least two high-quality studies

[25]. However, there were many studies that were classified as "poor-quality" with methodological limitations, including dropout rates and randomization methods.

Chronic headache pain, including tension-type and migraine, has also been studied extensively as a disorder that is responsive to biofeedback (EMG and thermal, respectively). The frontalis muscles of the forehead may be used as a site to place electrodes to teach an individual overall body relaxation for a goal of reducing tension and replacing anxiety with a sense of calming [26]. The other two muscle groups that are beneficial for monitoring include the masseter and the trapezius for chronic tension-type headaches. Electrodes on the fingertips may provide feedback on the temperature of the fingers as a method to teach about the autonomic activity related to blood flow for migraine headaches. A meta-analysis on interventions for pediatric migraine headaches revealed thermal biofeedback and interventions combining biofeedback and progressive muscle relaxation as more efficacious than other behavioral treatment modalities [27]. However, additional research has indicated that biofeedback may not increase benefits substantially over relaxation techniques used in adults with migraine and tension type headaches [28].

3.4 Hypnosis

Hypnotic techniques date back thousands of years to Egypt, Greece, and Rome. There are more than 220 years of clinical practice and an increasing interest over the years, in part due to a demand for non-pharmacologic interventions without side effects. Hypnosis, or hypnotherapy, is a trance-like state in which an individual has heightened focus or attention. When used to assist with chronic pain management, it usually involves an induction with suggestions for relaxation, comfort, and improvement in symptoms. Many times, an individual will be taught post-hypnotic suggestions to aid with recreating the relaxed stated and thus producing analgesia or reducing pain sensations (how it is viewed or experienced). Most often, it appears that the benefits of hypnosis occur over time as the skill is learned and practiced, rather than as an immediate and automatic process [29].

An increased number of controlled studies related to hypnosis and chronic pain has been conducted and includes work with the following conditions: cancer, low-back pain, arthritis, sickle cell disease, temporomandibular pain, fibromyalgia, headaches, gastrointestinal pain, and physical disability. A review of these studies revealed consistency in the positive effects of hypnosis in reducing chronic pain as more effective than the control group/no treatment [30]. The effects, when compared with relaxation interventions, were not statistically different, alluding to the two interventions possibly having similar mechanisms of action and effects. This may support the other benefits of hypnosis, which include reducing anxiety and improving sleep. With regard to chronic back pain, there have unfortunately been very few controlled studies in the literature. The few available have revealed some improvement in sleep onset and a reduction in pain intensity [31].

Unfortunately, several studies combining hypnosis with guided imagery were found to be of poor-quality and underpowered, resulting in the inability to provide a recommendation for using these in treatment for chronic pain [25]. However, it appears that increasing standardization in the hypnotic process (induction and interventions) may provide more specific comparison data to other methods of pain management. Jensen and Patterson [29] reviewed several studies comparing hypnotic interventions with a no-treatment baseline, standard medical care, physical therapy, medication management, occlusal appliance, biofeedback, and attention control. Their findings indicate that hypnosis contributes to significant reductions in pain perception which maintain for several months. When compared with medication management, physical therapy, and education, hypnosis appears to be more effective and appears to be just as effective as autogenic training and progressive muscle relaxation.

3.5 Acupuncture

The recorded use of acupuncture has been documented more than 5000 years ago in China, but concerted research attempts related to its efficacy did not begin until the 1970s. *The Yellow Emperor's Classic of Internal Medicine* is the first identified book describing an organized method now recognized as acupuncture, and *The Great Compendium of Acupuncture and Moxibustion*, which dates back to the Ming dynasty (1368–1644), has been used as the basis for modern techniques [32]. As a key component of Chinese medicine, acupuncture eventually spread to other countries and became more accepted in the United States after NIH reported positive evidence for its effectiveness in postoperative and chemotherapy side effects, nausea during pregnancy, and postoperative dental pain [33].

Acupuncture requires the insertion of thin, solid, metallic needles into specific points on the body which then stimulate Qi (vital energy or life force). Blockages in Qi may occur along meridians, which the needles unblock to bring about a healthy state in an individual. The goal is to obtain a delicate balance of two forces, known as the yin and yang. Throughout time, the traditional concept involving Qi and meridians has been challenged by a neurological model where the needles are thought to stimulate nerve endings and alter brain functioning [34]. The needles may also release neurotransmitters and produce changes in the hypothalamus and amygdala. Although these effects are relevant to analgesia, there has been little understanding to the mechanism of action related to chronic pain, resulting in acupuncture being a controversial therapy.

Acupuncture has been studied to determine its efficacy for many different disorders, not inclusive of the following: anxiety, depression, low back pain, insomnia, cancer-related pain, headaches, fibromyalgia, osteoarthritis, and schizophrenia. There are initial, positive findings for anxiety, but they are inconclusive for depression [35], two emotional responses that can co-occur with and intensify chronic pain. Improvements in outcome measures related to sleep (quality and duration) and headache pain have been reported. Specifically, a Cochrane review [36] revealed a small to moderate size effect for use of acupuncture with migraine prophylaxis. Unfortunately, the research could also be complicated by the possible placebo effect of sham acupuncture when this intervention produces positive results as well. It appears that both sham acupuncture (insertion of needles without stimulation and in non-acupuncture points) and real acupuncture may be equally effective for chronic low-back pain. Another systematic review (31 eligible studies) supported the use of acupuncture compared to control groups with no intervention in patients with musculoskeletal pain, osteoarthritis, and chronic headache [37]. Overall, there was support for the use of acupuncture for chronic pain as more than a placebo and with larger benefits when coupled with ancillary care, such as physical therapy.

3.6 Conclusion

Use of alternative methods of chronic pain management is recommended on the basis of the biopsychosocial model incorporating biological, psychological, interpersonal, and social functioning. These methods of treating and managing chronic pain have empirical support for several different pain disorders and presentations. They tend to have fewer or no side effects when compared with pharmacologic interventions and can work well as adjunct to other methods. The nonpharmacologic modalities presented here (CBT, ACT, biofeedback, hypnosis, and acupuncture) have collective research with small to moderate size effects, primarily related to increasing function, improving coping with pain, and overall quality of life. There is also an impact on sleep, anxiety, and depression, which can co-occur with chronic pain and contribute to exacerbating or maintaining pain episodes. Further research to detail mechanisms of action is suggested via larger sample sizes, controlled settings, and overall improvement in the rigor of study methodology.

References

1. Thienhaus O, Cole BE. The classification of pain. In: Weiner RS, editor. Pain management: a practical guide for clinicians. 6th ed. Boca Raton: CRC; 2002. p. 27–36.
2. Engel GL. The need for a new medical model: a challenge for biomedicine. Science. 1977;196:129–36.
3. Kerns RD, Jacob MC. Toward an integrative diathesis-stress model of chronic pain. In: Goreczny AJ, editor. Handbook of health and rehabilitation psychology. New York: Plenum Press; 1995. p. 325–40.
4. Chambless DL, Baker MJ, Baucom DH, Beutler LE, Calhoun KS, Crist-Christoph P, et al. Update on empirically validated therapies, II. Clin Psychol. 1998;51:3–16.
5. Ehde DM, Dillworth TM, Turner JA. Cognitive-behavioral therapy for individuals with chronic pain. Am Psychol. 2014;69(2):153–66.
6. Melzack R, Wall PD. Pain mechanisms: a new theory. Science. 1965;150:971–9.
7. Turk DD, Meichenbaum D, Genest M. Pain and behavioral medicine: a cognitive-behavioral perspective. New York: Guilford Press; 1983.

8. Williams D. Pain and painful syndromes (Including rheumatoid arthritis and fibromyalgia). In: Suls JM, Davidson KW, Kaplan RM, editors. Handbook of health psychology and behavioral medicine. New York: Guilford Press; 2010. p. 476–93.
9. Caudill M. Managing pain before it manages you. New York: Guilford Press; 2009.
10. Williams AC, Eccleston C, Morley S. Psychological therapies for the management of chronic pain (excluding headache) in adults. Cochrane Database Syst Rev. 2012;11:CD007407.
11. Hoffman BM, Papas RK, Chatkoff DK, Kerns RD. Meta-analysis of psychological interventions for chronic low back pain. Health Psychol. 2007;26(1):1–9.
12. Duarte MA, Penna FJ, Andrade EM, Cancela CS, Neto JC, Barbosa TF. Treatment of nonorganic recurrent abdominal pain: cognitive-behavioral family intervention. J Pediatr Gastroenterol Nutr. 2006;43(1):59–64.
13. Weydert JA, Ball TM, Davis MF. Systematic review of treatments for recurrent abdominal pain. Pediatrics. 2003;111(1):1–11.
14. Hayes SC, Strosahl K, Wilson KG. Acceptance and commitment therapy: an experiential approach to behavior change. New York: Guilford Press; 1999.
15. Dahl J, Lundgren T. Acceptance and commitment therapy (ACT) in the treatment of chronic pain. In: Baer R, editor. Mindfulness-based treatment approaches: a clinician's guide to evidence base and applications. Oxford: Elsevier; 2006. p. 285–306.
16. Pull CB. Current empirical status of acceptance and commitment therapy. Curr Opin Psychiatry. 2008;22:55–60.
17. Vowles KE, Wetherell JL, Sorrell JT. Targeting acceptance, mindfulness, and values-based action in chronic pain: findings of two preliminary trials of an outpatient group-based intervention. Cogn Behav Pract. 2009;16:49–58.
18. Johnston M, Foster M, Shennan J, Starkey NJ, Johnston A. The effectiveness of an acceptance and commitment therapy self-help intervention for chronic pain. Clin J Pain. 2010; 26(5):393–402.
19. Thorsell J, Finnes A, Dahl J, Lundgren T, Gybrant M, Gordh T, Burhman M. A comparative study of 2 manual-based self-help interventions, acceptance and commitment therapy and applied relaxation, for persons with chronic pain. Clin J Pain. 2011;27(8):716–23.
20. Powers MB, Vording MB, Emmelkamp PM. Acceptance and commitment therapy: a meta-analytic review. Psychother Psychosom. 2009;78:73–80.
21. Veehof MM, Oskam MJ, Schreurs K, Bohlmeijer ET. Acceptance-based interventions for the treatment of chronic pain: a systematic review and meta-analysis. Pain. 2011;152:533–42.
22. Selye H. Stress without distress. Philadelphia: Lippincott; 1974.
23. Schwartz NM, Schwartz MS. Definitions of biofeedback and applied psychophysiology. In: Schwartz MS, Andrasik F, editors. Biofeedback: a practitioner's guide. New York: Guilford Press; 2003. p. 27–39.
24. Schwartz MS. Intake decisions and preparation of patients for therapy. In: Schwartz MS, Andrasik F, editors. Biofeedback: a practitioner's guide. New York: Guilford Press; 2003. p. 105–27.
25. Lee C, Crawford C, Hickey A. Mind-body therapies for the self-management of chronic pain symptoms. Pain Med. 2014;15:S21–39.
26. Catalano EM, Hardin KN. The chronic pain control workbook: a step-by-step guide for coping with and overcoming pain. New York: MJF Books; 1996.
27. Hermann C, Kim M, Blanchard EB. Behavioral and prophylactic pharmacological intervention studies of pediatric migraine: an exploratory meta-analysis. Pain. 1995;60:239–56.
28. Mullally WJ, Hall K, Goldstein R. Efficacy of biofeedback in the treatment of migraine and tension type headaches. Pain Physician. 2009;12:1005–11.
29. Jensen M, Patterson DR. Hypnotic treatment of chronic pain. J Behav Med. 2006;29(1): 95–124.
30. Elkins G, Jensen MP, Patterson DR. Hypnotherapy for the management of chronic pain. Int J Clin Exp Hypnosis. 2007;55(3):275–87.
31. Wellington J. Noninvasive and alternative management of chronic low back pain (efficacy and outcomes). Neuromodulation. 2014;17:24–30.

32. White A, Ernst E. A brief history of acupuncture. Rheumatology. 2004;43:662–3.
33. Acupuncture. NIH consensus statement online. 1997 Nov 3–5; 15(5):1–34.
34. Han J, Terenius L. Neurochemical basis of acupuncture analgesia. Annu Rev Pharmacol Toxicol. 1982;22:193–220.
35. Barnett JE, Shale AJ, Elkins G, Fisher W. Complementary and alternative medicine for psychologists. Washington, DC: American Psychological Association; 2014.
36. Linde K, Allais G, Brinkhaus B, Manheimer E, Vickers A, White AR. Acupuncture for migraine prophylaxis. Cochrane Database Syst Rev. 2009;1, CD001218. doi:10.1002/14651858. CD001218.pub2.
37. Vickers AJ, Cronin AM, Maschino AC, Lewith G, MacPherson H, Foster NE, Sherman, KJ, Witt, CM, Linde, K. Acupuncture for chronic pain., Archives of Internal Medicine, 2012;172(19):1444–1453.

Chapter 4
Evaluating the Biopsychosocial Milieu of Chronic Pain

Mary Elizabeth Turner and Marian Fireman

4.1 Introduction

The biopsychosocial model was developed in the 1970s and is now considered part of the standard of care in psychiatric and chronic pain assessments. The model incorporates three elements—biological, social, and psychological—and enforces the idea that medical illness is shaped by the combination of each of these three domains. In this chapter, we will discuss the history of the biopsychosocial model in evaluations, evidence for its usage, and tips for performing this assessment.

4.2 Background

George Engel, a psychiatrist, proposed the biopsychosocial model in 1977. He saw the model as a solution to the crisis in the field of psychiatry regarding its relationship with the rest of the medical field. Engel claimed psychiatry was divided between two groups—advocates of separating psychiatry from the medical field and its focus on treatment of "diseases" and advocates of having psychiatry focus on "biological" psychiatric "diseases." Engel believed the purely biomedical model hindered diagnosis. Patients can report symptoms in different ways depending on social and psychological factors, and we do not always have clear laboratory or other biological markers indicating the presence of disease. He advocated a biopsychosocial model that he claimed was more in keeping with the historical practice of medicine, arguing that this model would lead to improved diagnosis and treatment [1].

M.E. Turner, M.D., J.D. • M. Fireman, M.D. (✉)
Oregon Health & Science University,
3181 SW Sam Jackson, UHN80, Portland, OR 97239, USA
e-mail: mary.turner31@gmail.com; firemanm@ohsu.edu

© Springer International Publishing Switzerland 2016   35
A.M. Matthews, J.C. Fellers (eds.), *Treating Comorbid Opioid Use Disorder in Chronic Pain*, DOI 10.1007/978-3-319-29863-4_4

In promoting the benefit of a biopsychosocial model beyond psychiatry, Engel published an article describing the biopsychosocial assessment in a patient with chest pain. He constructed diagrams showing the interactions between an individual, their perceptions and history, and the molecular mechanisms of disease. He stated that the ultimate benefit of his model was to see a patient as a human [2]. Engel's ideas were rapidly adopted. By the late 1990s, nearly half of all medical schools incorporated the biopsychosocial model into their curriculum with up to 10 % of their curriculum being devoted to biopsychosocial issues [3]. Today, the American Psychiatric Association recommends that all psychiatry assessments include a biopsychosocial formulation [4].

Beyond psychiatry, Engel's ideas were incorporated into notions of patient-centered care [5] and have become especially prominent in medical specialties dealing with chronic pain and substance usage. Most treatment guidelines recommend that a biopsychosocial assessment be performed for these population groups [6–8]. According to the Institute of Medicine's 2011 report on pain management, "interdisciplinary, biopsychosocial approaches are the most promising for treating patients with chronic pain" [9].

4.3 Potential Concerns

Although the biopsychosocial model is now an institutional framework of psychiatry and general medicine, both philosophical and technical problems have appeared. Engel was accused of creating a "strawman" out of biomedical medicine and of forcing doctors to be "too good" by assessing and understanding patients in ways that were essentially too complex and time-consuming [10]. Even in psychiatry where trainees are taught to think in a biopsychosocial framework from internship onward, residents show poor ability to do a biopsychosocial assessment [11]. Determining the depth to be explored for each component is challenging as a full assessment in all three domains of the biopsychosocial model can be exhaustive, especially when coupled with limited clinical resources and time.

4.4 Examination of the Evidence

The broad scope of the biopsychosocial model results in challenges in researching its efficacy. Evidence for it in the chronic pain setting varies based on different pain modalities and on different patient populations. The Cochrane Review looked at studies on multidisciplinary biopsychosocial programs for chronic neck and shoulder pain and found only two low-quality studies that met their inclusion criteria [12]. For subacute back pain, they again found only two limited quality studies that met inclusion criteria, but determined there was moderate evidence for positive efficacy of a multidisciplinary biopsychosocial assessment, especially if it included a workplace evaluation [12, 13]. Forty-one qualifying randomized controlled trials were included in their review of chronic low back pain. The evidence did support a reduction in both pain intensity and disability in patients who received multidisciplinary biopsychosocial rehabilitation, although the effects were modest. More intensive interventions did not appear to result in significantly better improvement than less intensive interventions [14]. For repetitive strain injuries, they found only two low-quality studies, noting a need for higher-quality studies [15]. Of note, all of their studies focused solely on working age adults. There is a paucity of data for pediatric patients [16].

Although studies showing the efficacy of a comprehensive multidisciplinary biopsychosocial assessment are limited, there is strong evidence of a relationship between psychosocial factors and chronic pain. Many mechanisms are proposed and some are validated. For example, fear inhibits pain in the short run, but chronic fear leads to anticipatory anxiety, which worsens chronic pain. People who anticipate pain experience increased pain, and activation of the dopamine system, which increases positive emotions, reduces the subjective experience of pain ([17], p. 6).

Population studies show that people who suffer from chronic pain report higher rates of childhood adversity (divorce, sexual abuse, family conflict, etc.). Childhood abuse and neglect predict pain when compared with healthy controls. Alexithymia, the inability to describe one's feelings, is found in higher rates in people with chronic pain conditions, including low back pain and temporomandibular joint pain. Alexithymia has a positive correlation with pain severity ([17], p. 6). Pain catastrophizing, ruminating and feeling hopeless about pain, is associated with greater reported pain. Patients who catastrophize about pain are more likely to have a history of trauma ([17], p. 13). Patients with increased pain-related anxiety are more likely to avoid rehabilitation tasks, hindering recovery from injuries and procedures ([17], p. 13). There is growing evidence that people with a history of insecure parental attachment have increased pain. This association is theorized to have a role in the colloquial usage of pain language to describe interpersonal losses (e.g. "brokenhearted") ([17], p. 6).

Patients with chronic pain have a higher incidence of mental illness. Depression rates in chronic pain patients are as high as 85 % in dental clinics addressing chronic pain and 52 % in general chronic pain clinics, compared with depression rates of 5–10 % in the general population [18]. Anxiety disorders may be twice as common in chronic pain patients as in the general population, and Panic Disorder and Post Traumatic Stress Disorder occur three times as frequently in this population [19]. Addiction and substance use disorders are frequently comorbid in chronic pain. Treatment with opioids increases the risk of addiction. Estimates of rates of addiction among chronic pain patients range from 3 to 40 % [20].

Psychosocial treatments for pain can result in improved outcomes. Various psychological interventions have been studied, ranging from insight-oriented to psychodynamic to cognitive–behavioral therapies. Cognitive behavioral treatments and self-regulatory treatments have the strongest evidence base for efficacy [21] and can result in reduced pain and disability and improved overall functioning [22]. Other treatment modalities for chronic pain with less accumulated evidence than CBT include meditation, motivational interviewing, guided imagery, and hypnosis [22]. A biopsychosocial assessment may be helpful in determining which patients would benefit from therapy.

Table 4.1 Major treatment guideline recommendations

Institute of Medicine [9]	Assessment of emotional aspects of pain is essential; failure to adopt biopsychosocial model can result in increased disability
Institute for Clinical Systems Improvement [6]	Assess for biopsychosocial factors including psychiatric illness and trauma history
American Society for Anesthesiologists [23]	Assess for psychosocial factors that can contribute to pain
Institute of Health Economics (Canada) (IHE 2011) [46]	Assess for psychosocial factors with back pain; increase intensity of assessment if patients fail to improve with early interventions
Scottish Intercollegiate Guidelines Network (SIGN 2013) [37]	Use biopsychosocial frame to assess functional impact of pain, potentially spreading evaluation over several visits. Intensity of evaluation depends on severity of pain and responsiveness to early interventions. Refer to multidisciplinary pain clinic if patient fails to improve or if patient has significant social or occupational impairment from pain
National Institute for Health and Care Excellence (United Kingdom) [24]	No significant recommendation for biopsychosocial assessment for back pain; recommend treating identified causes of psychological distress before surgical referral
European Guidelines for Evidence-Based Management [25]	Strong evidence that low workplace support leads to chronicity in low back pain; moderate evidence that psychosocial distress leads to low back pain chronicity. Recommends an evaluation of work issues, psychological distress, and patient expectations

4.5 Current Recommendations for Chronic Pain Assessments

In spite of limitations in studies for chronic pain, a biopsychosocial assessment is recommended by most treatment guidelines. See the table below for a summary of current recommendations both from North America and Europe. In general, guidelines recommend assessing for psychosocial factors and considering a multidisciplinary biopsychosocial assessment if patients fail to improve with routine treatment (Table 4.1).

4.6 Performing the Assessment: The Biological Assessment

General elements of this part of the assessment include obtaining a thorough history of the pain, including its location, character, duration, intensity, exacerbating, and relieving factors. A physical examination should focus on looking for obvious deformities, atrophy, asymmetry, cyanosis, effusion, or pallor. A focused neurological exam including assessment of language and cognitive functioning, gait, strength, sensation, and reflexes should be included. Allodynia and hyperalgesia should be assessed as these are particularly prominent in chronic pain syndromes [6]. Interestingly, there is limited data to support the utility of most physical tests routinely done in a low back pain examination, both those assessing lumbar hernia-tion [26] and chronic low back pain [25].

Diagnostic testing is complicated in a chronic pain assessment. Individuals with identical imaging findings can have different subjective experiences of pain because of the complex and multifactorial nature of pain [27]. MRIs are the most frequent imaging test ordered in chronic pain assessments, but plain X-rays, electromyogra-phy, and nerve conduction studies may be used as well [6]. European guidelines recommend against electromyography in chronic low back pain assessments and against imaging in general unless there is strong clinical suspicion of need for imag-ing [25]. Imaging and diagnostic testing recommendations change over time and providers should remain updated on the latest recommendations and evidence regarding these tests to minimize the risk of excessive testing and iatrogenic harm.

Other elements of a biological assessment include determining the biological mechanism of the pain, dividing it into four types—neuropathic, inflammatory, muscle, and mechanical/inflammatory—with the understanding that there might be multiple types of pain in one presentation. This is important because the mechanism of pain can suggest the most appropriate pharmacologic treatment. This information should be obtained from the history, physical examination, and possibly diagnostic imaging [6].

4.7   The Social Assessment

Basic elements of a social history include developmental history, marital and rela-tionship status, occupational history, legal history, and access to treatment, which includes financial, insurance, and regional factors. Obtaining history about a per-son's work and home setting is a critical part of this assessment, and one should always be aware of the possibility for secondary gain [28]. Motivation to return to work or to obtain disability might affect a patient's presentation and engagement in treatment, and job dissatisfaction is a predictor of poor outcomes [29]. To under-stand the impact of the pain, determine premorbid and post-morbid social function-ing as chronic pain can negatively impact social functioning by leading to work and income loss, family stress, and social isolation [30].

The social assessment should be organized in a chronological manner, starting with childhood and moving through different stages of adulthood. Particular devel-opmental concerns can affect chronic pain, including early attachment to caregivers and abuse and neglect during childhood [31]. Attachment patterns can be ascer-tained by asking about early childhood figures and for a description of a person's childhood. Descriptions that are overly vague or idealized can be an indicator of an insecure attachment pattern [32]. Assessing the quality and duration of childhood and adult relationships also provides insight into social functioning and can give an idea of how well a person will engage in treatment. A person with a pattern of struggles with dependency may seek to find their own treatment rather than follow-ing medical advice, whereas a person with a history of dependent relationship needs might have an incentive to be perceived as sick or disabled [33].

An occupational history is particularly useful for a chronic pain assessment. Questions include how invested has the person been in work, what are the physical requirements of the job, and are work modifications possible. Once a person is out of work for an extended period for a disability, their odds of successfully returning to work falls precipitously [34]. Cultural factors are also important although it is difficult to make generalizations about culturally based responses [35]. There is limited indication that people of different cultures experience pain differently, although culture can influence expressions of pain [36].

4.8   The Psychological Assessment

The psychological assessment is often combined with the social assessment, and even in this chapter, we periodically refer to the psychosocial assessment, but a psychological assessment focuses on one's thoughts and feelings. It includes an assessment of one's psychiatric history including substance use disorders, and of a patient's coping skills and psychological defenses. This assessment can be conducted in many ways, but screening tools are often particularly helpful [29], as are serial assessments over time [37].

Screening intensity should vary based on the chronicity and severity of pain with an indication for increased screening when patients fail to respond to standard interventions [6, 25, 37]. Even non-specialty providers should assess for depression and substance use disorders [6, 25, 37]. There are multiple brief screening tools of proven validity, including the CAGE and AUDIT for substance use disorders and PHQ-9 for depression [38]. Simply asking a patient if they have experienced depression, hopelessness, or anhedonia in the past month has high sensitivity for depression [39].

If more screening is indicated, longer psychological screening tools include the Battery for Health Improvement (BHI 2), Brief Battery for Health Improvement (BBHI 2), and the Pain Patient Profile (P3) [29]. These tests are all under copyright and require licensing fees. The P3 screen may be able to detect malingering [40] and has been found to have high construct validity for depression, anxiety, and somatization in pain patients [41]. The BHI 2 was designed specifically with a bio-psychosocial assessment in mind with a goal to produce a graphical model of a biopsychosocial formulation. It has been accepted in evidence by different court systems and has been described as one of the "best" tools available for a pain assessment [42]. The BBHI 2 is a shorter version of the BHI and can be administered quickly in the office. It has validity measures for exaggerating and concealing information and can be used serially to assess for improvement over time [43].

Other psychological screening tools include the Million Behavioral Medicine Diagnostic (MBMD), which is designed for general medical patients and general psychological tests such as the Minnesota Multiphasic Personality Inventory (MMPI) and the Personality Assessment Inventory (PAI) [29]. The MBMD can be useful for assessing psychological issues in patients who do not have clear

Table 4.2 Psychological tests

psychological tests	Advantages	Disadvantages
Battery for Health Improvement (BHI 2)	Produces graph of biopsychosocial formulation; accepted as evidence in court hearings	Must pay fee to administer
Brief Battery for Health Improvement (BBHI 2)	Short, can be administered in office; can be used serially; validated for finding exaggerated responses and concealing information	Must pay fee to administer
Pain Patient Profile (P 3)	Can detect malingering; construct validity for depression, anxiety, and somatization	Must pay fee to administer
Million Behavioral Medicine Diagnostic (MBMD)	Designed for general medicine patients; might be useful for patients without clear psychopathology	Questionable reliability; not specifically designed for chronic pain; lengthy; must pay fee to administer
Minnesota Multiphasic Personality Inventory (MMPI)	General psychological screening; extensive	Needs to be combined with other testing for chronic pain; must pay fee to administer; time-consuming
Personality Assessment Inventory (PAI)	Useful for detecting psychopathology in chronic pain patients	Must pay fee to administer

psychopathology [43]. The MMPI is lengthy and would need to be combined with other instruments in performing a chronic pain assessment [43]. The PAI has been found to be useful for detecting psychopathology in chronic pain patients [44]. While all these tests have potential benefits, we do not have evidence to support the use of one screening tool over another or to suggest that one screening tool would work better than another in a specific population (Table 4.2).

4.9   Special Considerations for the Substance Using Patient

Substance abuse presents unique challenges in patient evaluations. Providers should be aware of red flags, including lost prescriptions, requests for early refills, belligerent, demanding or erratic behavior, and positive urine drug screens. Most treatment guidelines recommend a thorough assessment for substance using patients, including referral to multidisciplinary treatment centers. Unique biopsychosocial factors in substance using patients include the effects of tolerance and withdrawal, potential for overdose, legal consequences, diversion risk, and psychologically reinforcing effects of substances.

Providers should obtain collateral information from family members and previous providers and check any available prescription drug-monitoring databases. A thorough substance use history should be obtained, including tobacco and caffeine usage, as well as an assessment of consequences of usage. In performing an assessment, providers should be particularly aware of patients who focus exclusively on opioids as treatment for their condition. In the physical exam, look for signs of substance use (track marks, skin infections, nasal or oral pathology) and assess patients for signs of intoxication or cognitive impairment. Quick screening tools are available, including the CAGE adapted for drug usage, AUDIT-C and Michigan Alcoholism Screening Test (MAST), but no screening tool replaces a thorough clinical interview. The Substance Abuse and Mental Health Services Administration (SAMHSA) recommends that pain providers have a strong referral network for substance use providers [45].

SAMHSA recommends drug screening for chronic pain patients on opioid treatment with frequency determined based on clinical assessment. What tests to include in the urine drug screens and whether to do less-sensitive point of care testing depend on the situation and clinical assessment. Point of care testing is limited by the potential for false positives and poor ability to detect synthetic and semisynthetic opioids, but is convenient and allows quick, affordable screening. Providers should be aware of the strengths and limitations of testing and should have a close relationship with the testing laboratory. One caveat of random drug testing is that physicians should be aware of the risk of disproportionately testing minority or marginalized populations [45].

4.10   Summary

The biopsychosocial model started in psychiatry and spread to other medical disciplines, picking up special resonance in chronic pain evaluations. Performing a biopsychosocial assessment in chronic pain patients is a standard of care in most treatment guidelines, although recommendations for how thorough this assessment should be are less clear. Generally, more thorough assessments in multidisciplinary settings are indicated for patients who fail to respond to usual treatment, who show signs of poorly controlled psychiatric conditions, and who have substance use disorders, especially unacknowledged ones. However, randomized controlled trials testing the efficacy of a biopsychosocial assessment are lacking, while the evidence for the connection between chronic pain and psychosocial impairment is much stronger.

References

1. Engel GL. The need for a new medical model: a challenge for biomedicine. Science. 1977;196:129–36.
2. Engel GL. The clinical application of the biopsychosocial model. J Med Philos. 1981;6(2):101–24.
3. Adler RH. Engel's biopsychosocial model is still relevant today. J Psychosom Res. 2009;67(6):607–11.

4. American Psychiatric Association. Practice guidelines for psychiatric evaluation of an adult. June 2006. http://psychiatryonline.org/pb/assets/raw/sitewide/practice_guidelines/guidelines/psychevaladults.pdf.
5. Smith RC. The biopsychosocial revolution. J Gen Intern Med. 2002;17(4):309–10.
6. Hooten WM, Timming R, Belgrade M, Gaul J, Goertz M, Haake B, Myers C, Noonan MP, Owens J, Saeger L, Schweim K, Shteyman G, Walker N. Assessment and management of chronic pain. Bloomington: Institute for Clinical Systems Improvement (ICSI); 2013. p. 105.
7. Management of Opioid Therapy for Chronic Pain Working Group. VA/DoD clinical practice guideline for management of opioid therapy for chronic pain. Washington, DC: Department of Veterans Affairs, Department of Defense; 2010 May.
8. SAMHSA. Managing chronic pain in adults with or in recovery from substance use disorders. HHS publication no. (SMA) 12-4671. Rockville: Substance Abuse and Mental Health Services Administration; 2011.
9. Institute of Medicine. Relieving pain in America: a blueprint for transforming prevention care, education and research. Washington, DC: National Academies Press; 2011.
10. Kantos N. Biomedicine—menace or strawman? Reexamining the biopsychosocial argument. Acad Med. 2011;86(4):509–15.
11. McClain T, O'Sullivan PS, Clardy JA. Biopsychosocial formulation: recognizing educational shortcomings. Acad Psychiatry. 2004;28(2):88–94.
12. Karjalainin KA, Malmivaara A, van Tulder MW, Roine R, et al. Multidisciplinary biopsychosocial rehabilitation for neck and shoulder pain among working age adults. Cochrane Database Syst Rev. 2003;2, CD002194.
13. Karjalainen KA, Malmivaara A, van Tulder MW, Roine R, Jauhiainen M, Hurri H, Koes BW. Multidisciplinary biopsychosocial rehabilitation for subacute low-back pain among working age adults. Cochrane Database Syst Rev. 2003;2, CD002193.
14. Kamper SJ, Apeldoorn AT, Chiarotto A, Smeets RJ, Ostelo RWJG, Guzman J, van Tulder MW. Multidisciplinary biopsychosocial rehabilitation for chronic low back pain. Cochrane Database Syst Rev. 2014;9, CD000963.
15. Karjalainen K, Malmivaara A, van Tulder M, Roine R, Jauhiainen M, Hurri H, Koes B. Biopsychosocial rehabilitation for upper limb repetitive strain injuries in working age adults. Cochrane Database Syst Rev. 2000;3, CD002269.
16. Seshia SS, Phillips DF, Von Baeyer CL. Childhood chronic daily headache: a biopsychosocial perspective. Dev Med Child Neurol. 2008;50:541–5.
17. Lumley MA, Cohen JL, Borszcz GS, Canno A, Radcliffe AM, Porter LS, Schubiner H, Keefe FJ. Pain and emotion: a biopsychosocial review of recent research. J Clin Psychol. 2011;67(9):942–68.
18. Bair MJ, Robinson RL, Katon W, Kroenke K. Depression and pain comorbidity: a literature review. Arch Intern Med. 2003;163(20):2433–45.
19. Okifuji A, Turk DC. Assessment of patients with chronic pain with or without comorbid mental health problems. In: Marchard S, Gaumand I, Saravane D, editors. Mental health and pain: somatic and psychiatric components of pain in mental health. Paris: France. Springer-Verlag; 2014. p. 227–59.
20. National Institute of Drug Abuse. Chronic pain treatment and addiction. Nov 2014. http://www.drugabuse.gov/publications/research-reports/prescription-drugs/chronic-pain-treatment-addiction
21. Hoffman BM, Papas RK, Chatkoff DK, Kerns RD. Meta-analysis of psychological interventions for chronic low back pain. Health Psychol. 2007;26(1):1–9.
22. Turk DC, Swanson KS, Tunks ER. Psychological approaches in the treatment of chronic pain patients—when pills, scalpels and needles are not enough. Can J Psychiatry. 2008;53(4):213–24.

23. American Society of Anesthesiologists Task Force on Chronic Pain Management, American Society of Regional Anesthesia and Pain Medicine. Practice guidelines for chronic pain management: an updated report by the American Society of Anesthesiologists Task Force on Chronic Pain Management and the American Society of Regional Anesthesia and Pain Medicine. Anesthesiology. 2010;112(4):810–33.
24. National Institute for Health and Care Excellence. Low back pain: early management of persistent non-specific low back pain. May 2009. http://www.nice.org.uk/guidance/cg88/chapter/1-guidance#assessment-and-imaging.
25. Airaksinen O, Brox JI, Cedraschi C, Hildebrandt J, et al. European guidelines for the management of chronic nonspecific low back pain. Eur Spine J. 2006;15(Supp2):S192–300.
26. van der Windt DAWM, Simons E, Riphagen II, Ammendolia C, Verhagen AP, Laslett M, Devillé W, Deyo RA, Bouter LM, de Vet HCW, Aertgeerts B. Physical examination for lumbar radiculopathy due to disc herniation in patients with low-back pain. Cochrane Database Syst Rev. 2010;2, CD007431.
27. Robinson ME, Straud R, Price DD. Pain measurement and brain activity: will neuroimages replace pain ratings? J Pain. 2013;14(4):323–7.
28. patient.co.uk. Chronic Pain. http://www.patient.co.uk/doctor/chronic-pain.
29. Disorbio JM, Bruns D, Barolat G. Assessment and treatment of chronic pain: a physician's guide to a biopsychosocial approach. Pract Pain Manage. 2006;6(2):11–27.
30. American Chronic Pain Association. ACPA resource guide to chronic pain medication and treatment. 2013. http://www.theacpa.org/uploads/ACPA_Resource_Guide_2013_Final_011313.pdf.
31. Davis DA, Luecken LJ, Zuetra JA. Are reports of childhood abuse related to the experience of chronic pain in adulthood? A meta-analytic review of the literature. Clin J Pain. 2005;21(5):398–405.
32. Main M, Hesse E, Goldwyn R. Studying differences in language usage in recounting attachment history. In: Steele H, Steele M, editors. Clinical applications of the adult attachment inventory. New York: The Guildford Press; 2008. p. 31–68.
33. Dersh J, Polatin PB, Gatchel RJ. Chronic pain and psychopathology: research findings and theoretical considerations. Psychosom Med. 2002;64(5):773–86.
34. New York State Workers' Compensation Board Return to Work Program. http://www.wcb.ny.gov/content/main/ReturnToWork/RTW_Handbook.pdf.
35. Comas-Diaz L. Feminist therapy with Hispanic/Latina women. In: Fulani L, editor. The psychopathology of everyday racism and sexism. New York: Harrington Press; 2009. p. 51.
36. Finley GA, Kristjansdottir O, Forgeron PA. Cultural influences on assessment of children's pain. Pain Res Manag. 2009;14(1):33–7.
37. Healthcare Improvement Scotland. Sign 136: Management of Chronic Pain. 2013. Scottish Intercollegiate Guidelines Network (SIGN 2013). http://www.ckp.scot.nhs.uk/Published/PathwayViewer.aspx?id=609.
38. Spitzer RL, Kroenke K, Williams JBW. Validation and utility of a self report version of prime-MD: the PHQ primary care study. JAMA. 1999;282(18):1737–44.
39. Arroll B, Khin N, Kerse N. Screening for depression in primary care with two verbally asked questions: cross sectional study. BMJ. 2003;327:1144–6
40. McGuire BE, Shores EA. Pain patient profile and the assessment of malingered pain. J Clin Psychol. 2001;57(3):401–9.
41. Scott GW, Hailey BJ, Wheeler LC. Pain patient profile: a scale to measure psychological distress. Arch Phys Med Rehabil. 1999;80(10):1300–2.
42. Bruns D, Disorbio JM. The psychological evaluation of patients with chronic pain: a review of BHI 2 clinical and forensic interpretive considerations. Psychol Injury Law. 2014;7(4):335–61.
43. Bruns D, Disorbio JM. The psychological assessment of patients with chronic pain. In: Deer T, editor. Treatment of chronic pain by integrative approaches. New York: Springer; 2015. p. 71.

44. Karlin BE, Creech SK, Grimes JS, Clark TS, Meagher MW, Morey LC. The personality assessment inventory with chronic pain patients: psychometric properties and clinical utility. J Clin Psychol. 2005;61:1571–85.
45. Center for Substance Abuse Treatment. Managing chronic pain in adults with or in recovery from substance use disorders, Treatment Improvement Protocol (TIP) Series, vol. 54. Rockville: Substance Abuse and Mental Health Services Administration; 2012.
46. Toward Optimized Practice. Guideline for the evidence-informed primary care management of low back pain. Edmonton, AB: Toward Optimized Practice; 2011. Institute of Health Economics (Canada).

Chapter 5
Clinical Measurement of Pain, Opioid Addiction, and Functional Status

Veronica L. Rodriguez and Teni Davoudian

Learning Objectives
- To identify aberrant opioid-related behaviors
- To understand the relationships among opioid misuse, effect, cognitions, suicide, and chronic pain
- To recognize the diagnostic criteria for opioid use disorder as well as clinical indicators of opioid misuse
- To screen for opioid misuse and the psychological factors related to chronic pain

5.1 Introduction

Chronic pain is a complex and multifaceted condition influenced by biological, psychological, and social factors [1]. Due to its complicated nature, the assessment of chronic pain and its underlying factors is often approached from medical, psychological, and substance use disorder perspectives. Recent studies suggest that prescription opioid misuse occurs in up to 45 % of chronic pain patients [2]. Risk factors for opioid misuse include being of a younger age, history of a substance use

V.L. Rodriguez, Ph.D. (✉)
Mental Health and Clinical Neurosciences Division, VA Portland Health Care System,
3710 SW US Veterans Hospital Rd. (V3SATP), Portland, OR 97239, USA
e-mail: Veronica.Rodriguez@va.gov

T. Davoudian, Ph.D.
VA Portland Health Care System,
3710 SW US Veterans Hospital Rd. (V3SATP), Portland, OR 97239, USA
e-mail: Teni.Davoudian@va.gov

© Springer International Publishing Switzerland 2016
A.M. Matthews, J.C. Fellers (eds.), *Treating Comorbid Opioid Use Disorder in Chronic Pain*, DOI 10.1007/978-3-319-29863-4_5

disorder, family history of legal difficulties, and anxiety [3–5]. This chapter offers primary care providers and pain physicians with a greater understanding of the available assessment tools that examine the full pain experience, including physical sensations, psychological appraisals, and possible aberrant opioid-related behaviors.

5.2 Overview of Chronic Pain

From a psychological perspective, patients' cognitive and affective responses to their chronic pain are the focus of assessment and treatment. The co-occurrence of chronic pain and psychological disorders, such as depression, anxiety, insomnia, and posttraumatic stress disorder [1,6–8], necessitate the use of assessments that examine both the psychological distress and physical disabilities associated with chronic pain.

The experience of persistent pain along with a comorbid mental health conditions can result in a cycle of maladaptive coping resulting in further pain [1]. While it is difficult to determine whether emotional distress leads to greater vulnerability to chronic pain or if chronic pain predisposes patients to mental health issues, there is a clear interaction between affect and pain [7]. The psychological assessment of chronic pain extends far beyond patients' reported emotions. In addition to considering patients' reported affect, a thorough evaluation often includes examination of the cognitive styles, motivation, avoidance behaviors, and self-efficacy of those living with chronic pain. Many measures of chronic pain are closely related to the specific modality of treatment and indicate pre- and posttreatment coping. In addition, some assessments are utilized as educational tools, highlighting the interrelations between emotions, cognitions, and pain levels.

5.3 Measurement of Chronic Pain

5.3.1 Intensity and Functional Status

With the competing demands in most primary care clinics, efficient and thorough assessment of pain intensity is essential. The pain Numeric Rating Scale (NRS) offers a brief and unidimensional measure of pain intensity. The most commonly utilized version is the 11-item NRS. The items are rated on a numeric scale ranging from 0 to 10 (0 = no pain to 10 = worst pain imaginable). This measure is available at: www.partneragainstpain.com/prints/A7012AS2.pdf [9] (see Table 5.1).

The Brief Pain Inventory (BPI) evaluates pain intensity and interference. This measure offers rapid assessment of pain intensity and the impact of chronic pain on a patients' overall functioning. The short form of the BPI can be completed within

Table 5.1 Chronic pain

Instruments	Domain assessed
Pain measures	
Numeric Rating Scale (NRS) 11	Pain intensity
Brief Pain Inventory (BPI) 12	Pain intensity, pain interference, and functional status
Short Form McGill Pain Questionnaire (SF-MPQ-2) 13	Affective and sensory aspects of pain
Functional status instruments	
Pain Catastrophizing Scale (PCS) 19	Automatic negative pain thoughts and negative pain schemas
Tampa Scale for Kinesiophobia (TSK) 22	Fear of movement
Pain Acceptance Questionnaire (CPAQ) 25	Willingness to experience pain
Opioid misuse instruments	
Pain Medication Questionnaire (PMQ) 31 32	Opioid misuse
Rapid Opioid Dependence Screen (RODS) 33	Opioid misuse
Current Opioid Misuse Measure (COMM) 34	Aberrant medication behaviors of chronic pain patients
The Opioid Compliance Checklist (OCC) 35	Adherence to opioid agreements and/or contracts

a few minutes and is available in many languages. Because the experience of chronic pain can vary greatly throughout the day and time, the BPI assesses pain intensity over time, such as now, least, average, and over the last 24-h. In addition to measuring pain intensity longitudinally, the BPI also queries patients about the extent to which pain interferes with functional activities in their daily life, including walking, relationships with others, work, mood, sleep, and quality of life [10].

5.4   Measure of Affective and Sensory aspects of Pain

Chronic pain is often associated with diverse experiences, characteristics, and qualities. Comprehending the many aspects of pain is helpful in identifying pain treatment targets and efficacy of pain treatment(s). In addition, assessment of the affective and sensory aspects of pain can assist in identifying patients who may be prone to pain magnification. The Short Form McGill Pain Questionnaire (SF-MPQ-2) is a valid and reliable tool for the assessment of nonmalignant chronic pain. The measure has been revised and consists of 22-items that evaluate pain quality including the perception, emotional, and sensory aspects of pain. The SF-MPQ-2 provides a list of words that described various pain aspects and other related symptoms on an 11-point numeric rating scale (0=none to 10=worst possible). The SF-MPQ-2 is comprised of four summary scales: (1) continuous descriptors (throbbing, cramping, gnawing aching, heavy, and tender pain); (2) intermittent descriptors (shooting, stabbing, sharp, splitting, electric shock, and piecing pain); (3) neuropathic descriptors (hot-burning pain, cold freezing pain, pain caused by light touch, itching, and/or tingling); and (4) affective descriptors (fearful, exhausting, sickening, and punishing cruel). A total score is computed by averaging the numerical ratings across the questions. Information regarding permission to reproduce the SF-MPQ-2 can be obtained at www.immpact.org [11].

5.5 Neurocognitive or Communication Problems

When patients present with communication problems, proxy approaches are highly recommended. Proxy assessments include observing pain behaviors and/or reactions that may suggest that a patient is suffering or is in pain. The use of proxy methods may also be utilized for critically ill patients [12].

While the above instruments indicate the patients' general pain experience, there are additional assessment tools that examine the functional elements of chronic pain. The psychological aspects of pain are highly predictive of pain treatment outcomes [13], and thus, deserve equal attention and merit. Therefore, the subsequent section purposefully presents background and rationale to the psychological measurement of chronic pain.

5.6 Psychological and Functional Assessment of Chronic Pain

5.6.1 Pain Catastrophizing

Evidence-based psychotherapies for chronic pain target patients' appraisals of pain and their resulting behavioral responses [13]. Whether delivered through individual or group therapy modalities, the goals of treatment focus on improving functional performance, increasing coping skills, and preventing secondary disability from the psychological correlates of chronic pain, such as insomnia and anger [7]. For example, cognitive behavioral therapy (CBT) aims to restructure patients' maladaptive and catastrophic cognitions related to their pain [14]. Catastrophizing, which refers to the magnification of the threat of pain, feelings of helplessness, and difficulties inhibiting pain-related thoughts, is associated with increased pain intensity, psychosocial dysfunction, and pain-related disability [8,15,16]. In addition, the tendency to catastrophize has been linked to poor treatment outcomes [7,13].

While it is difficult to decipher if catastrophizing is driven by or a determinant of chronic pain, this construct can be assessed through the use of validated self-report measures. The Pain Catastrophizing Scale (PCS) is a brief psychological assessment of negative pain schemas [17]. Given the profound influence of catastrophizing on the cognitive, affective, and behavioral responses to pain, it is important to identify patients who may benefit from psychological interventions targeting their cognitive appraisals of pain.

5.6.2 Kinesiophobia

In addition to reducing pain catastrophizing, another goal of CBT is behavioral activation through the use of realistic, goal-directed physical activities. Patients are often encouraged to set small, attainable goals as they work toward larger goals. Engagement in physical activities can be especially helpful for chronic pain patients who also demonstrate a consistent fear of movement and reinjury, known as kinesiophobia. This fear of movement leads to avoidance of activities that are perceived to contribute to further pain or nerve damage, which, in turn, results in deconditioning and the perpetuation of chronic pain [18]. Overall, kinesiophobia is strongly associated with functional limitations and self-reported physical disability [18,19].

The most widely utilized assessment of kinesiophobia is the Tampa Scale for Kinesiophobia [20]. This brief, self-report measure allows providers to identify patients whose fear of movement and activity may negatively impact their process of rehabilitation. By conducting such screenings during medical visits, patients who may benefit from concomitant cognitive-based psychotherapies can be identified and referred to appropriate providers.

5.7 Acceptance of Pain

While CBT is one of the most commonly utilized modalities of psychotherapy for targeting maladaptive pain-related cognitions, other types of approaches can also aid in the assessment and treatment of chronic pain. For example, Acceptance Commitment Therapy (ACT), which examines the influence of pain on psychological suffering and the resulting disengagement from personally meaningful activities, is gaining empirical support [21]. ACT aims to disentangle patients from their threatening pain-related cognitions, foster acceptance of the chronic nature of their pain, and encourage commitment of values-based actions [6]. The acceptance of chronic pain is emerging as an important factor to assess and cultivate in treatment [6].

In the context of chronic pan, acceptance is defined as willingness to experience pain and its associated cognitive and affective components without attempts to control or avoid pain sensations [6,21,22]. In addition, acceptance entails continued engagement in meaningful and functional activities, even in the presence of chronic pain. Higher rates of acceptance of chronic pain are associated with less depression, pain-related anxiety, reductions in healthcare use, higher quality of life, and increased levels of activity [21,22].

The acceptance of chronic pain can be quantified through the use of the Pain Acceptance Questionnaire (CPAQ) [23]. Data gathered from the CPAQ can inform providers of their patients' willingness to experience pain and attempts to reduce or avoid the thoughts and emotions associated with pain. Similar to other psychological processes, acceptance is an ongoing and dynamic process. In order to fully cultivate acceptance, one must continue engagement in life activities despite the experience of chronic pain [23]. Therefore, it is important for healthcare professionals to provide ongoing encouragement of active coping and acceptance of chronic pain while discouraging maladaptive cognitions regarding patients' inabilities to function in the presence of pain.

5.8   Chronic Pain and Risk of Suicide

As previously noted, clinically significant psychological distress is frequently observed in chronic pain patients [1,7,24]. In fact, depression commonly co-occurs with chronic pain [16,24]. The assessment of depression and its multiple symptoms, such as insomnia and suicidal ideation, is of paramount importance when working with chronic pain patients. According to a number of studies, chronic pain is associated with higher rates of suicidal ideation, self-harm behaviors, and deaths by suicide [8,16,24]. Possible mediators between pain and suicidal ideation include catastrophizing [16,24], avoidance of the pain experience, and the desire to escape from pain [24]. These moderators underscore the importance and utility of assessing patient's catastrophizing and acceptance of pain. The association between chronic pain and suicidal ideation is further complicated by patients' access to opioid analgesics [16]. A recent study found drug overdose to be the most commonly reported plan for committing suicide among chronic pain populations [25].

When treating chronic pain patients, it is important for medical providers to be cognizant of possible mental health issues, particularly when prescribing opioids or benzodiazepines [16]. Brief screening tools, such as the Patient Health Questionnaire—9 (PHQ-9), rapidly provide information on depression severity and the presence of suicidal ideation. Brief mental health screeners allow for the identification of patients in need of psychological and/or psychopharmacological interventions.

5.9   Opioid Use Disorder in Chronic Pain Patients

Chronic pain patients have higher rates of substance use disorders [26] and may be at greater risk for misusing opioids [27]. Thus, valid and reliable assessment of opioid medication adherence and potential misuse is essential for effective management of chronic pain treatment planning and outcomes. A recent study found that of the patients with a substance use disorder history, those who were at greater risk for opioid misuse were more likely to report higher levels of pain, symptoms of depression, and pain impairment. Moreover, pain catastrophizing, which was discussed above, is significantly associated with risk for pain medication misuse [26]. A recent study found that cognitive tasks have prognostic value in identifying patients at risk for musing opioids. Addiction attentional biases toward drug-related cues as well as cue-elicited cravings are strong predictors of opioid misuse. Results from this recent study suggest that chronic pain patients who reported opioid misuse exhibited greater addiction attentional bias [27].

5.10 Opioid Use Disorder Defined

The Diagnostic and Statistical Manual of Mental Disorders (5th ed.; DSM–5; American Psychiatric Association, 2013) is the most widely accepted manual used by clinicians and researchers for the classification of mental disorders [28]. The DSM 5 defines an opioid use disorder as a pattern of use associated with significant life impairment and/or distress within a 12-month period. Opioid use disorder is classified on a range of severity varying from mild, moderate, or severe. Features of an opioid use disorder include the following: (1) Taking greater amounts of opioids than planned or taking opioids over a longer period of time than was intended; (2) Being unsuccessful efforts to cut down or control opioid use; (3) Spending a great deal of time in activities necessary to obtain, use, or recover from the effects; (4) Having a craving or experience a strong desire to use opioid; (5) The use of opioids despite failure to fulfill major or important roles at work, school, or home; (6) Ongoing use opioids regardless of experiencing persistent or recurrent social or interpersonal problems caused or exacerbated by the effects of opioids; (7) Giving up important social, occupational, or recreational activities as a result of opioid use; (8) Continuous opioid use in situations that are physically hazardous; (9) Continuing to use opioids even with knowledge of having persistent or recurrent physical or psychological difficulties that are likely to have been caused or exacerbated by opioid use; (10) Tolerance, as defined by either a need for markedly increased amounts of opioids to achieve intoxication or a desired effect or a markedly diminished effect with continued use; and (11) Withdrawal, as noted by either the characteristic opioid withdrawal syndrome, or taking opioids to relieve or avoid withdrawal symptoms. Of importance, the criterion for tolerance and withdrawal is not considered to be met when chronic pain patients are taking opioids solely under appropriate medical supervision [28].

In addition to the DSM 5 criteria, other behavioral indicators, such as requests for early refills, taking pain medication from others, focusing on obtaining additional opioids, running out of pain medication earlier than indicated, reporting loss of pain medication, and obtaining pain medication from multiple providers, may also signal opioid misuse [2].

5.11 Assessing Risk of Aberrant Behaviors and Opioid Misuse

Many physicians appreciate the relevance of monitoring problematic medication-related behaviors among chronic pain patients to improve the management of pain. While evaluating patients for opioid adherence may be a challenge, there are assessment tools that have been developed to monitor and assess possible opioid misuse. Various screening tools are identified and discussed below.

5.12 Ongoing Misuse of Pain Medication

The Pain Medication Questionnaire is a 26-items assessment tool that evaluates the inappropriate use of pain medication. The PMQ has demonstrated good reliability and validity and is predictive of early termination from treatment. It can help to identify chronic pain patients who are more likely to complete and benefit from a pain management program [29,30]. High PMQ scores have been associated with a history of substance abuse, psychosocial distress, and lower level of functioning.

The Rapid Opioid Dependence Screen (RODS) is another helpful brief assessment tool. The RODS is an 8-item measure to evaluate potential opioid dependence. While this measure is based on the *Diagnostic and Statistical Manual of Mental Disorders*, Fourth edition, criteria, it does offer a quick and targeted screening. Items are rated on a dichotomous scale of "yes" or "no." A total score is computed by adding the number of "yes" responses. A total score greater than 3 is highly suggestive of opioid misuse [31].

Long-term use of opioids among chronic pain patients may increase the risk of misuse of opioids [32]. The Current Opioid Misuse Measure (COMM) is a 17-item measure that demonstrates reliable and valid prediction of aberrant medication behaviors of chronic pain patients being prescribed opioid medication. Each item queries chronic pain patients on the occurrence of thoughts or behaviors related to opioid use within the past month on a 0–4 scale (0 = never to 4 = very often). Unlike other measures that identify potential traits based on past history, this assessment tool evaluates current behaviors and cognitions [33].

5.13 Adherence to Opioid Agreements

With the growing use of opioid treatment agreements, determining a patients' compliance is an important aspect of pain treatment planning. A new measure was recently developed that assesses adherence to opioid agreements and/or contracts. The Opioid Compliance Checklist (OCC) consists of 12-items, of which 5 showed to be most useful in identifying potential noncompliance. Because the measure contains items that are often recognized and contained within an opioid agreement, physicians and/or clinicians may prefer to include 10 of the original items, excluding items 9 and 11. OCC items query patient about their use of medication over the past month and any endorsement ("yes") on an item may suggest problems with adherence to opioids. Although this measure may require additional validation, it is a simple and brief assessment tool to administer [34].

5.14 Conclusion

Given the complicated nature of chronic pain, thorough assessment requires comprehensive approaches. The use of reliable and valid instruments to assess chronic pain is of importance in clinical practice and in furthering our understanding of the interconnections between pain, functional status, and opioid misuse. Assessment tools not only screen for important psychosocial moderators of pain, but they can also identify patients who may benefit from psychological, psychiatric, and/or specialized substance use disorder treatment. Since opioid misuse may be otherwise difficult to detect, assessment of aberrant opioid-related behaviors is especially meaningful within medical settings. Overall, efficacious treatment of chronic pain hinges on the holistic and robust assessment of the pain experience.

References

1. Grieve K, Schultewolter D. Chronic pain, current issues and opportunities for future collaborations. Br J Health Manag. 2014;20(12):563–7.
2. Robinson RC, Gatchel RJ, Polatin P, Deschner M, Noe C, Gajraji N. Screening for problematic opioid misuse. Clin J Pain. 2001;17(3):200–8.
3. Ives TJ, Chelminiski PR, Hammett-Stabler CA, Malone RM, Perhac SJ, Potiske NM, et al. Predictors of opioid misuse in patients with chronic pain: a prospective cohort study. BMC Health Serv Res. 2006;6:46.
4. Reid MC, Engles-Horton LL, Weber MB, Kerns RD, Rogers EL, O'Conner PG. Use of opioid medication in noncancer pain syndromes in primary care. J Gen Intern Med. 2002;17:173–9.
5. Michna E, Ross EL, Hynes WL, Nedeljkovic SS, Soumekh S, Janfaza D, et al. Predicting aberrant drug behavior in patients treated for chronic pain: importance of abuse history. J Pain Symptom Manage. 2004;28(3):250–8.
6. Vowles KE, McCracken LM. Acceptance and values-based action in chronic pain: a study of treatment effectiveness and process. J Consult Clin Psychol. 2008;76(3):397–407.
7. Gatchel RJ, Peng YB, Peters ML, Fuchs PN, Turk DC. The biopsychosocial approach to chronic pain: scientific advances and future directions. Psychol Bull. 2007;133(4):581–624.
8. Quartana PJ, Campbell CM, Edwards RR. Pain catastrophizing: a critical review. Expert Rev Neurother. 2009;9(5):745–8.
9. Farr JT, Young JP, LaMoreaux L, Werth JL, Poole MR. Clinical importance of changes in chronic pain intensity measured on an 11-point numerical pain rating scale. Pain. 2001;94:149–58.
10. Mendoza T, Mayne T, Rublee D, Cleeland C. Reliability and validity of a modified Brief Pain Inventory short form in patients with osteoarthritis. Eur J Pain. 2006;10:353–61.
11. Dworkin RH, Turk DC, Revicki DA, Harding G, Coyne KS, Peirce-Sander S, et al. Development and initial validation of an expanded and revised version of the Short-form McGill Pain Questionnaire (SF-MPQ-2). Pain. 2009;144:35–42.
12. Breivik H, Borchgrevink PC, Allen SM, Rosseland LA, Romundstad EK, Breivik EK, et al. Assessment of pain. Br J Anaesth. 2008;101(1):17–24.
13. Jensen MP, Turner JA, Romano JM. Changes in beliefs, catastrophizing, and coping are associated with improvement in multidisciplinary pain treatment. J Consult Clin Psychol. 2001;69(4):655–62.
14. Vlayen JW, Morley S. Cognitive-behavioral treatments for chronic pain: what works for whom? Clin J Pain. 2005;21(1):1–8.
15. Turner JA, Jensen MP, Warms CA, Gardenas DD. Catastrophizing is associated with pain intensity, psychological distress, and pain-related disability among individuals with chronic pain after spinal cord injury. Pain. 2002;98(1):127–34.
16. Chcatle MD. Depression, chronic pain, and suicide by overdose: on the edge. Pain Med. 2011;12(s2):43–8.
17. Sullivan ML, Bishop SR, Pivik J. The Pain Catastrophizing Scale: development and validation. Psychol Assess. 1995;7(4):524–32.

18. Thomas EN, Pers YM, Mercier G, Cambiere JP, Frasson N, Ster F, et al. The importance of fear, beliefs, catastrophizing and kinesiophobia in chronic low back pain rehabilitation. Ann Phys Rehabil Med. 2010;53(1):3–4.
19. Lundberg M, Larsson M, Ostlund H, Styf J. Kinesiophobia among patients with musculoskeletal pain in primary healthcare. J Rehabil Med. 2006;38(1):37–43.
20. Miller R, Kori S, Todd D. The Tampa Scale for Kinesiophobia. Unpublished report. 1991
21. McCracken LM, Eccleston C. Coping or acceptance: what to do about chronic pain? Pain. 2003;105(1):197–204.
22. McCracken LM, Eccleston C. A prospective study of acceptance of pain and patient functioning with chronic pain. Pain. 2005;118(1):164–9.
23. McCracken LM, Vowles KE, Eccleston C. Acceptance of chronic pain: component analysis and a revised assessment method. Pain. 2004;107(1):159–66.
24. Tang NK, Crane C. Suicidality in chronic pain: a review of the prevalence, risk factors and psychological links. Psychol Med. 2006;36(5):575–86.
25. Smith MT, Edwards RR, Robinson RC, Dworkin RH. Suicidal ideation, plans, and attempts in chronic pain patients: factors associated with increased pain. Pain. 2004;111(1):201–8.
26. Morasco BJ, Turk DC, Donovan DM, Dobscha SK. Risk for prescription opioid misuse among patients with a history of substance use disorder. Drug Alcohol Depend. 2013;127(1-3):193–9.
27. Garland EL, Howard MO. Opioid attentional bias and cue-elicited craving predict future risk of prescription opioid misuse among chronic pain patients. Drug Alcohol Depend. 2014;144:283–7.
28. American Psychiatric Association. Diagnostic and statistical manual of mental disorders. 5th ed. Arlington, VA: American Psychiatric Publishing; 2013.
29. Adams LL, Gatchel RJ, Robinson RC, Polatin P, Gajraj N, Deschner M, et al. Development of a self-report screening instrument for assessing potential opioid medication misuse in chronic pain patients. J Pain Symptom Manage. 2004;27(5):440–9.
30. Holmes CP, Gatchel RJ, Adams LL, Stowell AW, Hatten MS, Noe C, et al. An Opioid Screening Instrument: long-term evaluation of utility of the Pain Medication Questionnaire. Pain Pract. 2006;6(2):74–8.
31. Wickersham JA, Azar MM, Cannon CM, Altice FL, Springer SA. Validation of a brief measure of opioid dependence: the rapid opioid dependence screen (RODS). J Correct Health Care. 2015;21(1):12–26.
32. Solanki DR, Koyyalagunta D, Shah RV, Silverman S, Manchikanto L. Monitoring opioid adherence on chronic pain patients: assessment of risk of substance misuse. Pain Physician. 2011;14:119–31.
33. Butler SF, Budman SH, Fernandez KC, Houle B, Benoit C, Katz N, et al. Development and validation of the current opioid misuse measure. Pain. 2007;130:144–6.
34. Jamison RN, Martel MO, Edwards RR, Qian J, Sheehan KA, Ross E. Validation of a brief opioid compliance checklist for patient with chronic pain. J Pain. 2014;15(11):1092–101.

Chapter 6
Methadone and Buprenorphine: The Place of Opiate Replacement Therapies

Jonathan R. Buchholz and Andrew J. Saxon

6.1 Methadone

Methadone is a schedule II medication which requires care through a federally licensed clinic when being used to treat opioid use disorder. Requirement for admission into such clinics includes at least one year of documented opioid use disorder. This can be waived for patients who are pregnant, were recently released from incarceration, or had previous treatment within the past two years in a licensed clinic. Early in care, patients must have observed doses dispensed daily and eventually can earn take-home doses based on time in treatment and stability. Regulations state that medical, counseling, and education services be available as part of care (Saxon - Treatment of Opioid Dependence). The above regulations do not exist when methadone is used in the treatment of pain disorders.

6.1.1 Pharmacology

Methadone is unique in its pharmacokinetics and dynamics. It has good oral bioavailability, gradual onset, and long half-life. It also has various drug–drug interactions and safety considerations including a black box warning concerning respiratory

J.R. Buchholz, M.D. (✉) • A.J. Saxon, M.D.
VA Puget Sound Health Care System (S-116 ATC), 1660 S. Columbian Way,
Seattle, WA 98108, USA

Department of Psychiatry & Behavioral Sciences, University of Washington,
1660 S. Columbian Way, Seattle, WA 98108, USA
e-mail: jonathan.buchholz@va.gov; andrew.saxon@va.gov

© Springer International Publishing Switzerland 2016
A.M. Matthews, J.C. Fellers (eds.), *Treating Comorbid Opioid Use Disorder in Chronic Pain*, DOI 10.1007/978-3-319-29863-4_6

depression and QT interval prolongation. Oral methadone is available as a tablet, rapidly dissolving wafer and liquid. All formulations have generally equivalent bio-availability of around 80 % though inter-individual variation ranges from 41 to 95 % [2]. Initial effects occur within 30 min, but peak plasma levels and effects appear approximately 4 h after ingestion. The average half-life of methadone is 22 h with wide ranges reported from 5 to 130 h [3]. Metabolism is mainly catalyzed by the liver enzyme CYP 450 3A4, though other CYP enzymes may contribute as well. Methadone can induce its own metabolism, particularly during the first month of treatment. It has no active metabolites and has primarily renal excretion with some elimination in the feces. Methadone serves as an agonist at the μ-opioid receptor as well as an antagonist at the N-methyl, D-aspartate (NMDA) receptor while also blocking serotonin and norepinephrine transporters [1].

Methadone has a number of drug–drug interactions, many of which are mediated within the CYP 450 enzyme system. Generally, drugs that inhibit CYP enzymes can cause elevations in methadone serum levels and potentially clinically observable effects. For example, signal case reports have noted fluconazole or fluvoxamine co-administration leading to methadone toxicity [4, 5]. Conversely, drugs that induce these enzymes can lead to decreased methadone levels and opioid withdrawal or cravings. Drugs associated with such effects include anticonvulsants, phenytoin and carbamazepine; the antibiotic, rifampin; and antiretroviral medications, lopinavir, efavirenz, and nevirapine [6].

Side effects of methadone include those which are associated with full opioid agonists including miosis, decreased gut motility, analgesia sedation, and respiratory depression. Methadone is known to cause QT interval prolongation. As such, other medications which prolong QT co-administered with methadone could have additive effects and should be used with caution. Lastly, other substances which act as CNS depressants such as benzodiazepines and alcohol can potentiate risks for respiratory depression when used with methadone; patients should be counseled accordingly. Overall, it is important for clinicians to know that methadone is highly variable in its absorption, metabolism, and elimination among patients and within an individual over time. As such, dosing calculators and algorithms are often not reliable. Patients require personalized monitoring and management over time.

6.1.2   Clinical Use for Opioid Use Disorder

Prior to initiating the dose, a thorough medical history and physical exam along with appropriate laboratory tests and urine toxicology should be obtained. Informed consent should be provided including risks, benefits, and the fact that physiologic dependence will occur. Patients do not have to be in physiologic withdrawal to begin treatment, but should not display evidence of sedation or intoxication on opioids. Initial doses can range from 5 to 30 mg, with 30 mg being the highest first dose allowed by federal standards. A number of factors should be considered when choosing initial dosing including amount, frequency, last use, and type of opioid being abused. Patient's other medications and substance use should be taken into account since metabolism and respiratory drive, as noted above, is impacted by co-ingested substances and medications. For instance, comorbid medical conditions and age should be considered as well as older patients may metabolize methadone slower. Ideally, patients should receive an additional assessment 2–4 h following the initial methadone dose to determine if ongoing withdrawal vs. intoxication is observed. If withdrawal symptoms persist, the clinician may administer additional doses of methadone to a maximum of 40 mg total for day 1. If a patient exhibits sedation or intoxication at that reassessment, the patient should stay in clinic until the effects have resolved or, if necessary, receive emergency intervention such as naloxone administration and airway protection [1]. A number of treatment goals should be considered when assessing optimal stabilization doses of methadone. The dose should (1) eliminate opioid withdrawal symptoms throughout the 24-h following administration; (2) abolish cravings or urges to use other opioids; (3) establish adequate tolerance to preclude euphoria caused by use of illicit opioids; (4) eradicate use of illicit opioids as demonstrated by self-report and urine toxicology testing; and (5) minimize side effects so that the patient does not experience any intoxication and can function normally. All goals cannot always be achieved by doses that are safely attained during the induction period. It is important to remember that due to its long half-life and potential for "stacking" in the system, titrating by increments of 5–10 mg every 5–7 days is recommended. After the daily dose exceeds 40 mg, 10 mg increments usually are quite safe. Achieving the optimal dose requires the balance between establishing a sufficient tolerance and discouraging illicit opioid use while dealing with side effects. Clinical trials show that methadone doses of 80–100 mg per day have advantages over lower doses in reducing illicit opioid use and retaining patients in treatment [7]. For most patients, a stable dose will range from 80 to 120 mg per day, though due to inter-individual differences, some will require higher or lower doses. This can usually be achieved within the first 3 months of treatment [1]. Once patients reach an optimal dose of medication as assessed by criteria 1–5 above, routine medical evaluation may occur less frequently. However, if changes occur in the patient, such as signs of instability in the program, changes in medical problems, or initiation of new medications, the patient requires assessment and potential dose adjustments.

6.1.3   Pain and Opioid Use Disorder

Single daily dosed methadone as typically used in treatment of opioid use disorder does not provide adequate pain control for patients with chronic pain. Though it has a long half-life and can be very effective at preventing withdrawal and reducing cravings, leading to its efficacy in opioid use disorder, methadone's analgesic effects last only about 6 h [8]. Unfortunately, chronic pain is common among methadone-maintained patients and is associated with poorer functioning in social, work, physical, and daily activity realms. This can lead to a higher likelihood of continued drug abuse during and after treatment while having poorer treatment retention [9]. Regrettably, providers treating patients in the substance use setting may not be trained to deliver pain management treatments, and there are limited data to guide providers in such circumstances.

The practice of splitting a methadone dose into twice daily doses for pain management has been implemented in some clinics, but no studies have shown data to support this approach [10]. Although there are studies reporting efficacy of short-acting opioids for treatment of acute pain in patients undergoing methadone substitution for opioid use disorder [9], only one randomized control trial, discussed later in this chapter, has been published evaluating pain management in patients with opioid use disorder and chronic pain [11]. More often, studies are retrospective. One study showed that the addition of methadone for pain can be administered safely and effectively every 6–8 h to patients maintained on stable, daily doses of methadone for opioid use disorder. It is important to note this study was limited to patients with HIV/AIDS and included multiple non-opioid medications for adjunctive pain management [12].

Both analgesic tolerance and hyperalgesia have been described in association with chronic use of methadone [13]. Tolerance is expected and can manifest with decreased analgesic sensitivity over time, whereas opioid-induced hyperalgesia is defined as increased sensitivity to pain resulting from the use of the opioid. It is very difficult to distinguish between these two conditions in the clinical setting, and they may coexist [8]. However, the clinical implications of these findings are unclear, as studies indicate that opioid-induced hyperalgesia may develop with some measures of pain (cold presser), but not to others (pressure) [14]. There are no studies to support the idea that reductions in methadone dosing would decrease opioid-induced hyperalgesia and may well increase the risk of relapse to illicit opioid use [10].

More studies are required to guide providers of patients receiving methadone substitution for opioid use disorder in order to treat concurrent chronic pain and opioid use disorder. Though patients with under-treated pain problems are more likely to have worse substance use outcomes, much of the guidance for treatment of these patients is limited to retrospective and "model care" descriptions in the literature. Clark and colleagues in a 2008 review showed that substance abuse treatment programs offering integrated care for patients with opioid use disorder and chronic pain improved outcomes, with programs tailoring the level of care to the individual patient's needs being the best [15].

6.2 Buprenorphine

Buprenorphine is a schedule III medication and, in contrast to methadone, can be prescribed by waivered physicians in any medical setting. Physicians obtain a wavier and DEA number by passing addiction specialty examinations or by completing 8 h of training offered by several medical specialty organizations. A provider may prescribe buprenorphine for up to 30 patients in the first year and request to increase this to 100 patients after that year.

6.2.1 Pharmacology

Buprenorphine has a complex pharmacology, but in contrast to methadone, buprenorphine has a better safety profile. It has poor oral bioavailability and as such is taken by alternative routes described below. Like methadone, buprenorphine is gradual in its onset and has a long half-life, making it effective in the treatment of opioid use disorder. However, it is a partial μ-opioid agonist and has a ceiling effect such that, at some point, increasing doses do not lead independently to increasing activity [16, 17]. As such, there is less risk of respiratory depression and overdose. In addition to its effects on the μ-opioid receptor, it also acts as an antagonist at the κ-opioid receptor and has agonist properties at the nociception/orphanin FQ (NOP) receptor [20, 21]. Buprenorphine also has fewer drug–drug interactions than methadone and lesser effects on cardiac conduction [1].

Buprenorphine comes in multiple formulations: (1) buprenorphine sublingual tablets; (2) buprenorphine/naloxone sublingual tablets: (3) buprenorphine/naloxone sublingual film; (4) buprenorphine/naloxone buccal film; (5) buprenorphine IM/IV (mainly used for acute pain); and (6) buprenorphine transdermal patch (approved for use in management of pain). The combined buprenorphine/naloxone formulation is intended to prevent parenteral misuse of the medication. Since naloxone has minimal sublingual and buccal bioavailability, its μ-opioid antagonist effects are negligible when taken in the appropriate route. But if buprenorphine/naloxone is injected, the simultaneous effects of both buprenorphine and naloxone are experienced. This would blunt effects of buprenorphine and possibly precipitate opioid withdrawal [1]. The combined formulation is the most commonly prescribed formulation for opioid use disorder in the US due to this safety profile. One exception to this practice is that buprenorphine alone is the current recommended treatment in pregnancy to prevent potential exposure of naloxone to the fetus. There is, however, growing evidence that buprenorphine/naloxone may be safe in pregnancy [22].

Buprenorphine/naloxone tablet formulations come in two varieties, the 2 mg (buprenorphine)/0.5 mg (naloxone) and the 8 mg (buprenorphine)/2 mg (naloxone) versions, while the film is also available in the 4 mg/1 mg and 12 mg buprenorphine/3 mg naloxone version. Alternative formulations are now available to treat opioid use disorder including another sublingual tablet and buccal film, which both have higher bioavailability than the formulations described above. As such, these medications have alternative doses. These formulations along with the IM/IV and transdermal formulations will not be discussed in detail in this chapter. Package inserts on newer medications give approximate dose equivalents to buprenorphine/naloxone sublingual tablets and can be used by the clinician for guidance in prescribing.

Buprenorphine absorption occurs rapidly after administration, with bioavailability around 35 % for the tablet. There are significant inter-individual differences in bioavailability with buprenorphine in any formulation [18, 19]. Initial onset of action is around 30 min with peak effects and plasma levels occurring about 1 h after ingestion [18]. The average terminal half-life of buprenorphine is about 32 h, although again there are significant variations among individuals [18]. Metabolism occurs in the liver where the CYP 450 3A4 enzyme catalyzes N-dealkylation, which produces the active metabolite norbuprenorphine. Elimination is primarily fecal with some excretion by the kidneys [18].

Since buprenorphine is metabolized primarily by the CYP450 3A4 system, drugs that induce or inhibit this enzyme may impact blood levels of buprenorphine. It is important to note, however, that these interactions have not translated to clinically meaningful adverse effects in most situations [6]. One proposed explanation of this phenomenon is that buprenorphine's strong affinity for the μ-opioid receptor allows it to remain bound to the receptor, despite changes in the plasma levels of the drug. Exceptions to this finding are: (1) atazanavir which may increase buprenorphine levels and lead to over-sedation in some individuals and (2) rifampin which may reduce buprenorphine levels and lead to symptoms of withdrawal [23, 24]. As with methadone, substances that reduce respiratory drive may act synergistically with buprenorphine and lead to overdose. Fatal overdoses have been reported in cases where benzodiazepines or sedative hypnotics were used in combination with buprenorphine, particularly those situations where the substances were injected [25]. With its partial μ-opioid agonist effects and high affinity for the receptor, use of other opioids concurrently with buprenorphine is problematic. For instance, administration of buprenorphine in patients already on full μ-opioid agonists can lead to precipitated withdrawal. Addition of full agonists with a patient already maintained on buprenorphine may not be harmful, but also may not produce the desired effect as buprenorphine may occupy a majority of the μ-opioid receptors.

Buprenorphine, like methadone, can produce typical opioid-related side effects such as constipation, nausea, and sweating, but headaches may be more common in buprenorphine-treated patients [1]. Though some case reports suggested that buprenorphine had the potential to cause transaminitis, a recent randomized clinical trial did not show any difference between methadone and buprenorphine in rates of elevated liver transaminases. Further, results suggested that viral hepatitis, rather than the medications, were likely responsible for transaminase elevations during treatment with these medications [26]. Like methadone, buprenorphine, when taken regularly for opioid use disorder, will result in physiologic tolerance and dependence. Patients should be counseled accordingly.

6.2.2 Clinical Use for Opioid Use Disorder

The buprenorphine/naloxone formulation and buprenorphine alone formulation are very similar in their effects. For ease of reading, the following discussion will refer to the "buprenorphine" formulation, though in practice the combination medication is used more frequently. Due to the partial μ-opioid agonist effects and good safety profile, buprenorphine doses can be escalated with less worry for overdose than initial methadone dose increases. However, this partial μ-opioid agonist effect also means that there is a risk for precipitating opioid withdrawal in patients who are taking substances which act as full agonists.

A thorough medical history and at least a targeted physical exam (checking for signs of drug injection, intoxication, withdrawal, and gross motor impairment) along with appropriate laboratory tests and urine toxicology should be obtained prior to initiating dose. Informed consent should be provided including risks, benefits, and the fact that physiologic dependence will occur. Unlike with methadone, precipitated opioid withdrawal is a concern and, as such, a patient needs to have abstained from opioids long enough to display an objective state of moderate opioid withdrawal prior to the administration of the first dose of buprenorphine. Use of an objective measurement tool such as the Clinical Opiate Withdrawal Scale can be helpful in identifying moderate opioid withdrawal [27].

After objective signs of withdrawal are observed, the induction can begin with a dose of 2–4 mg of buprenorphine. The patient will likely have at least a partial response and alleviation of withdrawal symptoms within 30–60 min. From there, administration of up to 8 mg of buprenorphine (total daily dose) the first day and up to 16 mg of buprenorphine (total daily dose) the second day can be administered. Once withdrawal symptoms are fully alleviated, the induction is complete. This can usually be accomplished within the first few days of treatment.

In the unusual circumstance that buprenorphine is given prior to sufficient opioid withdrawal, precipitated withdrawal can ensue. As one would expect, this manifests with more severe opioid withdrawal symptoms as opposed to relief of symptoms. Unfortunately, since buprenorphine has a high affinity for the μ-opioid receptor, administration of full opioid agonists is not likely to relieve withdrawal symptoms. In this clinical situation, the provider has two options clinically (1) stop the induction and treat the withdrawal symptoms symptomatically using typical opioid withdrawal agents such as clonidine, benzodiazepines, anti-emetics, and anti-diarrheals, then retry induction after withdrawal is resolved; or (2) continuing ahead with induction knowing that the withdrawal will likely resolve over the next 24 h as buprenorphine will be fully on board by then. Option two can involve the use of adjuvant medications for management of withdrawal symptoms as well.

Once the induction is complete, finding a stable dose may require some days or weeks to achieve. There are no federal regulations specifying how often patients are required to be seen by providers during this period. Each physician must use his or her own best judgment, but many choose to have contact with patients weekly until a stable dose is reached, then decrease visit frequency thereafter. Like methadone, the goals of opioid substitution therapy are (1) eliminate opioid withdrawal symptoms consistently throughout the day; (2) abolish cravings or urges to use other opioids; (3) establish adequate tolerance to preclude euphoria caused by use of illicit opioids; (4) eradicate use of illicit opioids as demonstrated by self-report and urine toxicology testing; and (5) minimize side effects so that the patient does not experience any intoxication and can function normally. The optimal dose range can vary widely among individuals from as little as 2 mg per day to a maximum of 32 mg per day, with many patients stabilizing on doses between 12 and 24 mg per day. Even after initial stability, patients may require adjustments up or down over time. If a patient were to relapse onto a full agonist opioid at any time during treatment, he or she would require another induction phase as described above.

6.2.3   Pain and Opioid Use Disorder

Buprenorphine is dosed once daily for opioid substitution in many cases. Currently, sublingual buprenorphine/naloxone is not FDA-approved for the treatment of pain, but does have evidence for treatment of chronic pain and is acknowledged by the DEA as a legal off label treatment for pain disorders [28]. The analgesic duration of action of buprenorphine in the sublingual form has been approximated at 6–8 h, thus arguing for multiple dosing times throughout the day to address pain [29]. Sublingual buprenorphine has been shown effective in treating chronic pain conditions using this split dosing regimen [28, 30]. Further, buprenorphine/naloxone seems to benefit patients with chronic pain and physiologic opioid dependence. In one study, patients who were taking a full opioid agonist but experiencing tolerance with diminished analgesia or having side effects on their opioid medications were switched to buprenorphine/naloxone. They experienced an average 2.3-point pain reduction (0–10 pain scale) within 60 days of the switch [28]. Though studies show clinical efficacy in this population, the mechanism by which patients experience benefit is not fully known. Aside from its analgesic effects, buprenorphine exerts an antihyperalgesic effect and may reverse opioid-induced hyperalgesia associated with previous use of full opioid agonists [31].

Few studies have specifically looked at treatment of chronic pain in patients experiencing both chronic pain and opioid use disorder. One model of care described in the literature has been shown to have both good outcomes in retention and reduction in pain among patients at a Co-occurring Disorders Clinic embedded within the Primary Care Service of Raymond G. Murphy VA Medical Center in Albuquerque, NM. A retrospective chart review of 143 patients with co-occurring chronic non-cancer pain and opioid dependence showed retention rates of 65 %, defined as treatment >6 months without relapse to opioid use as well as a mean pain score reduction after induction onto buprenorphine/naloxone [32]. The mean total daily dose was 16 mg, which was split into BID or TID schedules. Buprenorphine dose adjustments were made based on four factors: cravings, pain relief, side effects, and opioid use/abstinence. Additionally, patients' pain conditions were treated with adjunctive measures such as non-opioid pain medications and physical therapy.

Transdermal buprenorphine has been shown to be effective in the treatment of chronic pain [33]. Aside from case reports, no studies have discussed the use of this formulation in patients with co-occurring chronic pain and opioid use disorder.

6.3   Methadone vs. Buprenorphine/Naloxone

At this time, only one randomized prospective trial has compared buprenorphine/naloxone and methadone among patients with chronic pain and coexistent opioid use disorder. Neumann and colleagues randomly assigned 54 patients with chronic pain and opioid addiction to treatment with either methadone or buprenorphine/naltrexone with the primary outcome measure being self-reported analgesia at 6-month follow-up. Other outcomes included retention, self-reported functioning, and self-reported substance use. Overall, treatment retention was 48 % and did not differ across groups. No difference in pain response between groups was noted, with an overall reduction in pain of 12.75 % among completers. In this study, patients in the methadone treatment condition reported less use of other opioids, but no differences in other measures were found. Average daily dose of methadone was 29 mg, while the average dose of buprenorphine was 14.9 mg. Medication doses were chosen based on pain literature and typically were delivered in 3–4 times per day dosing [11].

6.4 Summary

Patients with both opioid use disorder and chronic non-cancer pain (CNCP) pose a particular challenge to the treating clinician. As one article put it "although pain and addiction can and sometimes do exist as co-morbid conditions, they may also present as part of a dynamic continuum with pain at one end of the spectrum and addiction at the other" [34]. Distinguishing symptoms driven by underlying pain from symptoms associated with opioid use disorder can be a particular challenge in this population but clinically useful in directing care. As with any patient with opioid use disorder, if it is clear that the patient is experiencing withdrawal symptoms or cravings to use opioids, they would likely benefit from an increase in their methadone or buprenorphine substitution dose. But if pain is the primary complaint, there is little evidence that making such a change will have long-term benefits to the patient's experience of pain. As such, it is important to thoroughly discuss treatment goals and set reasonable expectations with patients prior to initiation of treatment with either methadone or buprenorphine for opioid use disorder.

Unfortunately, a considerable paucity of data exists to guide clinicians in how best to treat patients with co-occurring pain and opioid use disorders. Furthermore, clinicians are often not trained fully in both realms of care, leaving addiction doctors ill-equipped to deal with pain and pain physicians ill-equipped to deal with addiction. Models of care that attempt to address both conditions simultaneously may offer benefits over standard "silo" style approaches in treatment retention as well as overall addiction and pain management outcomes.

With the current evidence and in our clinical experience collectively, we would recommend the use of buprenorphine/naloxone therapy in patients with chronic pain and opioid use disorder as a first-line agent due to its safety profile and clinical efficacy. Additionally, if a patient does not respond to buprenorphine, it is easier to switch from buprenorphine to methadone than the other way around. Though published data has not established optimal schedules or dosing amounts, pharmacokinetic principals and clinical experience lead us to believe a minimum of BID and more optimally TID/QID dosing may be most beneficial so long as the patient can remain compliant with such a schedule. As with any pain management or opioid replacement dosing, each patient should be treated on a case-by-case basis using parameters described above. Average dosing among the few studies published has been 12–16 mg for the total daily dose. Patient compliance and efficacy should be considered closely at regular follow-up visits. If a patient is not benefiting from buprenorphine/naloxone, a provider may consider switching the patient to methadone. Again, TID or QID dosing may be more beneficial in addressing the patient's underlying pain and opioid use disorder. Ideally, care for these patients would be delivered using a multidisciplinary approach as these programs have better retention and outcomes in general. More randomized studies are required to further guide clinicians caring for these complex patients.

References

1. Saxon AJ. Treatment of opioid dependence. In: Ko M-C, Husbands SM, editors. Research and development of opioid-related ligands. New York: Oxford University Press; 2013. p. 61–102.
2. Ferrari A, Coccia CP, Bertolini A, Sternieri E. Methadone metabolism, pharmacokinetics and interactions. Pharmacol Res. 2004;50(6):551–9.
3. Eap CB, Buclin T, Baumann P. Interindividual variability of the clinical pharmacokinetics of methadone: implications for the treatment of opioid dependence. Clin Pharmacokinet. 2002;41(14):1153–93.
4. Armstrong SC, Cozza KL. Med-psych drug-drug interaction update. Psychosomatics. 2001; 42(5):435–7.
5. Tarumi Y, Pereira J, Watanabe S. Methadone and fluconazole: respiratory depression by drug interaction. J Pain Symptom Mange. 2002;23(2):148–53.
6. McCance-Katz EF, Sullivan LE, Nallani S. Drug interactions of clinical importance among the opioids, methadone and buprenorphine and other frequently prescribed medications: a review. Am J Addict. 2010;19(1):4–16.
7. Strain EC, Bigelow GE, Lievson IA, Stilzer ML. Moderate- vs high-dose methadone in the treatment of opioid dependence: a randomized trial. JAMA. 1999;281(11):100–5.
8. Abuse S, Administration MHS. Managing chronic pain in adults with or in recovery from substance use disorders. HHS publication No. (SMA) 12-4671, Treatment improvement protocol (TIP), vol. 54. Rockville: Substance Abuse and Mental Health Services Administration; 2011.
9. Eyler E. Chronic and acute pain and pain management for patients in methadone maintenance treatment. Am J Addict. 2013;22:75–83.
10. Dunn KE, Brooner RK, Clark MR. Severity and interference of chronic pain in methadone-maintained outpatients. Pain Med. 2014;15(9):1540–8.
11. Neumann AM, Blondell RD, Jaanimagi U, ct al. A preliminary study comparing methadone and buprenorphine in patients with chronic pain and co-existent opioid addiction. J Addict Dis. 2013;32(1):68–78.
12. Blinderman CD, Sekine R, Zhang B, et al. Methadone as an analgesic for patients with chronic pain in methadone maintenance treatment programs (MMTPs). J Opioid Manag. 2009; 5:107–14.
13. Angst MS, Clark DJ. Opioid-induced hyperalgesia: a qualitative systematic review. Anesthesiology. 2006;104:570–87.
14. Mao J. Opioid-induced abnormal pain sensitivity: implications in clinical opioid therapy. Pain. 2002;100:213–7.
15. Clark MR, Stoller KB, Brooner RK. Assessment and management of chronic pain in individuals seeking treatment for opioid use disorder. Can J Psychiatry. 2008;53(8):496–508.

16. Dahan A, Yassen A, Bijl H, Romberg R, Sarton E, Teppema L, et al. Comparison of the respiratory effects of intravenous buprenorphine and fentanyl in humans and rats. Br J Anaesth. 2005.
17. Walsh SL, Preston KL, Stitzer ML, Cone EJ, Bigelow GE. Clinical pharmacology of buprenorphine: ceiling effect at high doses. Clin Pharmacol Ther. 1994;55(5):569–80.
18. Chiang CN, Hawks RL. Pharmacokinetics of the combination tablet of buprenorphine and naloxone. Drug Alcohol Depend. 2003;70(2 Suppl):S39–47.
19. Nath RP, Upton RA, Everhart ET, Cheung P, Shwonek P, Jones RT, et al. Buprenorphine pharmacokinetics: relative bioavailability of sublingual tablet and liquid formulations. J Clin Pharmacol. 1999;39(6):619–23.
20. Chiou LC, Liao YY, Fan PC, Kuo PH, Wang CH, Riemer C, et al. Nociceptin/orphanin FQ peptide receptors: pharmacology and clinical implications. Curr Drug Targets. 2007;8(1):117–35.
21. Walsh SL, Eissenberg T. The clinical pharmacology of buprenorphine: extrapolating from the laboratory to the clinic. Drug Alcohl Depend. 2003;70(2 Suppl):S13–27.
22. Debelak K, Korrone WR, O'Grady KE, Jones HE. Buprenorphine + naloxone in the treatment of opioid dependence during pregnancy—initial patient care and outcome data. Am J Addict. 2013;22(3):252–4.
23. Bruce RD, Moody DE, Altice FL, Gourevitch MN, Friedland GH. A review of pharmacological interactions between HIV or hepatitis C virus medications and opioid agonist therapy: implications and management for clinical practice. Expert Rev Clin Pharmacol. 2013;6(3):249–69.
24. McCance-Katz EF, Moody DE, Prathikanti S, Friedland G, Rainey PM. Rifampin, but not rifabutin, may produce opiate withdrawal in burprenorphine-maintained patients. Drug Alcohol Depend. 2011;118(2-3):326–34.
25. Sanson RA, Sansone LA. Buprenorphine treatment for narcotic addiction: not without risks. Innov Clin Neurosci. 2015;12(3-4):32–6.
26. Saxon AJ, Ling W, Hillhouse M, Thomas C, Hasson A, Ang A, et al. Buprenorphine/Naloxone and methadone effects on laboratory indices of liver health: a randomized trial. Drug Alcohol Depend. 2013;128(1-2):71–6.
27. Wesson DR, Ling W. The Clinical Opiate Withdrawal Scale (COWS). J Psychoactive Drugs. 2003;35(2):253–9.
28. Daitch J, Frey ME, Silver D, Mitnick C, Daitch D, Pergolizzi Jr J. Conversion of chronic pain patients from full-opioid agonists to sublingual buprenorphine. Pain Physician. 2012;15(3 suppl):ES59–66.
29. Heit HA, Gourlay DL. Buprenorphine: new tricks with an old molecule for pain management. Clin J Pain. 2008;24(2):93–7.
30. Malinoff HL, Barkin RL, et al. Sublingual buprenorphine is effective in the treatment of chronic pain syndrome. Am J Ther. 2005;12(5):410–8.
31. Chen K, Chen L, Mao J. Buprenorphine-Naloxone therapy in pain management. Anesthesiology. 2014;120:1262–74.
32. Pade PA, Cardon KE, et al. Prescription opioid abuse, chronic pain, and primary care: a co-occurring disorders clinic in the chronic disease model. J Subst Abuse Treat. 2012;43:446–50.
33. Sittl R, Griessinger N, Likar R. Analgesic efficacy and tolerability of transdermal buprenorphine in patients with inadequately controlled chronic pain related to cancer and other disorders: A multicenter, randomized, double-blind, placebo-controlled trial. Clin Ther. 2003;25:150–68.
34. Gourlay DL, Heit HA. Pain and addiction: managing risk through comprehensive care. J Addict Dis. 2008;27(3):23–30.

Chapter 7
Interventional and Surgical Approaches to the Cervical and Lumbar Spine for Chronic Noncancer Pain

Andrew J. Engel

7.1 Introduction

After conservative therapies including medications and physical therapy have failed, more invasive treatments for lumbar and cervical spine pain are usually considered. Traditionally, injections are attempted to help patients avoid surgery. Yet, interventional pain procedures and surgical approaches to the lumbar and cervical spine are rarely used to treat the same diagnosis. Therefore, they will be discussed separately in this chapter.

The interventional spine injections will be divided into diagnostic and therapeutic procedures, whereas the surgical procedures are only therapeutic. Each interventional procedure will be discussed individually, and when there is a closely linked surgical procedure, it will be reviewed after the spinal injection. This order mirrors clinical practice since all non-surgical interventions are usually attempted prior to surgery. This summary of treatment options excludes the management of cancer, infection, and cauda equina syndrome.

7.2 Lumbar Interlaminar Epidural Steroid Injection

Historically, lumbar interlaminar (IL) epidural steroid injections have been used to treat low back pain or low back pain radiating into the leg(s). A patient will present with low back pain and leg pain or numbness radiating in a dermatomal pattern. The pathophysiology is a lumbar disc herniation irritating or compressing a passing or

A.J. Engel, M.D. (✉)
Affordable Pain Management, 5600 N Sheridan Rd,
Chicago, IL 60660, USA
e-mail: engel.andrew@gmail.com

© Springer International Publishing Switzerland 2016   69
A.M. Matthews, J.C. Fellers (eds.), *Treating Comorbid Opioid Use Disorder in Chronic Pain*, DOI 10.1007/978-3-319-29863-4_7

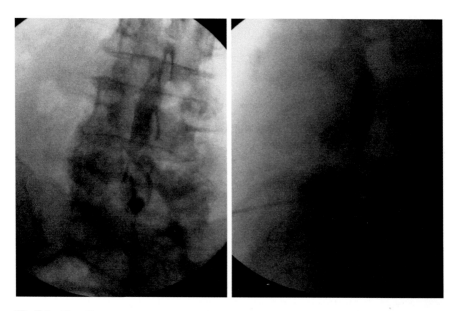

Fig. 7.1 AP and lateral views of epidural contrast medium spread (Courtesy of Savio D'Souza, M.D.)

exiting nerve causing lumbar radiculopathy (sciatica). In theory, steroid placed into the epidural space should decrease the inflammation around the nerve. With decreased inflammation, the pain should subside.

Accessing the epidural space under fluoroscopic guidance is very straightforward. The needle tip is placed between the lamina and advanced through the ligamentum flavum until there is a loss of resistance in the syringe attached to the needle. The epidural space is a potential space, which is why there is a loss of resistance. A lateral view is checked to confirm needle depth. Contrast medium is injected to confirm that the needle tip is in fact in the epidural space and not in an epidural vein. Epidural fat and cranial-caudal spread of the contrast medium is expected (Fig. 7.1). Steroid with or without local anesthetic is injected at that point.

Though this injection remains very common, the supporting literature is extremely weak. In a series of double-blind randomized controlled trials, Manchikanti et al. demonstrated that the addition of steroid to local anesthetic had no additional benefit [1–4]. In fact, there are no placebo-controlled trials demonstrating that IL epidural steroid injections provide benefit beyond the nonspecific effects of an injection or the natural history of the disease.

ILESI weak effect is highlighted by the number needed to treat (NNT) to reach 50 % improvement in pain score and disability. The NNT is the average number of patients that need to be treated before one person has success from the treatment itself (Table 7.1).

Since the NNT is either negative or double-digits, the efficacy of lumbar IL steroids is poor. Though this treatment is popular, currently the data does not support its continued use.

Diagnosis	NNT
Herniated disc	10
Discogenic pain	−20
Radiculitis	17
Post-lumbar surgery syndrome	10

Table 7.1 The number of patients that need steroid in an IL epidural injection to see 50 % improvement in pain and disability [1–4]

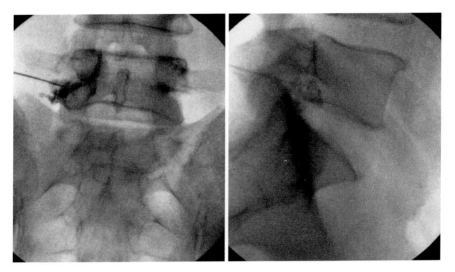

Fig. 7.2 AP and lateral views of a contrast medium spread during a lumbar transforaminal steroid injection (Courtesy of Andrew Engel, M.D.)

7.3   Lumbar Transforaminal Steroid Injection

Another access to the lumbar epidural space to treat a herniated disc causing radiculopathy exists: lumbar transforaminal steroid injection (LTFSI) under fluoroscopy. Rather than depositing steroid dorsally, a small gauge spinal needle can be advanced into the neuroforamen allowing placement of steroid at the dorsal root ganglion. For this injection, the foramen is approached obliquely. A lateral view confirms that the needle is in the foramen. Contrast medium will demonstrate a neurogram without vascular uptake confirming that the steroid will bathe the affected nerve (Fig. 7.2).

Depositing the steroid ventrally rather than dorsally dramatically changes the efficacy of the injection. In a five-arm double blind randomized placebo-controlled trial, patients with a lumbar herniated disc leading to radiculopathy who were scheduled for surgery were treated with one of five injections: transforaminal injection of steroid, transforaminal injection of local anesthetic, transforaminal injection of normal saline, intramuscular steroids, or intramuscular saline. Patients treated with LTFSI were more likely to improve than patients who received any of the placebo injections. With success defined as a 50 % reduction in pain and disability, the NNT is four. Importantly, the benefits of LTFSI are not due to nonspecific effects of an injection, but steroid decreasing the inflammation around the affected nerve. The benefits of this injection are independent of the nonspecific effects of an injection or natural history of the disease. One in three patients is able to avoid surgery because of this injection [5]. Non-compressive disc herniations respond best to this injection [6].

7.4 Lumbar Hemilaminectomy and Discectomy

Patients with large compressive disc herniations do not respond well to injections and usually progress to surgery. These patients typically present with motor, neurologic, or sensory changes that correlate with the compressed nerve. Surgery to decompress the nerve can resolve the radicular symptoms associated with the disc herniation. To achieve the goal of nerve decompression, there are microsurgical and open approaches to the lumbar intervertebral disc. Since both approaches achieve the same goal, surgeon and patient preference determine the type of surgery.

As described by the name, a hemilaminectomy involves shaving away or removing a portion of the lamina with the goal of creating additional space for the nerve roots. Once a portion of the lamina has been removed, the thecal sac is displaced to the side and the surgeon has access to the disc herniation. The herniated portion of the disc is excised, decompressing the nerve root. Depending on the condition of the disc, the anular tear can be repaired. The thecal sac and nerve root are allowed to relax to their anatomic positions, allowing a resolution of the radicular symptoms.

Patients with large disc herniations whose symptoms are severe enough to warrant surgery are more likely to improve with surgery than with conservative care including injections [7]. While patients with small disc herniations and less severe symptoms are more likely to improve with injections. Therefore, there is probably very little overlap in patients who will improve with injections and those who will improve with surgery. Patients with objective motor or neurologic changes typically do not even try injections; instead they progress immediately to surgery to avoid permanent nerve damage.

7.5 Lumbar Medial Branch Blocks

Patients who have axial low back or low back referred to the buttock or posterior thigh, but no radicular pain, could be suffering from pain that originates in the facet joint. Since the nerves exiting the spine are not irritated or compressed with facet pain, there is no radiculopathy. The pain can be referred as far caudally as the posterior thigh, but not in a dermatomal distribution, and signs of nerve root tension should not exist. Theoretically, patients with facet pain should have increased pain with maneuvers that stress the facet joint. Patients who have increased pain with lumbar extension and lateral rotation are usually considered appropriate candidates for testing the facet joint. Though facet arthropathy or spondylosis on MRI, CT scan, and X-rays are a common finding, these findings do not correlate with pain. Only medial branch blocks can accurately diagnosis facetogenic pain. Under fluoroscopic guidance, anesthetizing the nerves that innervates the facet joint makes the diagnosis. This injection is purely diagnostic.

Each facet joint is innervated from above and below; therefore, to anesthetize one facet joint, the superior and inferior medial branch nerves need to be blocked. If the patient has 100 % relief of the index pain, it could be argued that the pain originates in the facet joint. Diagnostic injections have a high false positive rate; patients seek out care to improve. Typically, medial branch blocks are repeated at another visit to confirm if the facet joint is causing the pain. If the patient has continued low back pain in a pattern consistent with the anesthetized joint after medial branch blocks, that joint is not causing the pain.

Technically, these injections appear very easy. In practice, precisely placing local anesthetic on the medial branch nerve can be very demanding; in addition, structures around the medial branch cannot be anesthetized since that would decrease the target specificity of these injections. The medial branch nerve sits in the sulcus between the superior articular process and the transverse process (Fig. 7.3). The L5 dorsal ramus (the caudal nerve that innervates the L5-S1 facet joint) sits in the sacral ALA. Again a lateral view is checked to confirm needle placement. A small amount of contrast medium is injected to confirm that the needle tip is not in a blood vessel. Since this injection is solely diagnostic, only local anesthetic is injected. Up to 0.5 mL of local anesthetic is injected at each nerve. This small volume is enough to anesthetize the nerve (positive target specificity), but not enough to anesthetize nearby structures (negative target specificity).

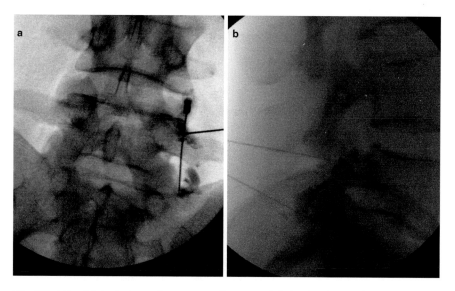

Fig. 7.3 AP and lateral views of contrast medium spread during lumbar medial branch blocks (Courtesy of Andrew Engel, M.D.)

If a patient has temporary 100 % pain relief, the facet joint is likely the pain generator. The best way to confirm that the facet joint is causing the pain is placebo-controlled blocks. On consecutive appointments, the medial branch nerves are blocked once with saline and once with local anesthetic in a double-blind fashion. If the patient has no pain relief with the saline and complete pain relief with the local anesthetic, the facet joint is causing the pain. To expedite treatment, an alternative diagnostic approach has been developed. After the initial local anesthetic block, a confirmatory local anesthetic block is performed. Traditionally, a local anesthetic with different duration of action is utilized. Patients should have a shorter duration of relief with short-acting local anesthetic and a longer duration of relief with the longer-acting anesthetic. Though concordant responses would be ideal, the duration of action of local anesthetics in the setting of pain has not been determined. Therefore, temporary relief that approximates the duration of action of the local anesthetic injected is appropriate. Since local anesthetics completely anesthetize the medial branch nerves, 100 % relief of the index pain is expected. Dual comparative medial branch blocks with complete relief is the diagnostic standard.

7.6 Lumbar Medial Branch Radiofrequency Ablation

Once the facet joint has been identified as the pain generator, lumbar medial branch radiofrequency ablation under fluoroscopy is the therapeutic procedure. A Teflon-coated needle with an active tip is placed parallel to the course of the medial branch nerve. Using radiofrequency energy, the needle tip is heated to 80 °C for 90 seconds. The needle is then repositioned and multiple ablations are made coagulating the nerve.

Lumbar medial branch radiofrequency ablations have not been tested against placebo; even though it is not clear why patients improve, the outcomes of this procedure are excellent. In an observational study, 55 % of patients experienced 100 % relief for an average of 15 months after this procedure. Patients who experienced 100 % pain relief used no further medical treatment for this problem and had a return of all activities of daily living. The pain relief was associated with functional benefit. Once the pain started to return, medial branch radiofrequency ablations could be repeated, thereby reinstating the pain relief [8].

7.7 Sacroiliac Joint Injection

Patients suffering from sacroiliac joint pain have back pain below L5 that radiates into the buttock, groin, or posterior thigh. Sacroiliitis is a common feature of spondyloarthropathies, but the majority of patients presenting with low back pain below L5 and over the buttock typically do not suffer from a spondyloarthropathy. Their pain could be emanating from the sacroiliac joint or the posterior ligaments of the sacroiliac joint. Differentiating these two sources of pain can be very difficult. Physical examination findings yield a diagnostic confidence of about 50 % and there is no radiologic examination that can determine if the sacroiliac joint or posterior

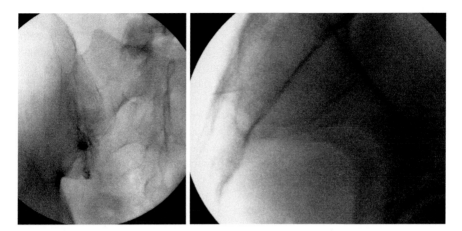

Fig. 7.4 AP and lateral views of contrast spread within the sacroiliac joint (Courtesy of Andrew Engel, M.D.)

complex is the pain generator; therefore, only local anesthetic injections can make the diagnosis of sacroiliitis. Fluoroscopically guided local anesthetic intra-articular sacroiliac joint injections can determine if the sacroiliac joint itself is causing the pain [9]. While multi-depth, multi-site lateral branch and L5 dorsal ramus blocks can diagnose pain from the posterior complex of the joint [10].

Fluoroscopically guided intra-articular sacroiliac joint injections are very straightforward and safe. Under fluoroscopic guidance, the needle tip is directed into the sacroiliac joint. A lateral view confirms depth. A small volume of contrast medium (approximately 0.2 mL's) is injected to outline the joint. A lateral image then confirms contrast medium within the joint (Fig. 7.4). For a diagnostic injection, local anesthetic is injected. If the sacroiliac joint were causing the pain, complete pain relief would be expected. Steroid-only intra-articular injections have been demonstrated to give therapeutic benefit beyond the placebo effect [9].

In contrast, multi-depth, multi-site lateral branch blocks are technically very challenging. When properly placed, these blocks can anesthetize the dorsal complex of the sacroiliac joint [11]. Unfortunately, the therapeutic treatment, radiofrequency ablation of the lateral branch nerves, has not been demonstrated to work [10].

Though intra-articular steroid injections can decrease the pain of the sacroiliac joint, this intervention is not usually curative. Patients traditionally need to return for injections, but repeat injections can reinstate pain relief.

7.8 Vertobroplasty/Kyphoplasty

Patients with a history of osteoporosis or metastatic cancer are at risk for vertebral compression fractures. Traditionally, these patients feel acute severe pain in the center of the back focused around the level of the fracture. Though an inciting event can occur, many of these fractures occur spontaneously. A vertebral body fracture is diagnosed with a spine X-ray. Prior to considering an intervention, an MRI can help determine the age of the fracture and if there is retropulsion (a potential contraindication to intervention) of the vertebral body into the spinal canal. No physical examination maneuver can accurately determine if the compression fracture is painful.

There are two interventional approaches to treating vertebral body compression fractures or painful metastatic lesions to the vertebral body: vertebroplasty and kyphoplasty. Both approaches involve stabilization of the fracture, but kyphoplasty also includes inflating a balloon in an attempt to expand the vertebral body. In both approaches, trocars are placed through the pedicles into the vertebral body under fluoroscopy. Using the access afforded by the trocars, vertebroplasty is accomplished by injecting polymethyl methacrylate (cement) into the vertebral body stabilizing the fracture. In addition to just injecting cement, kyphoplasty includes inflating a balloon before injecting cement with the hope of increasing vertebral body height.

Vertebral body compression fractures remain painful for approximately 2–3 months. Therefore, the indication for this procedure is not entirely clear: decreasing the time until the pain resolves or treating patients where the pain was not self-limited and became chronic. Traditionally, 3 weeks of non-surgical care is recommended prior to an intervention. Since the natural history of a compression fracture is favorable, finding benefit for these procedures has been difficult. Studies that compare vertebroplasty to sham injections have found no benefit, while studies that compare vertebroplasty/kyphoplasty to other methods of pain control have found benefit. It appears that this intervention provides more rapid pain relief compared to medication management, but any long-term benefit is not clear [12].

7.9 Discography

A spine X-ray, CT scan, or MRI can demonstrate that a disc has degenerated, but none of these imaging modalities can demonstrate if that disc is causing pain. Provocative discography is the only way to determine if a disc is painful. This diagnostic test may not lead to improved outcomes since the therapeutic treatments for disc disease have not been perfected, but more importantly, provocative discography can make a diagnosis.

Accessing a disc is relatively straightforward. Under an oblique fluoroscopic view, the superior articular process is placed in the midpoint of the intervertebral disc. An introducer needle follows the fluoroscopy beam until the anulus is reached. A smaller needle is passed into the middle third of the intervertebral disc. In both an AP and lateral view, the needle tip should be in the middle third of the disc. Under low pressure, the disc is injected with contrast medium under fluoroscopic vision and the patient's response is recorded. If disc stimulation causes no pain, that disc is not the pain generator. If the stimulated disc is painful, that disc is likely causing the patient's pain.

There is a theoretical high false positive rate associated with this injection [13]; therefore, multiple criteria are required for a stimulated disc to be considered the pain generator. The injection of contrast medium must be into the nucleus. An injection into the anulus is painful in itself. The pressure at which the disc is painful must be less than 50 psi above the internal pressure of the disc. The injected volume must be less than 3 mL for a lumbar disc. If the disc is painful, the pain should be 7/10 or higher and at least one neighboring disc should cause no pain (control level). The patient must have a postinjection CT scan to measure how far the contrast medium spreads into or through the anulus. For the disc to be the pain generator, the contrast medium must at least reach the outer third of the anulus (Dallas Grade III tear). When all of these measures are taken, the false positive rate of provocative discography is 0–3 % [14].

Since surgical outcomes for disc disease can be poor, operating on the basis of discography results is not encouraged. Discography is therefore used to determine if a disc is not the pain generator, thereby preventing a surgery that has no chance of helping the patient.

7.10 Lumbar Fusion

Lumbar fusion treats axial low back pain from disc disease or back and leg pain from spondylolisthesis. The goal of this surgery is to remove the offending disc and stabilize the spine (Fig. 7.5). Though approaching the disc posteriorly is traditional, there are multiple approaches (anterior, transforaminal, and posterior) to fuse the lumbar spine. An advantage of the posterior approach is the ability to decompress the spinal canal if symptomatic spinal stenosis is contributing to the pain. Decompressing the nerves can treat radicular symptoms or neurogenic claudication. In patients with spondylolisthesis, the vertebral bodies can be realigned.

To access the intervertebral disc, a posterior or transforaminal approach is taken. Using this method, the surgeon can decompress the lumbar spine by removing a portion of the lamina, the associated ligamentum flavum, and the intervertebral disc. The disc is replaced with a polyetheretherketone (PEEK) cage and bone fragments. Pedicle screws and rods are placed to keep the vertebral bodies in place while the vertebra fuse together. Once a solid fusion has been accomplished, the patient is free to pursue activities as tolerated.

Theoretically, since the disc has been removed, once the vertebral bodies fuse together, the patient should be pain-free. Unfortunately, the data for this surgery does not suggest that type of success. A randomized controlled trial of posterior lumbar fusion for pain versus continued conservative care favored lumbar fusion. At 2 years, the average pain relief in the lumbar fusion group was superior to the average pain relief in the conservative care group. Yet, the average pain relief in the lumbar fusion group was a minimal 30 % [15]. A more modern review of 3060 patients who underwent posterior lumbar fusion for degenerative disc disease demonstrated a 37/100 average reduction in VAS for back pain [16]. Again, the results were barely superior to the minimal clinically important change.

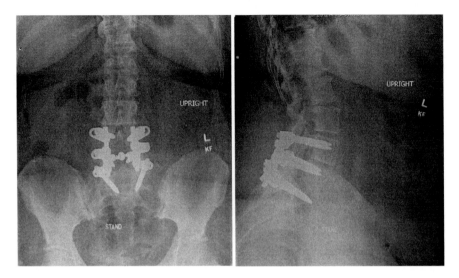

Fig. 7.5 AP and lateral views of a two-level posterior lumbar fusion (Courtesy of Purnendu Gupta, M.D.)

7.11 Cervical Interlaminar Epidural Steroid Injection

Analogous to LESI, cervical interlaminar epidural steroid injections (CESI) have been used to treat neck and neck pain with radicular symptoms to the arm and hand. The needle approach to the cervical epidural space is the same as the approach to the lumbar epidural space, except that the ligamentum flavum is thinner. Accordingly, the loss of resistance is not as clear and the risk of intrathecal or direct spinal cord injection is increased. To mitigate that risk, some physicians pass a catheter through the epidural space to the level that is causing pain.

Since a CESI deposits steroid in the dorsal aspect of the epidural space, the effectiveness data are poor (Table 7.2) [17–21].

With a negative NNT for all possible indications for CESI, offering steroids with this injection cannot help. Since inflammation is considered the root cause of pain caused by disc disease leading to radiculopathy, offering epidural injections of other substances would not address the pathophysiology.

7.12 Cervical Transforaminal Steroid Injection

Just as the dorsal cervical epidural space can be accessed by a CESI, the ventral epidural space can be reached by a transforaminal approach. As opposed to accessing the neuroforamen in the lumbar spine, cervical transforaminal steroid injections (CTFSI) are exceedingly dangerous. The vertebral artery and anterior spinal arteries

Table 7.2 The number of patients that need steroid in an IL epidural injection to see 50 % improvement in pain and disability

Diagnosis	NNT
Discogenic pain	−34
Disc herniation	−25
Disc herniation and radiculitis	−25
Spinal stenosis	−34
Post-surgery syndrome	−34

can be punctured with a transforaminal approach. Injection of particulate steroid leads to infarction, paralysis, and potentially death. When a CTFSI is offered for a foraminal disc herniation, the safe window between the vertebral artery and the nerve root is dramatically decreased down to 2 mm [22].

More than the potential catastrophic complications associated with CTFSI, the benefit of this injection has never been demonstrated. Any benefit that patients report could just as easily have occurred because of the natural history of the disease or the nonspecific benefits of an injection [23]. Currently, this injection is rarely offered as there is no way to guarantee safety.

7.13   Cervical Medial Branch Blocks

Axial neck pain stemming from the facet joint is the most common cause of pain in the cervical spine. The presence of cervical facet pain is up to 60 % [24]. Pain originating from the facet joint presents as neck pain that can radiate to the top of the shoulder or behind the shoulder blade. As with lumbar facet pain, there are no radiologic or physical examination tests that can diagnose the painful facet joint. Only medial branch blocks can determine if a facet joint is the pain generator.

Just as anesthetizing the cervical facet joints can diagnose the cause of neck pain, anesthetizing the third occipital nerve, which crosses the C2–3 facet joint, can diagnose the pain source for a cervicogenic headache.

As with lumbar medial branch blocks, placebo-controlled medial branch blocks have an infinite likelihood ratio, but are impractical because of the additional injection required. Therefore, comparative blocks are used as a surrogate. If the response to the local anesthetic is concordant, complete pain relief lasting for the expected duration of the local anesthetic, the likelihood ratio is 4.50. If the response is discordant, not the expected duration of the local anesthetic, the likelihood ratio falls to 2.86 [25]. Because of the high prevalence of cervical facet disease, the diagnostic confidences are 87 % and 78 %, respectively. Therefore, comparative cervical medial branch blocks are required to make the diagnosis of cervical facet disease.

Though seemingly more demanding than lumbar medial branch blocks, cervical medial branch blocks are very straightforward and safe. Under fluoroscopic guidance in a lateral view, the needle tip is placed at the centroid of the articular pillar. An anterior–posterior view is taken to confirm the depth of the needles (Fig. 7.6).

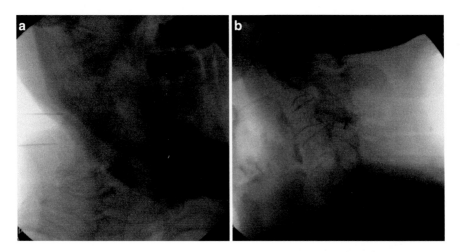

Fig. 7.6 An AP (**a**) and lateral (**b**) view of needle placement for cervical medial branch blocks (Courtesy of Andrew Engel, M.D.)

Contrast media is injected to confirm that there is no vascular uptake and a maximum of 0.3 mL local anesthetic is injected at each level. As with the lumbar facet joint, each joint is innervated from above and below, therefore two injections are required to anesthetize one joint. As with lumbar medial branch blocks, this injection is solely diagnostic; no steroid is used.

Since there is no partial response to local anesthetics, complete temporary relief of the index pain is the expected response. A patient with both shoulder pain and cervical facet pain may report shoulder pain after successful diagnostic cervical medial branch blocks as the injection can only diagnosis neck and referred pain from the cervical facet joints. Though the patient may not have 100 % pain relief, the patient had complete relief of the facet pain. The shoulder pain could independently come from the shoulder.

7.14   Cervical Medial Branch Radiofrequency Ablations

The therapeutic treatment for cervical facet disease is cervical medial branch radiofrequency ablations. Specialized needles placed parallel to the medial branch nerve under fluoroscopic guidance can coagulate the nerve preventing the nociceptive signal from reaching the brain.

When properly performed on appropriately selected patients, two thirds of patients can expect complete pain relief with restoration of all activities of daily living for approximately one and a half years [26]. If the pain returns, pain relief can be reinstated with a repeat radiofrequency ablation. This response is not because of the placebo effect [27]. The NNT is two when patients have complete relief of their index pain with dual comparative medial branch blocks progress to medial branch radiofrequency ablation.

7.15   Cervical Fusion

In contrast to the outcomes for cervical facet disease, the interventional outcomes for cervical disc disease and cervical radiculopathy are poor. Patients will present to the surgeon with neck pain radiating to the arm. The pain can radiate into the shoulder, all the way to the fingers, or anywhere in between. The patient will typically describe numbness and parathesias with associated sensory or deep tendon reflex changes. Patients have the option of conservative care or surgery. There are two common approaches to the cervical disc: anterior cervical discectomy (ACDF) and fusion or disc arthroplasty.

An ACDF involves removing the disc from an anterior approach. A PEEK cage with bone growth replaces the disc. An anterior plate is screwed into the cranial and caudal vertebral bodies holds the fusion construct together until the vertebral bodies fuse together (Fig. 7.7). Rather than fusing the bones together, disc arthroplasty involves replacing the diseased disc with an artifical disc. The outcomes from both surgeries are essentially equivalent [28].

Though cervical fusion or arthroplasty likely gives short-term pain relief more promptly than conservative care, there is no high-quality data to demonstrate that there are any long-term benefits from cervical spine surgery for the degenerative disc causing radiculopathy [29].

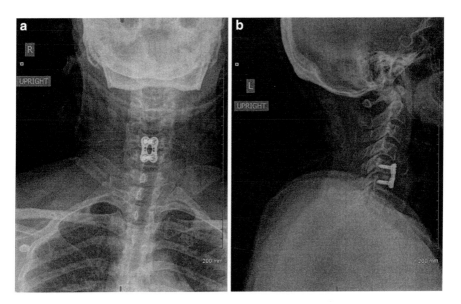

Fig. 7.7 An AP (**a**) and Lateral (**b**) views of ACDF (Courtesy of Purnendu Gupta, M.D.)

7.16 Spinal Cord Stimulation

Patients with intractable neuropathic pain may be candidates for spinal cord stimulation (SCS). This treatment does nothing to change the underlying condition, but it may be able to decrease pain. Traditionally, this treatment is offered for chronic noncancer pain, since SCS has not demonstrated appropriate efficacy for acute pain.

The exact mechanism by which SCS decreases pain is unclear, but several explanations exist. The original theory was based on the gate control theory. Antidromic activation of the collateral fibers of the dorsal columns would prevent the nociceptive signal in the dorsal horn from reaching the brain. If this were the only mechanism by which SCS worked, it should be effective for acute pain. Therefore, in addition to antidromic activation, there is also orthodromic stimulation, manifested as paresthesias in the affected area.

Additionally, SCS might increase GABA release leading to a decrease in the over-excitability of wide dynamic range neurons. Supporting that theory, extracellular glutamate concentration in the dorsal horn is also reduced. Beyond the GABA and glutamate effects, serotonergic descending pathways are involved in pain modulation. The effects of SCS might not be limited to the spinal cord. A dorsal column-brainstem-spinal loop might also help explain the pain-relieving mechanism [30]. Ultimately, SCS might work by more than one of the proposed pathways.

Though it would seem logical that preventing the pain signal from reaching the brain or masking it with parethesias would reduce pain in all patients, success is not universal. Trial SCS leads connected to an external generator are placed in the epidural space. The patient usually keeps the leads for 1 week, and during that time keeps a pain diary to determine if the SCS is helping. To be considered successful, patients need substantial pain relief (the definition of success varies) in addition to functional benefit.

If the trial SCS provides appropriate benefit, permanent leads can be placed in the epidural space percutaneously or surgically. To place the leads percutaneously, the epidural space is entered with a needle and the leads are placed in the appropriate position. If the leads are placed surgically, a laminotomy is performed and the leads are positioned in the epidural space (Fig. 7.8). Percutaneous insertion has a decreased recovery time, but takes longer for the leads to scar into place. If the leads migrate prior to scarring into place, the potential benefit of SCS could be lost. At the same time as the SCS leads are permanently placed, the SCS generator is inserted in a surgically formed pocket near the waist (Fig. 7.9). The pocket location is determined by patient and surgeon preference, as the SCS generator needs constant recharging.

Permanent implantation of the SCS is an outpatient procedure. Patients typically follow up for an incision check within a couple of weeks. A properly placed SCS will not need further follow-up with a physician as long as the leads don't migrate and the patient recharges the battery.

Fig. 7.8 Surgically placed SCS paddle leads (Courtesy of Andrew Engel, M.D.)

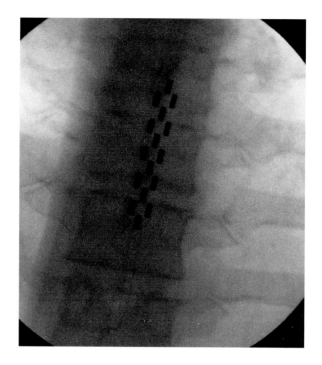

Fig. 7.9 Image of a surgically implanted SCS generator (Courtesy of Andrew Engel, M.D.)

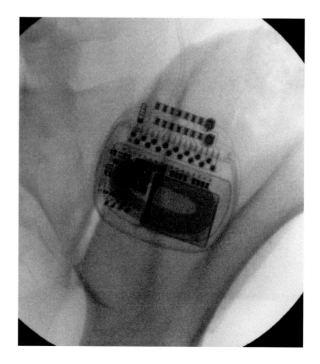

7.17   Intrathecal Opioid Pump

The use of opioids for the treatment of chronic noncancer pain is starting to fall out of favor because of their lack of efficacy and the risk of addiction. But when prescribing opioids for chronic noncancer pain was common, an intrathecal pump was an alternate way of delivering medication for patients who could not tolerate the side effects of opioids or were experiencing decreased efficacy even after opioid rotation.

Intrathecal opioids are 100 times as potent as intravenous opioids. Therefore, much smaller doses of medication can be prescribed minimizing side effects and potentially increasing pain relief. For patients who have increasing pain, newer pumps have a patient-activated bolus feature that can be triggered by a remote control.

Since intrathecal opioids are not beneficial for all patients, a trial is attempted to determine if the patient will benefit from this treatment prior to implantation of an intrathecal pump. There are two ways to trial intrathecal medications: single shot or a temporary catheter. A single intrathecal dose of morphine is the most efficient method of determining the percentage relief from intrathecal medications (Fig. 7.10). Patients do not need to stay in the hospital overnight and the single dose can help determine the efficacy and side effects of intrathecal medication for that patient. If the trial is unsuccessful, another single shot trial with a higher dose of medication can be attempted. In contrast, a temporary epidural or intrathecal cath-

Fig. 7.10 Image of a single shot intrathecal pump trial (Courtesy of Andrew Engel, M.D.)

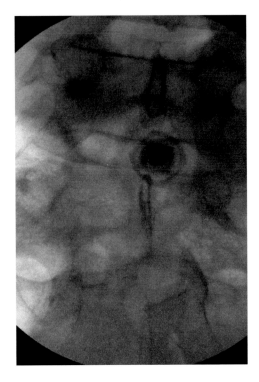

eter allows for dose titration, but requires hospitalization with connection to an external pump.

If the patient finds that intrathecal medications are more effective than oral or intravenous medications and there are no limiting side effects, an intrathecal pump can be placed. Under fluoroscopic guidance, the catheter is placed intrathecally below the level of the conus. The catheter is then tunneled under the skin to the abdomen where it is attached to the 20 or 40 mL pump that is placed in a subcutaneous pocket (Fig. 7.11). A pump can be implanted on an outpatient basis.

Ideally, the pump is programmed so that it needs to be refilled every 2–3 months. A physician-controlled remote programmer controls the rate of the pump. If refills of the intrathecal pump start to become too frequent, the concentration of the medication can be increased since intrathecal medication is compounded for the individual patient. Refilling the pump is a simple office procedure completed with a guide and specialized needle.

Intuitively, it would seem that intrathecal opioids would be the panacea for pain control: high efficacy and low complications. In reality, intrathecal opioids for chronic noncancer pain are falling out of favor because the long-term outcomes are generally poor [31]. As tolerance to opioids increases and the medication in the pump needs to be concentrated, there is an increased risk of granuloma formation. Patients exposed to long-term opioid therapy are at risk for hyperalgesia. The efficacy of this treatment is purely dependent upon patient selection.

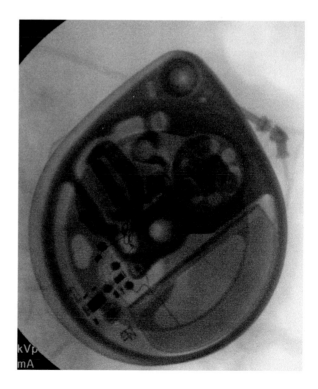

Fig. 7.11 Image of a surgically implanted intrathecal pump (Courtesy of Andrew Engel, M.D.)

7.18 Conclusion

Clearly, each of these topics deserves in-depth treatment, but this chapter was designed to give nonspecialists an idea of what types of interventional treatment are available for chronic pain. When conservative measures fail, appropriately selected interventional procedures can decrease pain and prevent patients from needing surgery. When patients fail interventional procedures, surgery remains an option. For all of the aforementioned treatments, the indications are very narrow and success is dependent upon patient selection.

References

1. Manchikanti L, Singh V, Cash KA, Pampati V, Falco FJ. A randomized, double-blind, active-control trial of the effectiveness of lumbar interlaminar epidural injections in disc herniation. Pain Physician. 2014;17:E61–74.
2. Manchikanti L, Cash KA, McManus CD, Pampati V, Benyamin RM. A randomized, double-blind, active-controlled trial of fluoroscopic lumbar interlaminar epidural injections in chronic axial or discogenic low back pain: results of 2-year follow-up. Pain Physician. 2013;16:E491–504.
3. Manchikanti L, Singh V, Cash KA, Pampati V, Falco FJ. The role of fluoroscopic interlaminar epidural injections in managing chronic pain of lumbar disc herniation or radiculitis: a randomized, double-blind trial. Pain Pract. 2013;13:547–58.
4. Manchikanti L, Singh V, Cash KA, Pampati V, Datta S. Fluoroscopic caudal epidural injections in managing post lumbar surgery syndrome: two-year results of a randomized, double-blind, active-control trial. Int J Med Sci. 2012;9:582–91.
5. Ghahreman A, Ferch R, Bogduk N. The efficacy of transforaminal injection of steroids for the treatment of lumbar radicular pain. Pain Med. 2010;11:1149–68.
6. Karppinen J, Ohinmaa A, Malmivaara A, Kurunlahti M, Kyllönen E, Pienimäki T, Nieminen P, Tervonen O, Vanharanta H. Cost effectiveness of periradicular infiltration for sciatica: subgroup analysis of a randomized controlled trial. Spine (Phila Pa 1976). 2001;26:2587–95.
7. Kreiner D, et al. Evidence-based clinical guidelines for multidisciplinary spine care. Diagnosis and treatment of lumbar disc herniation with radiculopathy. Spine J. 2014;14(1):180–91.
8. MacVicar J, Borowczyk J, MacVicar A, Loughnan B, Bogduk N. Lumbar medial branch radiofrequency neurotomy in New Zealand. Pain Med. 2013;14:639–45.
9. Kennedy DJ, Engel A, Kreiner D, Nampiaparampil D, Duszynski B, MacVicar J. Fluoroscopically-guided diagnostic and therapeutic intra-articular sacroiliac joint injections: a systematic review. Pain Med. 2015;16(8):1500–18.
10. King W, Ahmed S, Baisden J, Patel N, Kennedy DJ, MacVicar J, Duszunski B. Diagnosis and treatment of posterior sacroiliac complex pain: a systematic review with comprehensive analysis of the published data. Pain Med. 2015;16:257–65.
11. Dreyfuss P, Henning T, Malladi N, Goldstein B, Bogduk N. The ability of multi-site, multi-depth sacral lateral branch blocks to anesthetize the sacroiliac joint complex. Pain Med. 2009;10:679–88.
12. Savage JW, Schroeder GD, Anderson PA. Vertebroplasty and kyphoplasty for the treatment of osteoporotic vertebral compression fractures. J Am Acad Orthop Surg. 2014;22:653–64.
13. Carragee EJ, Tanner CM, Khurana S, Hayward C, Welsh J, Date E, Truong T, Rossi M, Hagle C. The rates of false-positive lumbar discography in select patients without low back symptoms. Spine (Phila Pa 1976). 2000;25:1373–80.

14. Bogduk N, Aprill C, Derby R. Lumbar discogenic pain: state-of-the-art review. Pain Med. 2013;14:813–36.
15. Fritzell P, Hägg O, Wessberg P, Nordwall A, and the Swedish Lumbar Spine Study Group. 2001 Volvo award winner in clinical studies: lumbar fusion *versus* nonsurgical treatment for chronic low back pain. Spine (Phila Pa 1976). 2001;26:2521–34.
16. Phillips F, Slosar P, Youssef J, Andersson G, Papatheofanis F. Lumbar spine fusion for chronic low back pain due to degenerative disc disease. Spine (Phila Pa 1976). 2013;38:E409–22.
17. Manchikanti L, Cash KA, Pampati V, Malla Y. Two-year follow-up results of fluoroscopic cervical epidural injections in chronic axial or discogenic neck pain: a randomized, double-blind, controlled trial. Int J Med Sci. 2014;11:309–20.
18. Manchikanti L, Cash KA, Pampati V, Wargo BW, Malla Y. A randomized, double-blind, active control trial of fluoroscopic cervical interlaminar epidural injections in chronic pain of cervical disc herniation: results of a 2-year follow-up. Pain Physician. 2013;16:465–78.
19. Manchikanti L, Cash KA, Pampati V, Wargo BW, Malla Y. Management of chronic pain of cervical disc herniation and radiculitis with fluoroscopic cervical interlaminar epidural injections. Int J Med Sci. 2012;9:424–34.
20. Manchikanti L, Malla Y, Cash KA, McManus CD, Pampati V. Fluoroscopic epidural injections in cervical spinal stenosis: preliminary results of a randomized, double-blind, active control trial. Pain Physician. 2012;15:E59–70.
21. Manchikanti L, Malla Y, Cash KA, McManus CD, Pampati V. Fluoroscopic cervical interlaminar epidural injections in managing chronic pain of cervical postsurgery syndrome: preliminary results of a randomized, double-blind, active control trial. Pain Physician. 2012;15:13–25.
22. Beckworth WJ, Sood R, Katzer AF, Wu B. Anomalous location of the vertebral artery in relation to the neural foramen. Implications for cervical transforaminal epidural steroid injections. Pain Med. 2013;14(8):1119–25.
23. Engel A, King W, MacVicar J, and on behalf of the Standards Division of the International Spine Intervention Society. The effectiveness and risks of fluoroscopically guided cervical transforaminal injections of steroids: a systematic review with comprehensive analysis of the published data. Pain Med. 2014;15:386–402.
24. Lord S, Barnsley L, Wallis BJ, Bogduk N. Chronic cervical zygopophysial joint pain after whiplash: a placebo-controlled prevalence study. Spine. 1996;21:1737–45.
25. Lord SM, Barnsley L, Bogduk N. The utility of comparative local anaesthetic blocks versus placebo-controlled blocks for the diagnosis of cervical zygopophysial joint pain. Clin J Pain. 1995;11:208–13.
26. MacVicar J, Borowczyk J, MacVicar A, Loughnan B, Bogduk N. Cervical medial branch radiofrequency neurotomy in New Zealand. Pain Med. 2012;13:647–54.
27. Lord SM, Barnsley L, Wallis BJ, McDonald GJ, Bogduk N. Percutaneous radio-frequency neurotomy for chronic cervical zygapophyseal-joint pain. N Engl J Med. 1996;335:1721–6.
28. Verhagen A, van Middelkoop M, Rubinstein S, Ostelo R, Jacobs W, Peul W, Koes B, van Tulder M. Effect of various kinds of cervical spinal surgery on clinical outcomes: a systematic review and meta-analysis. Pain. 2013;154:2388–96.
29. North American Spine Society. Evidence-based clinical guidelines for multidisciplinary spine care. Diagnosis and treatment of cervical radiculopathy from degenerative disorders. Burr Ridge: North American Spine Society; 2010.
30. Wolter T. Spinal cord stimulation for neuropathic pain: current perspectives. J Pain Res. 2014;7:651–63.
31. Ver Donck A, Vranken J, Puylaert M, Hayek S, Mekhail N, Van Zundert J. Intrathecal drug administration in chronic pain syndromes. Pain Pract. 2014;14:461–76.

Chapter 8
Special Issues in the Treatment of Women

Stacey Gramann

8.1 Pain in Women

In general, women experience more chronic pain compared to men. Research supports this finding as women have higher rates of pain reporting and functional impairment secondary to pain [1–3]. Women have a higher prevalence of chronic pain conditions including migraines/chronic tension headaches, temporomandibular disorders, interstitial cystitis, irritable bowel syndrome, fibromyalgia, osteoarthritis, rheumatoid arthritis, and musculoskeletal pain [1, 2, 4]. In addition, female-specific pain conditions exist including dyspareunia, chronic pelvic pain, menstrual pain, and vulvodynia [4]. Prevalence rates of chronic pelvic pain conditions in women are as high as 15 %, with such conditions being difficult to diagnosis and treat [5]. In the Danish National Health and Morbidity Survey ($N = 10{,}066$), women compared to men were found to have 1.2–1.6 higher odds of endorsing chronic pain. Female subjects in the study endorsed pain with greater intensity, frequency, duration, and distribution over a larger number of locations in the body. They also reported a higher level of functional impairment related to their pain [1]. Despite evidence that pain is more common in women, gender differences in pain sensitivity and severity have been more difficult to understand due to methodological issues in research. Reviews of experimental-induced pain studies suggest women experience higher pain sensitivity than men, but a statistically significant difference has been variable [2].

Appreciating this complexity, biological, psychological, and social factors have been theorized in an effort to explain such gender differences in pain experience (Table 8.1). With regard to biological factors, research suggests that female and

S. Gramann, D.O., M.P.H. (✉)
Mental Health Division, Portland VA Medical Center,
3710 US Veteran's Hospital Rd, Mail Code P3MHDC, Portland, OR 97207, USA
e-mail: Stacey.Gramann@va.gov

© Springer International Publishing Switzerland 2016
A.M. Matthews, J.C. Fellers (eds.), *Treating Comorbid Opioid Use Disorder in Chronic Pain*, DOI 10.1007/978-3-319-29863-4_8

Table 8.1 Factors in understanding gender differences in pain experience

Mechanism	Women
Biological	• Differences in endogenous opioid system
	• Genotype expression
	• Gonadal hormone (Estradiol) influence
	– Low estradiol, low progesterone phase of menstrual cycle associated with higher pain levels
	– May influence opioid receptor concentration
Psychological	• Pain-coping style
	• Social supports, positive self-affirmations, emotion-focused techniques, cognitive reframing/interpretation, and attentional focus
	• Cognitive schemas
	• Catastrophic thinking
Social	• Gender roles: Women more socially acceptable to have pain
	• Early exposure to stress/trauma (?)

male functional differences exist within the endogenous opioid system [2, 6]. In addition, genotype expression may alter pain response, along with the modulatory effects of gonadal hormones interacting with the endogenous opioid system [2, 7]. Pronociceptive and antinociceptive effects of estradiol and progesterone have been studied with varying results. Based on postmortem and functional neuroimaging studies, it has been suggested that estradiol influences pain through interaction with the endogenous opioid system and by influencing opioid receptor concentration [7]. In a small study using PET scan, the nociceptive effects of estradiol via the endogenous opioid system were studied. In low estradiol, low progesterone states, women demonstrated a lower capacity to activate the endogenous opioid system as evidenced by higher ratings of pain and negative affective state. Furthermore, the low estradiol, low progesterone (early follicular) phase of the menstrual cycle was associated with a reduction in baseline tonic activity at the level of the thalamus, nucleus accumbens, and amygdala resulting in higher pain ratings, influencing pain recall in both sensory and affective qualities [7]. Overall, the role of hormones estradiol and progesterone in pain is complex, with both exhibiting pronociceptive and antinociceptive effects. Of note, testosterone has been shown to be more antinociceptive and protective in nature [2]. Psychological factors include variations in pain-coping styles and cognitive patterns. In general, men use behavioral distraction and problem-focused strategies to cope with pain. Women rely more on social supports, positive self-affirmations, emotion-focused techniques, cognitive reframing/interpretation, and attentional focus. Research has also shown that women have a greater tendency to fall into patterns of catastrophic thinking with pain, which has been associated with a greater level of pain-related disability. Lastly, social factors include cultural gender roles and early life trauma. Sociocultural beliefs of masculinity and femininity are thought to influence pain expression, with women more commonly in the socially accepted role of experiencing pain. Early life exposure to stress including child abuse is thought to influence gender differences in pain experience, but the relationship has been less clear [2].

8.2 Opioid Treatment of Pain in Women

Various studies have explored the antinociceptive and rewarding effects of opioids in women [2, 8, 9]. However, studies of variation of opioid reward effect by menstrual cycle phase have not found a clear relationship between ovarian hormones and opioid effects [9, 10]. In regard to gender differences in specific opioid response, in a systematic review there was evidence suggesting that μ-opioids have greater analgesic effect for women compared to men. A significant effect was observed in intravenous patient-controlled analgesia (PCA) studies in which men consumed higher amounts of μ-opioids compared to women, indicating increased efficacy in women. More specifically, morphine had greater potency of effect for women, but a slower onset of action. No gender differences were shown with analgesic response to μ/κ-opioids [8].

Although there is limited knowledge of opioid analgesia in women, more is known about side effects, long-term consequences, and clinical management challenges encountered when providing medical care to women maintained on chronic opioid therapy. Female gender has been associated with higher opioid prescription rates and dosages, and specifically older women are at higher risk for long-term opioid use. However, research identifying gender differences in opioid tolerance, dependence, and opioid-induced hyperalgesia is lacking [4]. In general, women experience higher rates of side effects from opioids, including opioid-induced emesis and respiratory depression [8]. As women experience opioid-induced nausea more commonly, it has been theorized that women are at lower risk for nonmedical use of prescription opioids (NMUPO) with nausea deterring misuse [11]. Long-term opioid therapy for both chronic pain and substance use disorders can lead to side effects of infertility, loss of libido, fatigue, depression, anxiety, osteoporosis, sleep apnea, muscle wasting, and hyperalgesia [4, 12, 13]. The endocrine system is particularly vulnerable to chronic opioid therapy, and women, like men, can develop opioid-induced central, secondary, and hypogonadotropic hypogonadism [4, 12–14]. Central hypogonadism is characterized by central suppression of gonadotropin-releasing hormone (GNRH) production, leading to decreased gonadal hormone production (testosterone, estradiol, FSH, and LH) [12, 13]. Careful monitoring for the condition and treatment is recommended, as premenopausal women are at risk for premature osteoporosis, infertility secondary to amenorrhea, galactorrhea, and increased cardiovascular risk [13]. Monitoring gonadal hormone levels including estradiol and free testosterone is recommended along with routine bone density screening [12]. Guidelines for treatment of opioid-induced hypogonadism in women recommend a three-step approach as follows: (1) non-opioid therapy, (2) opioid rotation, and (3) hormone replacement therapy (HRT). When considering HRT, it is recommended to consult endocrinology first, as HRT is associated with an increased risk of cardiovascular disease and breast and ovarian cancers [13]. Lastly, women of reproductive age on chronic opioid therapy may be at risk for unplanned pregnancies. Menstrual cycle irregularities are caused by reduced ovarian and adrenal testosterone production and reduced conversion to estradiol with simultaneous opioid-induced reduction of FSH levels [12]. Consequently, women of reproductive age must be educated on the risks of unplanned pregnancy with discussion of contraception options.

Ultimately, when prescribing opioids for women, providers may encounter several challenges in their efforts to provide optimal care to patients. Women on long-term opioid therapy receive less preventative healthcare and basic screening. One theory is that the focus of primary care visits surrounds opioid management, limiting a provider's time to focus on basic preventative health. Further complicating the picture, women on long-term opioid therapy have higher rates of sleep apnea (up to 50 %), but are less likely to receive sleep studies resulting in undiagnosed and untreated breathing-related sleep disorders. Beyond these challenges, women receiving long-term opioid therapy are at higher risk for polypharmacy (drug–drug interactions) and frequent emergency room visits and medical hospitalizations, leading to increased risk of iatrogenic complications [4]. Therefore, efforts should be made to routinely perform preventative health screening, monitor for signs of breathing-related sleep disorders, and minimize polypharmacy in women maintained on chronic opioid therapy.

8.3   Opioid Use Disorders in Women

In general, men have higher rates of substance use disorders than women with use of nicotine, alcohol, and most illicit drugs. However, men and women have equivalent rates of NMUPO, spanning from adolescence to older age [1]. Similarly, men and women suffering from chronic pain conditions have equal rates of opioid use disorders [3]. However, research has shown a trend of increasing rates of opioid use among women [4, 15]. Based on survey findings from the Addiction Severity Index-Multimedia Version Connect prescription opioid database ($N=29,906$), women were 1.59 times more likely to report recent (past 30 days) prescription opioid use than men and 1.50 times more likely to report recent abuse of a prescription opioid than men [15]. With increasing rates of opioid use among women, there is reason for growing concern, as women are known to progress from use to dependence more rapidly than men, a phenomenon referred to as 'telescoping' [1, 16–18]. Consequently, they present to treatment with more severe medical, psychological, social, and behavioral issues [19]. In addition, women are more likely to underutilize substance treatment. In the National Survey of Drug Use and Health, a survey of 892 opioid-dependent, treatment-seeking subjects, rates of women presenting for an opioid-related, substance use issue rarely exceeded 35 % [16].

To better identify women at risk for opioid use disorders, both risk factors and prescription opioid aberrant behaviors for NMUPO will be reviewed and the influence of comorbid psychiatric conditions and the possible role of ovarian hormones in substance response. Women who have a history of childhood abuse (sexual or physical), family history of substance abuse, personal history of psychiatric or psychological issues, and single marital status were more likely to develop aberrant behaviors with prescription opioid use [1, 3]. Aberrant behaviors observed in women include hoarding of unused opioid medications, use of other sedative medications to enhance opioid effect, preoccupation with pill counts, and a pattern of use motivated by a desire to treat negative affective and somatic (pain) states [1, 3, 16, 20, 21].

Unlike men, women with opioid use disorders exhibit more treatment-compliant behaviors with a higher likelihood of receiving opioids through a prescription and use of an opioid via the intended route of administration and treatment indication [21]. It remains unclear whether aberrant behaviors with prescription opioid use have predictive validity as indicators for opioid dependence. Furthermore, it is difficult to screen and incorporate these female-specific risk factors and behaviors into substance treatment [1]. However, it is clear with the absence of traditional behaviors associated with misuse in men that it can be more challenging for the provider to detect women at risk. In addition, prescription of medications that are difficult to modify, such as Suboxone®, is less likely to be a deterrent for misuse in women [21]. Consequently, it is important to monitor closely for signs of opioid misuse, including use of alternative sedative medications, risk for drug–drug interactions, and potential for unintended overdose. Discussion and safety planning should occur with women to make sure access to stockpiled medications is restricted in an effort to minimize potential for a child or family member ingesting medication [1].

Comorbid psychiatric conditions including depression and anxiety have been identified as risk factors for prescription aberrant behaviors, as women with opioid use disorders report increased rates of psychiatric severity with major depressive disorder and PTSD [21]. As women have higher lifetime prevalence rates for depression than men (a ratio of 2:1), it has been observed that women presenting with a negative affective state or who have experienced a recent depressive episode are more likely to receive a prescribed opioid medication from their provider [4]. A theory is women experiencing anxiety and/or depression are less able to manage their opioid medications for pain, as they are more likely to self-medicate for affective and interpersonal distress [3, 4, 16, 20, 21]. To explain this, research has suggested that women have higher levels of 'anxiety sensitivity,' defined as negative perceptions of bodily sensations, leading to fear, a suspected motivator for sedative use. In a study comparing 68 opioid-dependent, mixed-gender subjects, women had significantly higher levels of anxiety sensitivity compared to men, even when controlling for PTSD, a disorder twice as common in women [20]. Furthermore, women with opioid use disorders have higher rates of impairment in occupational, social, and family functioning [21, 22]. Substance treatment for women with opioid use disorders and chronic pain should focus on distress tolerance interventions such as Acceptance and Commitment therapy (ACT) along with treatment of comorbid depression, anxiety, and sleep-related issues [2, 3, 20, 21]. Also, psychosocial interventions that provide vocational support along with financial and family services could help address barriers to access and enhance treatment compliance [21, 22].

As observed with pain sensitivity in women, it has been suggested that fluctuating levels of hormones and/or the progesterone-to-estrogen ratio may influence substance response in women to a greater degree than absolute hormone levels. More specifically, high endogenous progesterone levels may be protective against certain stress responses and drug-seeking behaviors in women with nicotine and cocaine use disorders [10]. Exogenous progesterone for treatment of women with substance use disorders has been trialed, but the influence of ovarian hormones in drug-seeking behavior in opioid use disorders continues to be overall poorly understood [10].

8.4 Pharmacologic Treatment of Opioid Use Disorders in Women

Prior to 1993, women of childbearing age were banned from participating in US investigational drug trials. Since that time, studies have begun to look at gender differences in response to opioid-agonist medication for treatment of opioid use disorders [23]. In general, pharmacotherapy in women compared to men requires consideration of unique differences related to pharmacology and the role of hormones. Progesterone and estrogen can affect absorption, hepatic metabolism, distribution, and excretion of medications, but the overall influence on medication levels is poorly understood [24]. Biological, pharmacodynamic, and pharmacokinetic differences with methadone and buprenorphine in nonpregnant women and men have not been identified. As a result, there are no gender-specific guidelines for either buprenorphine or methadone treatment in nonpregnant women with opioid use disorders [17, 25].

Gender differences in the efficacy of opioid maintenance therapies (OMT) for opioid use disorders have been studied. In a randomized-controlled trial (RCT), treatment outcomes were compared between levacetylmethadol (LAAM), methadone, and buprenorphine for men and women. For women, buprenorphine therapy resulted in less objective measures (urine drug screen confirmation) of illicit opioid use compared to methadone with longer treatment retention rates. However, the difference in retention rates between genders was not significant. This effect was not observed in the women's methadone group [23]. An earlier study conducted in 1993 by Johnson et al., produced conflicting results with women receiving buprenorphine therapy having higher rates of illicit opioid use. However, the study design was different with a shorter treatment period (14 days) compared to a longer treatment period (17 and 24 weeks) in the later study that showed a beneficial effect of buprenorphine in women [17]. It has been suggested that women of childbearing age may benefit more from buprenorphine due to a higher density of μ- and κ-opioid receptors, gender differences in opioid receptor signal transduction, and/or gonadal hormone-dependent differences in pharmacokinetics [17, 23]. However, women maintained on long-term opioid maintenance therapy (OMT) require close monitoring due to cardiac side effects and gonadal hormone suppression. First, women are at greater risk of developing drug-induced prolonged QT syndrome. This occurs via an estrogen-mediated reduction in repolarization within the cardiac muscle [26]. Thus, women across the reproductive life-cycle, including postmenopausal women receiving estrogen HRT, should receive routine cardiac monitoring with both methadone and buprenorphine treatment [17, 26]. It is important to note that studies comparing methadone and buprenorphine and risk of drug-induced prolonged QT syndrome show a higher risk with methadone [17]. Second, as occurs with long-term opioid therapy for pain in women, risks of neuroendocrine abnormalities leading to irregular menstrual cycles and fertility effects must be considered with methadone maintenance therapy (MMT). It has been shown that women with heroin and short-acting opioid misuse can develop blunting of pulsatile luteinizing hormone, resulting in menstrual cycle irregularities and infertility. Neuroendocrine function then normalizes within 1-year of steady-dose MMT with resumption of regular menstrual cycles and increased fertility in women of childbearing age [25, 27]. Thus, women must be educated regarding the risks of unplanned pregnancy with discussion of contraception options.

Based on the limited research to date, there may be enhanced efficacy with buprenorphine compared to methadone when treating opioid use disorders in non-pregnant women. Also, buprenorphine has lower potential for drug–drug interactions and drug-induced prolonged QT syndrome compared to methadone [17]. As women with opioid use disorders are at risk for polypharmacy and misuse of alternative sedative medications to enhance opioid effect, buprenorphine may be a safer option. However, MMT managed within the structure of a multidisciplinary psychosocial program may outweigh such benefits if psychosocial issues present as a barrier to accessing and engaging in treatment. Despite these results, further research is needed to better understand gender differences in outcomes with opioid-agonist medications for treatment of opioid use disorders.

8.5 Opioid Use Disorders in Pregnant Women

Prevalence rates of opioid use disorders in pregnant women vary [28]. However, national surveys show that up to 4.4 % of pregnant women (ages 15–44) reported NMUPO within the past year, with higher rates up to 15 % for pregnant adolescents (ages 15–17) [27]. Women with opioid use disorders have a greater likelihood of conceiving, with 54 % of women with opioid use disorders having four or more pregnancies in their lifetime compared to only 14 % in a representative sample of US women [29, 30]. In 2012, incidence rates of maternal opioid use at delivery had a fourfold increase and neonatal abstinence syndrome (NAS) had a threefold increase over the prior decade [31]. With a growing trend of opioid use in pregnancy, particularly in younger pregnant women, there has been a greater focus on treating opioid use disorders in pregnancy and lactation due to the potential risks to mother, fetus, and the high level of healthcare burden [32]. Intricate social, biological, and psychological factors complicate recovery of pregnant women with substance use issues. In particular, comorbid psychiatric conditions, prior trauma, family substance use history, and lack of education, housing, and employment can present barriers to accessing and complying with substance treatment [31, 33]. In an effort to better understand treatment of opioid use disorders in pregnancy, both fetal risks and maternal consequences of opioid use disorders in pregnancy along with recommendations for treatment and management in pregnancy and lactation will be reviewed.

Fetal risks of maternal opioid use in pregnancy extend from congenital defects with first trimester exposure to long-term developmental issues in the child. Risks include congenital heart defects with first trimester exposure and pregnancy complications of preeclampsia, intrauterine growth retardation/microcephaly, spontaneous abortion, intrauterine death, preterm birth, low Apgar scores, infections, third trimester bleeding, intrauterine passage of meconium, placental insufficiency, and premature rupture of membranes [27, 28, 34]. NAS is a common neonatal complication for neonates exposed to chronic opioids during pregnancy. Prevalence rates of NAS among neonates exposed to methadone or buprenorphine in pregnancy range from 40 to 90 % [27, 34, 35]. NAS is a syndrome marked by dysfunction of the autonomic, respiratory, central nervous, and GI systems with symptoms of hyperirritability in the neonate [14, 34, 35]. Additional neonatal complications include postnatal growth deficiency, microcephaly, neurobehavioral problems, and a 74-fold increase in the risk of sudden infant death syndrome [28]. Maternal consequences of opioid use in pregnancy include unplanned pregnancy, delayed initiation or lack of prenatal care, poor nutrition, interpersonal violence, comorbid psychiatric illness, polysubstance use, infectious disease exposure, housing instability, poverty, legal problems, and poor dentition [27, 34, 36]. Such consequences can complicate prenatal and obstetric care along with substance use treatment for opioid disorders in pregnant women.

8.6 Treatment of Opioid Use Disorders in Pregnant and Lactating Women

Treatment of opioid use disorders in pregnancy is based on a harm-reduction model, alternative to the abstinence-only model [27]. The standard of care for many years has been OMT with methadone, offered through a federally regulated clinic for pregnant women; however, buprenorphine has recently been studied as a reasonable option [27, 28, 35]. Newer agents like naltrexone, administered orally or via intramuscular injection, have been considered as an alternative to opioid agonist medication, but little is known regarding efficacy and safety in pregnancy [27, 29]. Therefore, this discussion will focus on methadone and buprenorphine, outlining management in pregnancy, labor and delivery, and lactation.

For pregnant women with opioid use disorders, optimal care is provided within an addiction program that specializes in pregnancy where a multidisciplinary approach is offered to address complex psychosocial needs. Methadone, a full μ-opioid receptor agonist, managed within the structure of a comprehensive prenatal program, has been shown to increase the number of prenatal visits, lengthen gestational periods, reduce pregnancy complications, decrease crime rates, and reduce HIV risk behaviors when compared to continued opioid use [27, 35]. Furthermore, the long half-life (24–36 h) maintains consistent blood levels in the fetus [27]. However, methadone has been associated with risks of altered fetal activity, heart activity, and NAS [17]. Recommended dosing is the same as nonpregnant adults; however, some adjustment may be required in pregnancy, as methadone clearance increases in late pregnancy due to elevated progesterone levels in the third trimester. Additional factors in pregnancy including decreased oral absorption, reduced plasma-protein binding, and increased volume of distribution may also affect serum levels. In an effort to avoid opioid cravings and withdrawal, it is recommended to increase methadone dosing and/or use split dosing in late pregnancy [25, 27].

Buprenorphine, a partial μ-opioid receptor agonist and κ-opioid receptor antagonist, has differing pharmacology and risk of precipitating opioid withdrawal in pregnancy. SAMHSA recommends avoiding buprenorphine/naloxone (Suboxone®) in pregnancy due to a risk of precipitating withdrawal when crushed and injected. Buprenorphine monotherapy (Subutex®) is recommended as the safer option [17, 27, 34, 37]. However, a more recent review of seven studies, comparing buprenorphine/naloxone with buprenorphine and methadone, did not identify any greater risk with buprenorphine/naloxone. Thus, further research is needed [34]. Dosing of buprenorphine in pregnancy, unlike methadone, requires no dose adjustment [27]. Careful monitoring is required at the time of induction due to risk of precipitating withdrawal if buprenorphine dosing is too high or low, or administered at too short an interval from last opioid use [17] (Table 8.2).

Table 8.2 Management of opioid maintenance therapy in pregnancy

	Methadone	Buprenorphine
Pregnancy	• Full μ-opioid receptor agonist	• Partial μ-opioid receptor agonist/κ-opioid receptor antagonist
	• ½ life 24–36 h, maintains consistent blood levels in fetus	• ½ life 24–60 h, maintains consistent blood levels in fetus
	• Dosing consistent with nonpregnant adults	• Dosing consistent with nonpregnant adults
	• Increased metabolism and clearance in third trimester requires increased dosing and/or split dosing	• No dose adjustment
	• Coordination of care with OB provider to plan intrapartum dosing	• Buprenorphine monotherapy only
	• Continue regimen in labor/delivery	• Coordination of care with OB provider to plan intrapartum dosing
Labor and delivery	• NSAIDs or non-opioid analgesics can be used for acute pain	• Continue regimen in labor/delivery
	• Anesthesiology consult if considering epidural anesthesia	• NSAIDs or non-opioid analgesics can be used for acute pain
Lactation	• Safe to breastfeed	• Reduce dosing or discontinue if analgesic requirements high. Reattempt induction when pain resolved.
	• Contraindicated if HIV risk status and/or active illicit drug use	• Anesthesiology consult if considering epidural anesthesia
		• Minimal amount excreted in breastmilk, generally safe, studies lacking
		• Contraindicated if HIV risk status and/or active illicit drug use

In comparing methadone, buprenorphine, and slow-release morphine, a Cochrane review was published by Minozzi et al. in 2013, comparing efficacy and safety in treating opioid-dependent, pregnant women. The review included four RCTs with a total of 271 pregnant women. Included within the review was the Maternal Opioid Treatment: Human Experimental Research (MOTHER) study, an eight site, international, double-blind, double dummy study comparing methadone and buprenorphine offered within a comprehensive prenatal program. Overall, based on the Cochrane review, methadone and buprenorphine had no significant differences to conclude that one treatment was superior. In terms of risks and benefits, methadone had higher treatment retention rates, and buprenorphine had less severe and shorter NAS. It was concluded that more studies were needed with larger sample sizes to determine an overall comparison [28]. In general, if a woman conceives and has responded well to a particular agent, either buprenorphine or methadone, the recommendation is to continue the medication to avoid risk of destabilization [17, 34, 38]. Transitioning from methadone to buprenorphine in pregnancy is possible, but not recommended, as this can precipitate opioid withdrawal, increasing risk of preterm birth, abortion, dysphoric mood, and illicit drug use [17, 27, 39]. Furthermore, opioid detoxification is in general avoided in pregnancy due to the high risk of relapse. If detoxification is attempted, it should occur in the second trimester (12–28 weeks) to avoid miscarriage in the first trimester and preterm delivery after 32 weeks [14, 17, 27, 40].

Lastly, when treating pregnant women with opioid use disorders, it is important to assess, diagnose, and treat comorbid psychiatric conditions; as pregnant women with opioid use disorders commonly experience anxiety and depression at rates of 65–73 %, compared to 20 % in nonpregnant, substance-using controls. These disorders can present as barriers to care, potentially leading to poorer maternal and neonatal outcomes with OMT [27, 32, 33]. In a secondary data analysis from the MOTHER study, women reporting anxiety symptoms compared to women reporting depressive symptoms had statistically significant differences in treatment discontinuation, with anxiety associated with a higher risk of premature termination of treatment. However, more research is needed to understand this complex relationship [32, 41].

During labor and delivery, women receiving OMT may experience hyperalgesia and opioid tolerance, requiring higher opioid dosing to manage pain. For this indication, opioid agents prescribed in addition to the outpatient OMT regimen have been shown to be safe in both vaginal and caesarian deliveries [35]. Nonopioid analgesics and non-steroidal anti-inflammatory medications may be used for management of acute pain during labor. If epidural anesthesia is considered, it is recommended to consult with the anesthesiologist beforehand, as certain opioid agents, when used with buprenorphine or methadone, can precipitate withdrawal due to a higher binding affinity for the μ-opioid receptor [27]. In patients with severe pain who are receiving buprenorphine, it is recommended to reduce regular buprenorphine dosing to 8 mg/daily, then account for the difference with a short-acting opioid administered in divided doses, in addition to routine dosing of opioids for the specific procedure. If pain persists in setting of high analgesic requirements for more than 2 days, the recommendation is to discontinue the buprenorphine with the goal of reducing opioid dose requirements over the subsequent days. Then restart buprenorphine induction when the pain issues have resolved [27, 33].

In 1993, the US Department of Health and Human Services concluded that breast-feeding was no longer contraindicated with methadone therapy. Exposure to methadone in breastmilk diminishes duration of methadone-associated NAS in the infant and facilitates bonding. This is generally recommended if no risk factors are present such as infectious diseases (including HIV) or active illicit drug use. Buprenorphine clinically follows a similar recommendation with breastfeeding; however, there are limited study cases to date. Minimal amounts of buprenorphine are excreted into the breastmilk with infant exposure being only 1/5–1/10 of total buprenorphine dose. Consequently, there is limited improvement of NAS symptoms with breastfeeding [17, 42].

8.7 Conclusion

With increasing opioid use and patterns of misuse among women, researchers have identified risk factors and aberrant behaviors that may help predict those women at greater risk of developing opioid dependence. However, more research is needed to develop screening tools and practice guidelines for safe opioid prescribing in women. There is some evidence supporting the role of ovarian hormones in pain experience, opioid response, and substance use disorders, with estrogen having some antinociceptive benefits and endogenous progesterone having protective effects against stress and substance-seeking behaviors in women. OMT continues to be the standard of care for pharmacologic treatment of opioid use disorder in women. Methadone or buprenorphine may be reasonable options in both nonpregnant and pregnant women; however, serious thought should be given to the risks and benefits of both medications, accounting for the side effects, psychosocial barriers, and long-term treatment risks reviewed in this chapter.

References

1. Back SE, Payne RA, Waldrop AE, Smith A, Reeves S, Brady KT. Prescription opioid aberrant behaviors. Clin J Pain. 2009;25(6):477–84.
2. Bartley EJ, Fillingim RB. Sex differences in pain: a brief review of clinical and experimental findings. Br J Anaesth. 2013;111(1):52–8.
3. Jamison RN, Butler SF, Budman SH, Edwards RR, Wasan AD. Gender differences in risk factors for aberrant prescription opioid use. J Pain. 2010;11(4):312–20.
4. Darnall BD, Stacey BR, Chou R. Medical and psychological risks and consequences of long-term opioid therapy in women. Pain Med. 2012;13:1181–211.
5. Stein SL. Chronic pelvic pain. Gastroenterol Clin North Am. 2013;42(4):785–800.
6. al'Absi M, Wittmers LE, Ellestad D, Nordehn G, Won Kim S, Kirschbaum C et al. Sex differences in pain and hypothalamic-pituitary-adrenocortical responses to opioid blockade. Psychosom Med. 2004;66:198–206.

7. Smith YR, Stohler CS, Nichols TE, Bueller JA, Koeppe RA, Zubieta J. Pronociceptive and antinociceptive effects of estradiol through endogenous opioid neurotransmission in women. J Neurosci. 2006;26(21):5777–85.
8. Niesters M, Dahan A, Kest B, Zacny J, Stijnen T, Aarts L. Do sex differences exist in opioid analgesia? A systematic review and meta-analysis of human experimental and clinical studies. Pain. 2010;151:61–8.
9. Terner JM, De Wit H. Menstrual cycle phase and responses to drugs of abuse in humans. Drug Alcohol Depend. 2006;84(1):1–13.
10. Moran-Santa Maria MM, Flanagan J, Brady K. Ovarian hormones and drug abuse. Curr Psychiatry Rep. 2014;16(11):511.
11. Zacny JP, Apfelbaum SM. Modulating roles of smoking status and sex on oxycodone-induced nausea and drug liking. Exp Clin Psychopharmacol. 2013;21(2):103–11.
12. Daniell HW. Opioid endocrinopathy in women consuming prescribed sustained-action opioids for control of nonmalignant pain. J Pain. 2008;9(1):28–36.
13. Katz N, Mazer NA. The impact of opioids on the endocrine system. Clin J Pain. 2009;25(2):170–5.
14. Wong D, Gray D, Simmonds M, Rashig S, Sobolev I, Morrish DW. Opioid analgesics suppress male gonadal function, but opioid use in men and women does not correlate with symptoms of sexual dysfunction. Pain Res Manag. 2011;16:311–6.
15. Green TC, Grimes Serrano JM, Licari A, Budman SH, Butler SF. Women who abuse prescription opioids: findings from the Addiction Severity Index-Multimedia Verson® Connect prescription opioid database. Drug Alcohol Depend. 2009;103: 65–73.
16. Back SE, Lawson KM, Singleton LM, Brady KT. Characteristics and correlates of men and women with prescription opioid dependence. Addict Behav. 2011;36:829–34.
17. Unger A, Jung E, Winklbaur B, Fischer G. Gender issues in the pharmacotherapy of opioid-addicted women: buprenorphine. J Addict Dis. 2010;29:217–30.
18. Zilberman ML, Blume SB. Substance use and abuse in women. In: Romans SE, Seeman MV, editors. Women's mental health a life cycle approach. Philadelphia: Lippincott Williams & Wilkins; 2006. p. 179–90.
19. Greenfield SF, Back SE, Lawson K, Brady KT. Substance abuse in women. Psychiatr Clin North Am. 2010;33:339–55.
20. Hearon BA, Calkins AW, Halperin DM, McHugh RK, Murray HW, Otto MW. Anxiety sensitivity and illicit sedative use among opioid-dependent women and men. Am J Drug Alcohol Abuse. 2011;37:43–7.
21. McHugh RK, DeVito EE, Dodd D, Carroll KM, Sharpe Potter J, Greenfield SF, Connery HS, et al. Gender differences in a clinical trial of prescription opioid dependence. J Subst Abuse Treat. 2013;45:38–43.
22. Back SE, Payne RL, Herrin Wahlquist A, Carter RE, Stroud Z, Haynes L, et al. Comparative profiles of men and women with opioid dependence: results from a National Multisite Effectiveness Trial. Am J Drug Alcohol Abuse. 2013;37:313–23.
23. Jones HE, Fitzgerald H, Johnson RE. Males and females differ in response to opioid agonist medications. Am J Addict. 2005;14:223–33.
24. Burt VK, Hendrick VA. Clinical manual of Women's mental health. 1st ed. Arlington: American Psychiatric Publishing Inc; 2005.
25. Kreek MJ, Borg L, Ducat E, Ray B. Pharmacotherapy in the treatment of addiction: methadone. J Addict Dis. 2010;29:200–16.
26. Li G, Cheng G, Wu J, Zhou W, Liu P, Sun C. Drug-induced long QT syndrome in women. Adv Ther. 2013;30:793–802.
27. Park EM, Meltzer-Brody S, Suzuki J. Evaluation and management of opioid dependence in pregnancy. Psychosomatics. 2012;53:424–32.
28. Minozzi S, Amato L, Bellisario C, Ferri M, Davoli M. Maintenance agonist treatments for opiate-dependent pregnant women. Cochrane Database Syst Rev. 2013;12.
29. Jones HE, Heil SH, Baewart A, Arria AM, Kaltenbach K, Martin PR et al. Buprenorphine treatment of opioid-dependent pregnant women: a comprehensive review. Addiction. 2012; (Suppl. 1) 5-27.

30. Jones HE, Chisholm MS, Jansson LM, Terplan M. Naltrexone in the treatment of opioid-dependent pregnant women: the case for a considered and measured approach to research. Addiction. 2012;108:233–47.
31. Jones HE. Treating opioid use disorders during pregnancy: historical, current, and future directions. Subst Abus. 2013;34:89–91.
32. Benningield MM, Dietrich MS, Jones HE, Kaltenbach K, Heil SH, Stine SM, et al. Opioid dependence during pregnancy: relationships of anxiety and depression symptoms to treatment outcomes. Addiction. 2012;107 Suppl 1:74–82.
33. Alto WA, O'Conner AB. Management of women treated with buprenorphine during pregnancy. Am J Obstet Gynecol. 2011;303–308.
34. Soyka M. Buprenorphine use in pregnant opioid users: a critical review. CNS Drugs. 2013;27:653–62.
35. Jones HE, Friedman CJ, Starer JJ, Terplan M, Gitlow S, American Society of Addiction Medicine, Women and Substance Use Disorders Work Group. Opioid use during pregnancy: an international road map for future research and clinical practice. Addict Disord Treatment. 2014;13:1.
36. Am H, Baxter JK, Jones HE, Heil SH, Coyle MG, Martin PR, et al. Infections and obstetric outcomes in opioid-dependent pregnant women maintained on methadone or buprenorphine. Addiction. 2012;107 Suppl 1:83–90.
37. SAMHSA. Clinical guidelines for the use of buprenorphine in the treatment of opioid addiction Treatment Improvement Protocol (TIP) Series 40. 2004 [cited 2015 Apr 22]. http://buprenorphine.samhsa.gov/Bup_Guidelines.pdf
38. Brandt L, Leifheit AK, Finnegan LP, Fischer G. Management of substance abuse in pregnancy: maternal and neonatal aspects. In: Galbally M, Snellen M, Lewis A, editors. Psychopharmacology in pregnancy. New York: Springer; 2014. p. 169–89.
39. Welle-Stand GK, Skurtveit S, Jones HE, Waal H, Bakstad B, Bjark Ø, et al. Neonatal outcomes following in utero exposure to methadone or buprenorphine: A national cohort study of opioid-agonist treatment for pregnant women in Norway from 1996-2009. Drug Alcohol Depend. 2013;127:200–6.
40. Wong S, Ordean A, Kahan M. Substance use in pregnancy. J Obstet Gynaecol Can. 2011;33(4):367–84.
41. Benningfield MM, Arria AM, Kaltenbach K, Heil SH, Stine SM, Coyle MG, et al. Co-occurring psychiatric symptoms are associated with increased psychological, social, and medical impairment in opioid dependent pregnant women. Am J Addict. 2010;19:416–21.
42. Hilton TC. Breastfeeding considerations of opioid dependent mothers and infants. Am J Matern Child Nurs. 2012;37(4):236–40.

Chapter 9
Managing Chronic Pain in Older Adults

Michael J. Yao and Katherine A. Tacker

9.1   Introduction

Persistent pain in older adults is a very complex challenge to manage effectively and safely. Among older adults 65 or over, chronic noncancer pain (CNCP) affects between 35 and 48 % of community dwelling and 45–85 % of nursing home residents [1–3]. CNCP is mediated by a number of comorbid chronic health conditions [3] and is associated with activity restriction, depressive symptoms, and increased functional disability [4–6]. Assessment of CNCP is complicated when older adults underreport CNCP symptoms because of coexisting sensory or cognitive impairments and stoic attitudes around pain tolerance [7, 8]. Additionally, clinicians may also inadequately communicate with these patients about pain concerns [4, 9]. Management of CNCP in older adults is complicated by age-related physiological changes, comorbid chronic health conditions, and widespread use of polypharmacy. This chapter addresses these complications and other special considerations in assessing, monitoring, and managing persistent pain among older adults.

M.J. Yao, M.D., M.P.H.
Mental Health and Neurosciences Division, Portland VA Health Care System,
3710 SW US Veterans Hospital Rd., V3CRS, Portland, OR 97239, USA
e-mail: Michael.Yao@va.gov

K.A. Tacker, M.D. (✉)
Department of Psychiatry, Oregon Health and Science University,
3818 SW Sam Jackson Park Rd., UHN 80, Portland, OR 97239, USA
e-mail: tackerk@ohsu.edu

© Springer International Publishing Switzerland 2016
A.M. Matthews, J.C. Fellers (eds.), *Treating Comorbid Opioid Use Disorder in Chronic Pain*, DOI 10.1007/978-3-319-29863-4_9

9.2   Complications of Pain Management in Older Adults

Pharmacologic changes with aging: Normal aging changes pharmacodynamic and pharmacokinetic effects. Both types of changes are important to acknowledge when considering pharmacologic treatment of CNCP. Older adults are more sensitive to the pharmacodynamic effects of medications, especially in patients with a multidrug regimen. This increased sensitivity could potentially result in more frequent falls and fractures secondary to orthostatic hypotension or in skin integrity problems from prolonged immobility secondary to oversedation [10]. Pharmacokinetic changes in older adults can also have noteworthy effects on medication management (Table 9.1) [10–12]. Taking both the pharmacodynamic and the pharmacokinetic changes into account, pharmacologic treatment should typically be initiated at lower doses and titrated more slowly in older adults to avoid adverse consequences.

Comorbid conditions of aging: Older adults have a higher prevalence of multiple chronic health conditions that cause or contribute to CNCP (Table 9.2) [3].

This CNCP is often treated with opioid and non-opioid analgesics. But the use or misuse of these drugs for pain relief in older patients is associated with additional risks, such as falls and hip fractures [13], anorexia [14], gastrointestinal motility issues [15], depression [16] and anxiety symptoms [17], delirium [18], cognitive impairment, and psychosocial dysfunction [19, 20]. Therefore, pharmacologic treatment of CNCP in patients with comorbid conditions requires careful consideration of all factors.

Polypharmacy in older adults: In the USA, nearly 37 % of people aged 60 or older take at least five medications. These patients have an 80 % chance of drug–drug interactions and increased frequency of adverse consequences such as respiratory depression and death [21, 22]. In one study of military veterans, hospitalizations due to adverse effects of medication quadrupled when they were taking five or more medications, often including both analgesic medications and benzodiazepines [23]. To minimize the untoward effects of polypharmacy, clinicians may find routine review of medications with the patient and engagement in care coordination with

Table 9.1 Pharmacokinetic changes in older adults

	Age-related changes	Consequences
Absorption	Decrease acid secretion, GI perfusion, membrane transport counterbalanced by longer transit time	Minimal impact to absorption capacity in healthy older adults
Volume of distribution	Loss of lean body mass and total body water; increase total body fat; decrease albumin	Increased accumulation of lipophilic drugs; change in availability of protein-bound drugs
Clearance rate	Decreased hepatic blood flow and metabolism via CYP450 system (oxidative > conjugation); decreased glomerular filtration rate (GFR) and creatinine clearance (CrCl)	Slower clearance depending on the degree of hepatic and renal impairment; elimination half-life prolonged in older adults

Table 9.2 Common chronic conditions in older adults that typically cause pain

Nociceptive pain	Coronary artery disease
	Low back pain from facet joint arthritis and spondylosis
	Osteoarthritis
	Osteoporosis
	Paget's disease
	Polymyalgia rheumatica
	Previous bone fractures
	Rheumatoid arthritis
Neuropathic pain	Central poststroke
	Nutritional neuropathies
	Peripheral neuropathies
	Postherpetic neuralgia
	Trigeminal neuralgia
Mixed pain	Fibromyalgia
	Myofascial pain

caregivers, prescribers, and pharmacists to be helpful. These reviews could potentially reduce redundant or unnecessary agents, mitigate high-risk drug–drug interactions, and support the lowest effective dosing of essential medications. Databases focusing on pharmacologic risks in older adults, such as the Beers criteria [24] or STOPP/START criteria [25], are useful guidelines for rational reduction of polypharmacy.

9.3 Assessment of Pain in Older Adults

The diagnosis and treatment of CNCP in older adults can be complex. Therefore, clinicians are advised to take a biopsychosocial approach in the assessment of pain to consider a broad array of potential contributing, ameliorating, and comorbid factors related to the presentation of pain complaints (Fig. 9.1) [26]. Behavioral observations, collateral informants, and formalized assessment tools, such as the Opioid Risk Tool (ORT) and the Current Opioid Misuse Measure (COMM) [27–29] or similar instruments [30–32], can help establish baseline characteristics, detect deviations from that baseline, stratify risk, guide treatment planning, and provide a framework for ongoing assessment of pain symptoms and response to treatment.

Pain can be assessed in cognitively intact older adults by using a variety of scales, such as the seven-point faces pain scale (FPS), the visual analogue scale (VAS), and the five-point verbal rating scale (VRS) [33]. However, assessments can be particularly challenging in older adults with neurocognitive disorders. One option is to use the Pain Assessment in Advanced Dementia scale (PAINAD). This uses the observations by a caregiver or provider to assess pain based on the patient's breathing, negative vocalizations, facial expressions, body language, and consolability.

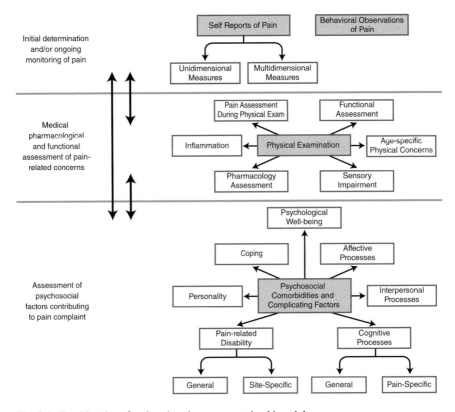

Fig. 9.1 Considerations for chronic pain assessment in older adults

Accurate completion does not depend on the patient's cognitive or language skills. Another option is the Pain Assessment Checklist for Seniors with Limited Ability to Communicate (PACSLAC) [34, 35]. While reduction of pain is an overarching goal, optimization of day-to-day functioning may be a higher priority than a reduced rating on a numerical pain scale [36]. Therefore, assessment of pain in older adults must also evaluate the loss of functioning and independence that has occurred with aging. Some useful metrics include changes in activities of daily living (ADLs) or in instrumental activities of daily living (IADLs), followed by screening tools like the Functional Independence Measure (FIM) and Physical Mobility Scale (PMS) [37].

9.4   Principles for Management of Pain in Older Adults

Clinicians must balance the goals of improving function and quality of life with the overall safety of using pain-treatment medications in the context of polypharmacy and comorbid conditions. Older adults are a heterogeneous group with variable responses to medication dosing and unpredictable manifestations of adverse effects. The following general principles may be useful for working with older adults.

Be realistic, educate, and have a plan. Because most persistent pain sufferers have no clearly identifiable cause to be treated or cured, it is important to help the older adult patient develop realistic expectations for pain management [38]. Even with opioid therapy, a 30 % reduction of pain severity and duration is considered a reasonably feasible analgesic response [39]. Educating the patient, their caregivers, and families about CNCP and the biopsychosocial factors related to pain may help them understand the symptoms and shift their goals from unattainable (e.g., total pain elimination) to feasible (e.g., regain function, increase activity, and participate in the community). The physician and patient should collaborate on a plan for pain management that personalizes goals and empowers the patient with a sense of self-efficacy, increased investment in the outcomes, and improved adherence. Effective implementation of any pain management plan depends on the coordinated efforts of the patient, providers, and in the case of older patients, their family, and caregivers [40, 41].

Assess comprehensively, treat holistically. The physical sensation of pain is but one component of CNCP. Pharmacotherapy alone provides only partial relief. Comprehensive assessment also includes considering how comorbid conditions may influence pain and vice versa. Comorbid conditions increase the odds of being initiated and maintained on chronic opioid therapy exceeding 6 months [42]. Assessment and treatment of older adults on chronic opioid therapy (COT) often must address psychological distress, sedentary lifestyles, social isolation, comorbid substance use, loss of independence [43], higher health-care utilization and a more restrictive level of care [44–47]. Clinicians who recognize these factors are better prepared to offer alternative therapies and nonpharmacological approaches to ameliorate pain and its comorbid conditions.

Start low and go slow, but go. When initiating pharmacotherapy for pain in older adults, starting doses of any drug should be lowered to half or one-third that of the starting doses typical for younger adults. Likewise, titration should proceed more slowly to minimize adverse effects. Some guidelines for using opioids in older adults suggest starting at 2.5–10 mg morphine equivalent dose (MED) four times per day (QID) for immediate-release opioids. Then increase the dose in increments of no more than 2.5–5 mg QID over the span of a week [10, 39]. Even though starting doses are low and increased slowly, the clinician must ensure that the trial of the pain medication is adequate through careful adjustments guided by frequent monitoring of pain response and medication tolerance. Meaningful variations in scores on 11-point pain numeric rating scales have been observed within the span of a month and can be predicted by baseline pain intensity, overall medical comorbidity, and non-partnered status [10, 48].

Timing is everything. The quality, duration, and frequency of pain guide pain management. For severe episodic pain, short-acting, rapid-onset analgesic drugs may be used as needed in those with low risk of abuse. For older adults with cognitive impairment who may not be able to communicate pain symptoms adequately or patients with anticipated pain episodes, medications can be scheduled [10]. In patients with continuous pain, around-the-clock coverage with scheduled dosing or longer-acting analgesic formulations can be considered, in combination with short-acting analgesics for breakthrough pain [10, 39].

Take universal precautions against misuse. Risk for misuse and abuse of analgesic medications, in particular opioids, among older adults without substance abuse history or family/genetic factors of risk are exceedingly low. Additionally, undertreatment with opioids is generally considered an equal if not greater problem than abuse among older adults [10, 39, 49]. However, the risk of misuse or abuse increases with COT that includes opioid-induced hyperalgesia, development of tolerance and physiological dependence, and experiencing symptoms of drug withdrawal [50].

Risk stratification can facilitate decision-making related to initiating analgesics with potential of abuse. This stratification ranges from lowest risk (without any history of substance use or comorbid psychiatric disorders) to those at highest risk (active substance use and major untreated psychiatric disorders). Additionally, active diversion of analgesics by the patient or their family/caregivers also increases risks [51]. Clinicians should recognize signs of addiction, including loss of control over use, preoccupation with obtaining the drug despite adequate analgesia, and continued use despite adverse consequences.

Clinicians can mitigate these risks by employing the universal precaution [52] approach to pain management. Documentation should reflect a comprehensive assessment of pain, psychiatric and addiction history, baseline urine drug screen, prescription database evaluation, informed consent, a pain management contract, clearly defined treatment goals, and monitoring of analgesic response, activity level, adverse effects, and aberrant use behaviors. Referral to a pain specialist is indicated if biopsychosocial factors are too complex for the primary care setting.

Avoid inappropriate prescribing. Inappropriate prescribing occurs when drugs pose more risk than benefit, particularly when good alternatives are available. Selection of appropriate analgesic options should consider the patient's comorbid conditions and potential drug–drug interactions based on a review of his or her medication list. For example, using tricyclic antidepressants (TCA) for neuropathic pain management in older adults is relatively contraindicated in the case of concurrent glaucoma, cardiac conductive abnormalities, history of stroke, or cognitive impairment. Nonsteroidal anti-inflammatory agents (NSAIDs) should not be routinely used in those with risk of GI bleeding, cardiovascular pathology, renal failure, or individuals on chronic steroids or serotonergic agents [26]. Dangerous polypharmacy, e.g., opiates and benzodiazepines, can lead to increased falls and bone fractures, respiratory suppression, and cognitive impairment, but unfortunately are often prescribed concurrently [39, 42, 50]. It is the clinician's responsibility to regularly engage in medication reconciliation to identify and avert inappropriate prescribing.

9.5 Nonpharmacological Approaches to Managing Pain

To address psychological factors involved in the experience of pain, cognitive behavioral therapy (CBT) is the most promising psychological technique to alter dysfunctional thinking about pain and to modify beliefs and attitudes to increase self-efficacy over pain. Small studies using group CBT among nursing home residents show 80 % improvement in chronic pain sustained at a 4-month follow-up vs. 33 % in controls [53]. However, further research is needed to demonstrate generalizability of these findings to community-dwelling older adults. Self-management techniques, including relaxation, meditation, coping strategies, and educational/support groups for chronic pain management, improve self-efficacy but show little long-term effect on pain reduction [54].

Theoretical models propose that acupuncture, massage, relaxation training, and aerobic exercise may activate opioid pathways and alter mu-opioid receptor binding. Theoretically this may enhance response to opioid analgesic medications and reduce the need for higher dosing [55]. Complementary therapies such as acupuncture, transcutaneous/percutaneous electrical nerve stimulation, and massage have shown modest improvement in persistent pain and have an additive effect when used with other modalities [56]. One randomized control trial showed that strengthening, flexibility, and endurance activities increased physical activity and improved function and reduced pain in older adults. Exercise regimens should take into account the individual's level of function, motivation, personalized goals, and availability of supervision.

9.6 Non-opioid Analgesics for Managing Pain in Older Adults

Non-opioid analgesics may be first line in treating mild to moderate pain in carefully selected older patients. Acetaminophen is widely used over the counter and in combination with opioid preparations for additive analgesic effect against osteoarthritis and lower back pain [10]. Acetaminophen is not associated with significant cardiovascular, gastrointestinal, or renal toxicity, although hepatotoxic effects have been observed in patients taking in excess of 3 g a day in older adults. Therefore, acetaminophen treatment requires careful monitoring of total daily dose from all sources. This medication is relatively contraindicated in those with hepatic insufficiency and those actively abusing alcohol [10].

Traditional NSAIDs and selective cyclooxygenase-2 (COX-2) inhibitors are more problematic for older adults because of their multiple, potentially severe adverse effects, including gastrointestinal bleeding and perforation, abnormal bleeding/clotting times, and cardiovascular, renal, and skin toxicities [49]. Contraindications to the use of NSAIDs and COX-2 inhibitors include peptic ulcer disease, *H. Pylori* infection, cardiovascular disease, and concurrent therapy with either corticosteroids or serotonin reuptake inhibitors [10].

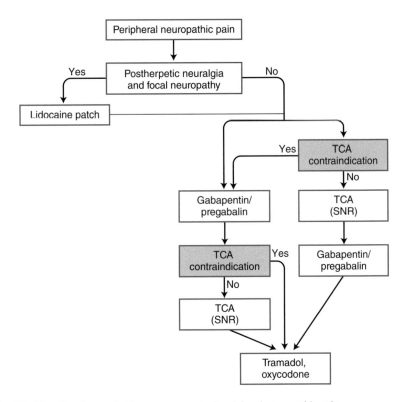

Fig. 9.2 Algorithm for medication management of peripheral neuropathic pain

9.7   Management of Neuropathic Pain in Older Adults

Neuropathic pain results from lesions or disease affecting the somatosensory nervous system and is more common in the older adult than the younger patient population [57]. Neuropathic pain can be classified as central or peripheral neuropathic pain [58], represented by the two different treatment algorithms (Figs. 9.2 and 9.3 [26]).

According to one recent meta-analysis [57], first-line agents for treating neuropathic pain include tricyclic antidepressants, serotonin–norepinephrine reuptake inhibitors, pregabalin, and gabapentin. There is weaker second-line support for the use of lidocaine patches and capsaicin patches and third-line support for tramadol and opioids, weaker in both cases because of significant safety concerns for long-term treatment. The second- and third-line drugs, however, may be used first line if shorter-term immediate relief is being sought [58]. Notably, few of the studies in the meta-analysis were more than 12–24 weeks in duration. Although TCAs can be very effective in treating pain in older adults, they should be used with caution due to increased risk for anticholinergic and cardio-conductive adverse effects in this age group. Anticonvulsants like carbamazepine, lamotrigine, and valproic acid had insufficient evidence to support the use in neuropathic pain among older adults (Table 9.3) [26, 57].

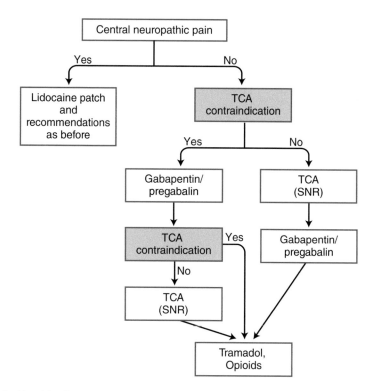

Fig. 9.3 Algorithm for medication management of central neuropathic pain

9.8   Opioid Pain Management in Older Adults

Opioid pain management may generally be used in those who have failed nonpharmacologic treatment and non-opioid analgesics [49], according to the American Geriatrics Society (AGS), American Pain Society (APS), American Academy of Pain Medicine (AAPM), American Society of Interventional Pain Physicians (ASIPP), and National Advisory Panel for the Federation of Medical Regulatory Authorities of Canada. Initiation of opioid analgesic treatment in a carefully monitored and risk-stratified older adult population must have clearly defined therapeutic goals and be part of a multimodal treatment plan with psychosocial and functional rehabilitative therapies as well as close management of comorbid chronic conditions contributing to pain [10].

Opioids are relatively contraindicated in those with significant cognitive impairment, respiratory disorders, or cardio-conduction disorders or in those who live alone and/or have a significant history of substance misuse. Careful and consistent monitoring becomes even more imperative in these situations [39]. Most commonly used opioid analgesics are metabolized through one or more cytochrome P450 systems and are subject to drug–drug interactions, particularly in the older patients on

Table 9.3 Medication management options for neuropathic pain in older adults

	Agents	Initial dose	Dose ranges	Limitations in use
First line: calcium channel alpha2-delta ligands	Gabapentin	100 mg bedtime	1200–3600 mg in three divided doses	Monitor for sedation, ataxia, and edema; adjust dose in renal impairment
	Pregabalin	50 mg bedtime	150–600 mg daily	
Serotonin–norepinephrine reuptake inhibitors	Duloxetine	20 mg daily	20–120 mg daily	Monitor blood pressure and heart rate (esp. venlafaxine), dizziness, cognitive effects, memory, and drug interactions
	Venlafaxine	37.5 mg daily	150–225 mg daily	
Tricyclic antidepressants	Amitriptyline	10 mg bedtime	Max 75–100 mg	Monitor for anticholinergic effects—blurry vision, urinary retention, and GI and cognitive imbalance; consider alternative if existing heart dz
	Nortriptyline			
	Desipramine			
Second line: topical	Capsaicin 8 % patches		1–4 patches to painful area 30–60 min every 3 months	For peripheral neuropathic pain
	Lidocaine topical (5 %)		1–3 patches 12 h/day	Monitor for skin rash
Third line: dual-action or strong opioids	Tramadol	12.5–25 mg	200–400 mg in two (ER) or three divided doses per day every 4–6 h	Monitor for seizures and serotonin syndrome with SSRI
	Strong opioids	Variable	Individual titration	Monitor for drowsiness, respiratory depression, constipation, nausea, and cognitive impairment

polypharmacy. Table 9.4 [10, 59–61] presents a partial listing of commonly used opioid analgesics. Starting doses and equivalent doses are extrapolated from data among younger adults.

Constipation is a common condition in older adults and is worsened by opioid use. Therefore, prophylactic laxative therapy is necessary when opioid pain management is considered. Respiratory depression effects of opioids are further complicated by age-related changes to baseline respiratory function, such as an abnormal ventilatory response to central hypercapnia and hypoxemia. Sleep-disordered breathing can worsen with the addition of opioid therapy. Benzodiazepines should ideally be tapered off prior to initiating opioid therapy in older adults because of the added risk for respiratory depression [42, 62].

Close monitoring for worsening impaired cognitive functioning is warranted whenever opioids are added to the regimen of a patient who already shows some degree of cognitive impairment at baseline. Another serious risk of opioid use is

Table 9.4 Select opioid management options for chronic pain in older adults

Drug	MED (mg/24 h)	Suggested starting dose in older adults	Metabolic pathway/elimination	Active metabolite	Clinical considerations
Codeine	200 mg	7.5–60 mg q4–6 h, NTE 360 mg/24 h	CYP2D6/renal	Morphine	In those with impaired CYP2D6 results in little to no analgesic effect
Tramadol	Not reliably established	12.5–25 mg q4–6 h, NTE 300 mg/day for those >75	CYP2D6 and CYP3A4	O-demethyl tramadol	Parent has higher monoaminergic activity, metabolite has higher mu-receptor affinity; drug interactions via CYP2D6 with potential seizure or serotonin syndrome
Morphine	30 oral	2.5–10 mg q4h(IR) / 15 mg q8–24 h (SR)	Glucuronidation/renal	Morphine-6-glucuronide	Morphine-3-glucuronide is a neurotoxic metabolite
Oxycodone	15–20 oral	2.5–5 mg q4–6 h (IR) / 10 mg q12h (ER)	CYP2D6/renal	Noroxycodone oxymorphone	Both parent and metabolite active, retains analgesic effect irrespective of impairment in CYP2D6
Hydromorphone	4–6 oral	1–2 mg q3–4 h	Glucuroconjugation; significant first-pass metabolism	No	Hydromorphone-3-glucuronide is a metabolite with potential neuroexcitatory effects
Fentanyl	12 µg/h patch	12–25 µg/h patch q72h	CYP3A4	No	Potential drug–drug interactions via CYP3A4
Methadone	Nonlinear dose equivalency	Not recommended as first-line agent	Hepatic N-demethylation to 2-ethylidene-1,5-dimethyl-3,3 diphenylpyrrolidine (EDDP), then CYP3A4 and CYP2D6 to inactive	Limited EDDP	Numerous drug–drug interactions via CYP3A4; highly variable half-life and unpredictable accumulation

balance dysregulation with ambulation, and this risk is amplified when opioids are used with other centrally acting medications. If opioid use is necessary or urgent, it would be prudent to provide supportive interventions such as physical therapy and/ or environmental balance and ambulation aids.

World Health Organization [63] and Canadian guidelines [39] recommend starting with lower potency analgesics, such as codeine or tramadol. Guidelines recommend the starting dose of opioids be one-third to one-half lower than the typical starting dose in younger adults [10]. Short-acting, rapid-onset opioid analgesics, e.g., hydrocodone, oxycodone, and hydromorphone, are preferred to manage severe episodic pain. Patients with continuous pain may be treated with scheduled long-acting formulations such as extended release oxycodone (OxyContin) or sustained release morphine (MScontin). Studies have shown individuals on scheduled long-acting opioids tend to be at higher MEDs overall [64], so clinicians may consider conversion to fentanyl transdermal patch for patients taking 60–100 mg MED per 24 h.

Opioid rotation: Older adults who have an inadequate pain response or had developed tolerance to or adverse effects from their current opioid analgesic may be appropriate for opioid rotation or switching [60].

The initial step when switching agents is to calculate the dose of the new opioid based on an equianalgesic dose table. To account for incomplete cross-tolerance, the new agent's equianalgesic dose from the table should then be decreased by approximately one-third to one-half for older adults or the medically frail [60]. Then the dose can be cautiously titrated by 15–30 % at a time based on pain severity. If only the route of administration of same agent is being modified, reduce the current dose by 25 % initially and then titrate as needed [60, 65]. When possible, avoid using methadone in older adults because it has unpredictable pharmacokinetics. Also, do not directly switch from a weak opioid like codeine to a high-potency opioid like fentanyl as there is an increased risk of overdose [39, 61].

Opioid tapering: Tapering down or off of opioids should be considered when there is increased risk versus benefit over long-term use on high MED. Even individuals with severe pain on high-dose COT experience less pain and improved mood with opioid tapering [39]. Withdrawal symptoms to watch for include anxiety, insomnia, chills, anorexia, muscle cramps, nausea, diarrhea, and elevated heart rate and blood pressure [50]. Providers should also use caution prescribing benzodiazepines or other hypnotic drugs for symptomatic management because of potential drug–drug interactions.

When tapering opioids, prescribe scheduled doses at frequent intervals, and reduce the dose by 5–10 % of the total daily dose every 1–4 weeks. Slower tapers over 3–6 months are recommended for those with anxiety or psychological dependence to mitigate risk of relapse or resumption of opioids [39]. Clinicians may consider switching to longer-acting formulations for the final 20 % of a dose taper due to metabolic and elimination considerations in older adults [39].

9.9 Conclusion

In closing, the assessment and management of CNCP in older patients can be complicated by the effects of aging. Clinicians treating CNCP in older patients need to take into account the effects of aging as they evaluate various aspects of the situation and develop a collaborative plan with realistic and clearly defined goals. Following the principles of pain management in older adults will help the clinician manage the treatment and, when necessary, make thoughtful changes. Keeping the effects of aging in mind when treating CNCP in an older adult will help the clinician minimize unnecessary complications and maximize the effects of treatment.

References

1. Zanocchi M, et al. Chronic pain in a sample of nursing home resident: prevalence, characteristics, influence of quality of life (QoL). Arch Gerontol Geriatr. 2008;47:121–8.
2. López-Lopez A, González JL, et al. Pain and symptoms of depression in older adults living in community and in nursing homes: the role of activity restriction as a potential mediator and moderator. Int Psychogeriatr. 2014;26(10):1679–91.
3. Herr K. Pain assessment strategies in older patients. J Pain. 2011;12(3):S3–13.
4. Monti DA, Kunkel EJS. Management of chronic pain among elderly patients. Psychiatr Serv. 1998;49(12):1537–9.
5. Kozma CM, Provenzano DA, Slaton TL, et al. Complexity of pain management among patients. J Manage Care Spec Pharm. 2014;20(5):455–66.
6. Lapane KL, et al. The association between pain and measures of well-being among nursing home residents. J Am Med Dir Assoc. 2012;13:344–9.
7. Yong HH. Can attitudes of stoicism and cautiousness explain observed age-related variation in levels of self-rated pain, mood disturbance and functional interference in chronic pain patients? Eur J Pain. 2006;10(5):399–407.
8. Turner JA, Ersek M, Kemp C. Self-efficacy for managing pain is associated with disability, depression, and pain coping among retirement community residents with chronic pain. J Pain. 2005;6(7):471–9.
9. Coupland J, Coupland N. "Old age doesn't come alone": discursive representations of health-in-aging in geriatric medicine. Int J Aging Hum Dev. 1994;39:81–95.
10. Ickowicz E, American Geriatric Society Panel on the Pharmacological Management of Persistent Pain in Older Persons, et al. Pharmacological management of persistent pain in older persons. J Am Geriatr Soc. 2009;57:1331–46.
11. Schatzberg A, Cole J, DeBattista C, editors. Pharmacotherapy in special situations manual of clinical psychopharmacology. 7th ed. Washington, DC: APA; 2010. p. 619.
12. Steffens DC, Blazer DG, Thakur ME, editors. Chapter 2: Physiological and clinical considerations of geriatric patient care—considerations in geriatric prescribing. Textbook of geriatric psychiatry. 5th ed. Arlington: APA; 2015.
13. Huang AR, Mallet L, Rochefort CM, Eguale T, Buckeridge DL, Tamblyn R. Medication-related falls in the elderly: causative factors and preventive strategies. Drugs Aging. 2012;29(5):359–76.
14. Chapman IM, MacIntosh CG, Morley JE, Horowitz M. The anorexia of ageing. Biogerontology. 2012;2(1-2):67–71.
15. Schmader K. Postherpetic neuralgia in immunocompetent elderly people. Vaccine. 1998;16(18):1768–70.

16. Schatzberg A, Cole J, DeBattista C, editors. Pharmacotherapy in special situations manual of clinical psychopharmacology. 7th ed. Washington, DC: APA; 2010. p. 635.
17. Koyyalagunta D, Bruera E, Aigner C, Nusrat H, Driver L, Novy D. Risk stratification of opioid misuse among patients with cancer pain using the SOAPP-SF. Pain Med. 2013;14(5):667–75.
18. Inouye SK, Westendorp RG, Saczynski JS. Delirium in elderly people. Lancet. 2014; 383(9920):911–22.
19. Weiner D, Karp J, Bernstein C, Morone N. Pain medicine in older adults: how should it differ? In: Der T, Ray A, Gordin V, et al., editors. Comprehensive treatment of chronic pain by medical, interventional and behavioral approaches. New York: Springer; 2012. p. 977.
20. Brown RT, Zuelsdorff M, Fleming M. Adverse effects and cognitive function among primary care patients taking opioids for chronic nonmalignant pain. J Opioid Manag. 2006;2(3): 137–46.
21. Gu Q, Dillon CF, Burt VL. Prescription drug use continues to increase: U.S. prescription drug data for 2007-2008. CDC. National Center for Health Statistics Data Brief No. 42,. http://www.cdc.gov/nchs/data/databriefs/db42.htm. Accessed March 31, 2015.
22. Maher RL, Hanlon JT, Hajjar ER. Clinical consequences of polypharmacy in elderly. Expert Opin Drug Saf. 2014;13(1):1–9.
23. Marcum ZA, Amuan ME, Hanlon JT, et al. Prevalence of unplanned hospitalizations caused by adverse drug reactions in older Veterans. J Am Geriatr Soc. 2012;60:34–41.
24. Davidoff AJ, Miller GE, Sarpong EM, Yang E, Brandt N, Fick DM. Prevalence of potentially inappropriate medication use in older adults using the 2012 Beers criteria. J Am Geriatr Soc. 2015;63(3):486–500.
25. Frankenthal D, Lerman Y, Kalendaryev E, Lerman Y. Intervention with the screening tool of older persons potentially inappropriate prescriptions/screening tool to alert doctors to right treatment criteria in elderly residents of a chronic geriatric facility: a randomized clinical trial. J Am Geriatr Soc. 2014;62(9):1658–65.
26. Fine PG. Chronic pain management in older adults: special considerations. J Pain Symptom Manage. 2009;38(2 Suppl):S4–14.
27. Meltzer EC, Rybin D, Saitz R, Samet JH, Schwartz SL, Butler SF, et al. Identifying prescription opioid use disorder in primary care: diagnostic characteristics of the Current Opioid Misuse Measure (COMM). Pain. 2011;152(2):397–402.
28. Webster LR, Webster RM. Predicting aberrant behaviors in opioid-treated patients: preliminary validation of the Opioid Risk Tool. Pain Med. 2005;6:432–42.
29. Butler SF, Budman SH, Fernandez KC, et al. Validation of the current opioid misuse measure. Pain. 2007;130:144–5.
30. Jones T, Lookatch S, Grant P, McIntyre J, Moore T. Further validation of an opioid risk assessment tool: the Brief Risk Interview. J Opioid Manag. 2014;10(5):353–64.
31. Moore TM, Jones T, Browder JH, Daffron S, Passik SD. A comparison of common screening methods for predicting aberrant drug-related behavior among patients receiving opioids for chronic pain management. Pain Med. 2009;10(8):1426–33.
32. Chou R, Fanciullo GJ, Fine PG, Miaskowski C, Passik SD, Portenoy RK. Opioids for chronic noncancer pain: prediction and identification of aberrant drug-related behaviors: a review of the evidence for an American Pain Society and American Academy of Pain Medicine clinical practice guideline. J Pain. 2009;10(2):131–46.
33. Pesonen A, Kauppila T, Tarkkila P, Sutela A, Niinisto L, Rosenberg PH. Evaluation of easily applicable pain measurement tools for the assessment of pain in demented patients. Acta Anaesthesiol Scand. 2009;53(5):657–64.
34. Apinis C, Tousignant M, Arcand M, Tousignant-Laflamme Y. Can adding a standardized observational tool to interdisciplinary evaluation enhance the detection of pain in older adults with cognitive impairment? Pain Med. 2014;15(1):32–41.
35. Horgas A, Mille L. Pain assessment in people with dementia. Am J Nurs. 2008;108(7):62–70; quiz 71.
36. Resnick NM, Marcantonio RO. How should clinical care of the aged differ? Lancet. 1997;350:1157.

37. Ozturk A, Simsek TT, Yumin ET, Sertel M, Yumin M. The relationship between physical, functional capacity, and quality of life (QoL) among elderly people with a chronic disease. Arch Gerontol Geriatr. 2011;53(3):278–83.
38. Panel AGS. The management of persistent pain in older persons. J Am Geriatr Soc. 2002;50:S205–24.
39. Kahan M, Mailis-Gagnon A, Wilson L, Srivastava A. Canadian guideline for safe and effective use of opioids for chronic noncancer pain. Clinical summary for family physicians. Part 1: general population. Can Fam Physician. 2011;57:1257–66.
40. Weiner DK. Office management of chronic pain in the elderly. Am J Med. 2007;120:306.
41. Weiner DK, Herr K. Comprehensive assessment and interdisciplinary treatment planning: an integrative overview. In: Weiner DK, Herr K, Rudy T, editors. Persistent pain in older adults: an interdisciplinary guide for treatment. New York: Springer; 2002. p. 18.
42. Dobscha SK, Morasco BJ, Dukart JP, Macey T, Deyo RA. Correlates of prescription opioid initiation and long-term opioid use in veterans with persistent pain. Clin J Pain. 2013; 29(2):102–8.
43. Windmill J, Fisher E, Eccleston C, Derry S, Stannard C, Knaggs R, Moore RA. Interventions for the reduction of prescribed opioid use in chronic non-cancer pain. Cochrane Database Syst Rev. 2013;9:CD010323.
44. Wallace LS, Wexler RK, McDougle L, Miser WF, Haddox JD. Voices that may not otherwise be heard: a qualitative exploration into the perspectives of primary care patients living with chronic pain. J Pain Res. 2014;7:291–9.
45. Benyamen R, Trescot AM, Datta S, Buenaventura R, Adlaka R, Sehgal N, et al. Opioid complications and side effects. Pain Physician. 2008;11(2):S105–20.
46. Kahan M, Wilson L, Mailis-Gagnon A, Srivastava A. Canadian guideline for safe and effective use of opioids for chronic noncancer pain clinical summary for family physicians. Part 2: special populations. Can Fam Physician. 2011;57:1269–76.
47. Deyo RA, Smith DH, Johnson ES, Donovan M, Tillotson CJ, Yang X, Petrik AF, Dobscha SK. Opioids for back pain patients: primary care prescribing patterns and use of services. J Am Board Fam Med. 2011;24(6):717–27.
48. Dobscha SK, Morasco BJ, Kovas AE, Peters DM, Hart K, McFarland BH. Short-term variability in outpatient pain intensity scores in a national sample of older veterans with chronic pain. Pain Med. 2014;16(5):855–65.
49. Gloth III FM. Pharmacological management of persistent pain in older persons: focus on opioids and nonopioids. J Pain. 2011;12(3):S14–20.
50. Miotto K, Kaufman A, Kong A, Jun G, Schwartz J. Managing co-occurring substance use and pain disorders. Psychiatr Clin North Am. 2012;35:393–409.
51. Cheatle M, Comer D, Wunsch M, Skoufasol A, Reddy Y. Treating pain in addicted patients: recommendations from an Expert Panel. Popul Health Manag. 2014;17(2):79–89.
52. Gourlay DL, Heit HA, Almahrezi A. Universal precautions in pain medicine: a rational approach to the treatment of chronic pain. Pain Med. 2005;6(2):107–12.
53. Cook AJ. Cognitive-behavioral pain management for elderly nursing home residents. J Gerontol B Psychol Sci Soc Sci. 1998;53:51–9.
54. Laforest S, Nour K, Gignac M, Gauvin L, Parisien M, Poirier M. Short-term effects of a self-management intervention on health status of housebound older adults with arthritis. J Appl Gerontol. 2008;27:539–67.
55. Bruel S, Apkarian AV, Ballantyne JC, Berger A, Borsook D, et al. Personalized medicine and opioid analgesic prescribing for chronic pain: opportunities and challenges. J Pain. 2013;14(2):103–13.
56. Abdulla A, Adams N, Bone M, Elliott AM, Gaffin J, Jones D, Knaggs R, Martin D, Sampson L, Schofield P, British Geriatric Society. Guidance on the management of pain in older people. Age Ageing. 2013;42:i1–i57.
57. Finnerup NB, Attal N, Haroutounian S, Mcnicol E, Baron R, et al. Pharmacotherapy for neuropathic pain in adults: a systematic review and metaanalysis. Lancet Neurol. 2015;162–73.

58. O'Connor AB, Dworkin RH. Treatment of neuropathic pain: an overview of recent guidelines. Am J Med. 2009;122:S22–32.
59. Huang AR, Mallet L. Prescribing opioids in older people. Maturitas. 2013;74(2):123–9.
60. Vissers KC, Besse K, Hans G, Devulder J, Morlion B. Opioid rotation in the management of chronic pain: where is the evidence? Pain Pract. 2010;10(2):85–93.
61. Knotova H, Fine PG, Protenoy RK. Opioid rotation: the science and the limitations of the equianalgesic dose table. J Pain Symptom Manage. 2009;38:426–39.
62. http://geriatricscareonline.org/toc/american-geriatrics-society-updated-beers-criteria-for-potentially-inappropriate-medication-use-in-older-adults/CL001
63. http://www.who int/cancer/palliative/painladder/en/
64. Von Korff MR. Long-term use of opioids for complex chronic pain. Best Pract Res Clin Rheumatol. 2013;27(5):663–72.
65. Fine PG, Protenoy RK. Establishing"best practices" for opioid rotation, conclusions of an expert panel. J Pain Symptom Manage. 2009;38:418–42.

Chapter 10
What Is Recovery?

Laura C. Moss

The definition of recovery depends on who is being asked. A limited definition could be the absence of illicit substance abuse. Many people in recovery circles call this abstinence rather than recovery. Most people in recovery and professionals that treat substance use disorders feel recovery is much more than just abstinence. People who are no longer using but are still behaving in the same dysfunctional manner they behaved in prior to becoming abstinent are often referred to as being on a "dry drunk." This state of being is thought to be as unpleasant for the individual who is abstinent as it is for the people around him or her. They are often described as being controlling, irritable, and discontent. If an abstinent person does not develop a new outlook about life, learn new coping skills, gain additional recovery supports, or utilize new behaviors, life can become very challenging. They are likely to return to substance abuse because life without their drug of choice can be miserable for them.

Another definition of recovery is a return to one's normal state of health, mind, or strength. I think anyone in recovery would say that a return to "normal" or one's previous pre-addicted state or function may not be possible. It is not unusual to hear people in 12-step recovery circles (Alcoholics Anonymous, Narcotics Anonymous, etc.) say, "once an addict always an addict." This statement simply summarizes a belief that something profound has happened to an addicted brain that makes it impossible to return to the previous recreational use without rapid loss of control and negative consequences. Another common concern by those in recovery is what is normal? The changes that occur in peoples' lives after addiction takes hold are often so life-changing that people in recovery cannot imagine a life without drugs or alcohol and at the same time cannot consider a life with alcohol and drugs. Another definition of recovery is the action or process of regaining control or

L.C. Moss, M.D. (✉)
Hazelden Springbrook, Part of the Hazelden Betty Ford Foundation,
1901 Esther Street, Newberg, OR 97132, USA
e-mail: lmoss@hazeldenbettyford.org

© Springer International Publishing Switzerland 2016
A.M. Matthews, J.C. Fellers (eds.), *Treating Comorbid Opioid Use Disorder in Chronic Pain*, DOI 10.1007/978-3-319-29863-4_10

possession of something that was lost or stolen. People in early recovery often experience grief about multiple losses- lives, time, ambitions, and innocence. There is often accompanying shame and guilt about the behaviors and events that occurred while using. In order to recover from substance abuse, one must abstain from a drug of choice and change how one approaches life. Some call this a spiritual change.

The Substance Abuse and Mental Health Services Administration's (SAMHSA) working definition of recovery: "Recovery is a process of change whereby individuals work to improve their own health and wellness and to live a meaningful life in a community of their choice while striving to achieve their full potential." SAMHSA describes four major dimensions that support a life with recovery—health, home, community, and purposeful life. Health is found by abstaining from use of alcohol, illicit drugs, and non-prescribed medications and making informed, healthy choices that support physical and emotional well-being. Home is a safe place to live. Community is having a social network and relationships that provide support, friendship, love, and hope. A purposeful life is a life that has meaningful daily activities such as work, school, volunteering, caring for family or creative endeavors, as well as independence, income, and resources that allow participation in society. SAMHSA also describes ten principles that support recovery. The principles include providing hope, individualizing options, being aware there are many pathways to recovery, remaining holistic, providing peer-support, keeping the process relational, being aware of culture, addressing trauma, creating treatment plans that capitalize on individual strengths, and maintaining respect.

Theories about change speak of it as a process where one has to first have awareness there is a problem and then becoming willing to change. Primary healthcare providers can play a pivotal role in moving patients towards change by providing kind, nonjudgmental feedback about health concerns associated with aberrant use of substances. Primary care providers may not see change in that moment of feedback, but once informed, a patient can never completely return to their previous naivety or denial about their substance use. Once an individual is interested in change, there is a golden opportunity to intervene. Reducing barriers to treatment and providing recovery supports allows people to move into action. In addition to reducing barriers for recovery, promoting hope is one of the key elements that often moves people from the contemplation stage of change into action. Many people in recovery have tried to quit using drugs or alcohol in the past, often multiple times, before they succeed. Remember that no one starts out using substances with a desire to become addicted. People often stop trying to quit using because they lose hope that they can recover. A few encouraging words from loved ones or from a provider can make the difference in motivating a person to try again. For example, "I know you have tried to quit using in the past and not succeeded. It often takes people multiple times before they succeed. We can learn from our relapses and I believe you can do this." Maintaining hope for change and a better future can be the catalyst for change.

Self-determination and self-direction are the foundations for recovery. If providers and loved ones allow individuals to define their own goals and processes for achieving those goals, we empower individuals. Our role is to provide information, resources, and help individuals find their own paths to recovery. This does not mean we do not encourage change. There is evidence that even brief interventions by physicians who endorse concern for a patient offer an opportunity to talk, and then discussing possible options for solutions can lead to contemplation about change or can even be a catalyst for change. It can be very helpful to sit with a patient and explain what you have noticed in a non-judgmental manner. For example, "Jim I have noticed that you seem to be using greater quantities of pain medication and your pain does not seem to be improving. I also notice that you seem anxious and that you report you are struggling at work. I am worried about you." If the patient is also concerned, you have an opening to ask if you can provide them with some suggestions and/or resources. Give the patient time to respond and share their thoughts. Ask permission if you can share some of the things you have learned about pain management or whatever topic you are discussing and ask how you can be helpful. Look for common goals. Ask if the patient has ideas and provide suggestions for additional options if the patient seems to be struggling. Ask what the patient would like to do and try to support the likelihood that the patient will take action by asking what barriers might interfere with achieving the goal. See what the patient will commit to doing and make a plan [1, 2]. It will be helpful if you explore what the local resources are and try to develop a network of recovery supports for assisting your patients.

People can find recovery in many ways, so having a basic understanding of local recovery support options will be very helpful. There are many pathways to recovery and people stop using drugs or alcohol in many different ways. Some people just stop using without treatment or recovery support groups like Alcoholics Anonymous (AA), Narcotics Anonymous (NA), Rational Recovery, Smart Recovery, Celebrate Recovery, etc. This is sometimes called Natural Recovery. These folks may never come to a medical provider's attention. If an individual seeks out additional support, the type of support to select depends on the individual's preference, the severity of the addiction, whether there are co-occurring medical/psychiatric issues, and whether the individual has succeeded with a previous level of support. Not everyone needs treatment, but formalized substance abuse treatment may be helpful for patients who have not been able to maintain abstinence using lower levels of intervention, for patients whose substance use is associated with medical comorbidity, or when withdrawal is complex or life-threatening. Substance use disorder treatment can be used to interrupt use in a more supportive environment than the individual has at home and also creates some distance from relapse triggers (people, places, and things associated with use). There are varying intensities of treatment from outpatient to residential to therapeutic communities where a person can live long term while doing treatment and working on their recovery.

Some patients find recovery with the use of 12-step programs, such as Alcoholics Anonymous (AA) and Narcotics Anonymous (NA). Attendance in AA and NA is free with the only requirement being a desire to stop using. There is a donation basket that gets passed around towards the end of 12-step meetings, but it is a voluntary donation of $1 or 2 if the individual is able. The 12-step support groups are available in most communities and sometimes available online. The 12-step support groups advocate for abstinence, not using one's drug of choice and not using any other intoxicating substances, even if not a drug of choice. It is not unusual for people to switch abuse of one substance to another in an effort to change how they feel or alter their consciousness. Use of any intoxicant, which may work through the brain's reward system, can trigger cravings for one's drug of choice. Finally, intoxication reduces one's inhibitions and could increase the risk of impulsive relapse to a drug of choice.

The 12-step programs started with Alcoholics Anonymous (AA) and the 12 steps of AA have been applied to multiple different types of addictions and compulsive behaviors, for example Narcotics Anonymous. Some opioid-dependent folks feel that NA is more welcoming to them or they feel more comfortable in NA than AA. Anyone who starts attending 12-step programs will want to attend many meetings and find one meeting that they can commit to attending on a weekly basis, one's "Home Group." A Home Group provides a supportive community and also provides some accountability around showing up for support and to support others. The 12-step attendee will also want to find a sponsor, a person with a long period of recovery, who is knowledgeable about the 12 steps, has completed the 12-step work themselves, and can guide the attendee through the program. The 12 steps allow the recovering person to review the chaos associated with their use and recognize their powerlessness over their drug of choice when they continue to use. People can share their story with a sponsor or other spiritual advisor, which reduces shame. Additionally, making amends or apologizing to others reduces shame and creates accountability. Continued participation in a recovery lifestyle allows the recovering individual to carry the message of hope to others who still suffer.

People who are seeking abstinence or recovery sometimes take offense to the word "God" in much of the 12-step literature. It is important to realize that the word "God" is another word for one's "Higher Power", something greater than oneself that will help one to accomplish the goal of recovery even if unsuccessful in the past. A Higher Power can be anything that is meaningful to the individual, nature, their NA group, etc. Below are the 12 steps of NA and "HOW" it works is by going to meetings, working the steps, and having "Honesty, Open Mindedness and Willingness [3]."

1. We admitted that we were powerless over our addiction, that our lives had become unmanageable.
2. We came to believe that a Power greater than ourselves could restore us to sanity.
3. We made a decision to turn our will and our lives over to the care of God as we understood Him.
4. We made a searching and fearless moral inventory of ourselves.
5. We admitted to God, to ourselves, and to another human being the exact nature of our wrongs.
6. We were entirely ready to have God remove all these defects of character.
7. We humbly asked Him to remove our shortcomings.
8. We made a list of all persons we had harmed, and became willing to make amends to them all.

9. We made direct amends to such people wherever possible, except when to do so would injure them or others.
10. We continued to take personal inventory and when we were wrong promptly admitted it.
11. We sought through prayer and meditation to improve our conscious contact with God as we understood Him, praying only for knowledge of His will for us and the power to carry that out.
12. Having had a spiritual awakening as the result of these steps, we tried to carry this message to addicts, and to practice these principles in all our affairs.

Additional non-12-step supports include Celebrate Recovery®, Rational Recovery®, Smart Recovery®, as well as other programs. Celebrate Recovery® appears to be one of the more popular group recovery support options after the 12-step groups. It is a Christ-based ministry that was established at Saddleback Church. Celebrate Recovery® utilizes facilitated groups that exclusively follow the Celebrate Recovery® curriculum and the Bible. The curriculum includes a Leader's Guide, four Participant Guides, and the Celebrate Recovery Journal. There are five small group guidelines that are utilized every meeting. Celebrate Recovery® groups can be complimentary to 12-step group attendance (Table 10.1).

Rational Recovery is a program that was developed by Jack Trimpey that utilizes AVRT®, Addictive Voice Recognition Technique®. AVRT® is a thinking skill based upon the experiences of people who have independently recovered from addiction. The essential beliefs associated with Rational Recovery include: It is solely up to the individual to decide if they are an addict and we are not powerless over our body or instincts. We all possess a moral conscience with the ability to choose right from wrong. When an individual becomes addicted, they are allowing the animal or instinctual body to run the show. Addiction is a voluntary behavior that persists against one's own better judgment. Addiction interferes with our connection to our moral conscience. The individual is free to choose between using or not. The addictive voice in one's head is any thinking that supports or suggests the future use of substances. The addictive voice is always wrong, immoral, and individuals can separate the voice from themselves. Twelve-step programs are believed to undermine the individual's identity and independence. Through logging onto the Rational Recovery Website, one can review the Declaration of Personal Independence, learn about the essentials of AVRT®, and have access to more in-depth information by purchasing additional educational materials. The program is abstinence-based and the Rational Recovery literature states that it is not compatible with other recovery-based programs.

SMART Recovery is an offshoot of Rational Recovery. It is a self-empowerment recovery support organization. The SMART Recovery 4-Point Program® endorses that it helps people recover from all sorts of addictive substances and behaviors by focusing on four areas. The first area is building and maintaining motivation. The second area is coping with urges to use. The third area is managing one's thoughts, feelings, and behaviors and the fourth area is living a balanced life. Their approach is to teach self-empowerment, self-reliance, and self-directed change to facilitate

Table 10.1 Community recovery supports

	Cost	Philosophy approach	Face to face meetings	Web-based meetings	Literature	Compatible with other programs
12 Step AA/NA	Meetings free ($1–2 donation if able)	Spiritual	Yes	Yes	Books and online	Yes
	Books low cost	Powerless over addiction and reliance on higher power (Group, Nature, Spirit, God, etc.)				
Rational Recovery	Cost for online materials training	Cognitive (thinking) (AVRT®) addictive voice	No	Yes	online	No
		Recognition to change behaviors. Addiction is voluntary animal instincts driving behavior				
Smart Recovery	Meetings free	Cognitive/behavioral (offshoot of rational recovery)	Yes	Yes	Online	Yes
	Cost for advanced online training	Self-empowerment, skills-based, recovery support organization				
Celebrate Recovery	Depends on church	Christian-based Ministry group support	Yes	No	Books	Yes

recovery from addiction and promote satisfying lives. They offer face-to-face and online meetings. They support scientifically informed use of psychological treatments and use of legally prescribed psychiatric medications and medication-assisted treatment (MAT). The SMART Recovery Website has free meeting facilitator manuals and offers facilitator training sessions.

Recovery is a process that unfolds over time in stages and looks different in different stages. Early recovery or abstinence is a tenuous time. The brain of an addicted individual has experienced neuroadaptation. Psychoactive drugs and alcohol cause exocytosis or block reuptake of neurotransmitters in the brain resulting in unusually high levels of these euphorigenic chemicals. The brain cells, in an effort to find homeostasis, reduce production of the neurotransmitters or downregulate receptors for the neurotransmitters. With continued abuse, there are long-term physiologic changes that occur at a nuclear and protein transcription level. Over time, addicts often use their drug of choice to feel normal because, if not using, they experience dysphoria due to the brain being out of its new baseline state [4]. Early abstinence or recovery is a time where individuals often experience a state of physiologic withdrawal and intense cravings to use in order to correct the dysphoric state. People withdrawing from opioids often return to use because the withdrawal is so uncomfortable. There are well-documented medication treatment options that can provide some comfort and reduce the suffering associated with opioid withdrawal, such as clonidine [5]. Once the acute withdrawal is complete, there is often a period of time where the person is not having severe withdrawal symptoms, but they continue to experience dysphoria and milder protracted symptoms such as depressed mood, irritability, anxiety, and insomnia. This is often called PAWS, post-acute withdrawal symptoms. Cravings, a strong desire or fantasies about using, for opioids may continue during this period of protracted withdrawal and the risk of relapse can remain high without a lot of individual motivation and support.

Medication-assisted therapy (MAT) utilizes medications that support ongoing abstinence from use of the drug of choice. Options for opioid-dependent patients include the mu opioid receptor antagonists, Naltrexone and Vivitrol®, a mu opioid agonist called methadone, and several partial mu opioid agonists buprenorphine hydrochloride (Subutex) and buprenorphine hydrochloride with naloxone hydrochloride (Suboxone®). There is debate among the public, some medical providers, and even within recovery communities about whether using MAT is really being in recovery from opioids. If patients are not abusing their drug of choice, are engaged in meaningful activities, are not engaged in criminal behavior, and are reconnecting with family or community while on MAT, I would argue that this is indeed recovery. Would one say that a patient who was previously in diabetic ketoacidosis and now compliant with their insulin with stable blood sugars is not in recovery?

Please notice that the key concept is recovery, not cure. What about the previously depressed and suicidal patient who is now euthymic on antidepressants? The morbidity and mortality rates associated with opioid abuse or dependence are staggering. The risk of relapse is highest during the first 12–18 months. Use of MAT may help with reducing the risk of relapse, accidental overdose, and death.

It can be challenging for a person who is using MAT to find AA or NA meetings that support the use of medications, especially buprenorphine or methadone. The belief can be that using a medication means you are still active in your addiction or not in recovery, especially if using the opioid substitution options, methadone or buprenorphine. It will be helpful if providers who utilize medication-assisted therapies have some ideas about which meetings are more supportive of MAT by asking their colleagues or their patients. It is also important to alert their patients about where to find friendlier meetings. One can also advise patients that the use of MAT is part of their medical care and a topic that is part of their personal medical record to be discussed with their physicians. Of note, some opioid-dependent people in recovery find NA to be more supportive and more welcoming than AA meetings to opioid addicts.

Early recovery often is associated with a lot of dysphoria related to altered brain chemistry and multiple loses. The recovering individual needs to find new friends, new activities, and a new way of life. Triggers from the sights, sounds, smells, and emotions associated with the previous drug using lifestyle can worsen cravings and add to the dysphoria. Many opioid-addicted individuals have lost friends due to overdose or through being rejected by previous friends or family due to their substance use. Often times, there is excitement and danger associated with use of illicit substances, so early recovery can seem rather dull. The early period of opioid recovery can be associated with depressed mood, anxiety, hopelessness, and even suicide ideation. It is important to provide mental health support, which could include therapy and medication. Formalized treatment and 12-step or other recovery support groups can provide community support and reduce isolation during the difficult times. Individual or group treatment also helps to provide new coping skills for dealing with life issues previously managed by drinking and using drugs.

Over time, the brain chemistry stabilizes and the emotional ups and downs become less intense. The recovering individual starts to gain confidence in their ability to negotiate the challenges of life without using alcohol or drugs. Hopefully, they have found a recovery community to spend time with for socialization and support. They start to look at their life and think about goals that they may have previously given up on, like finishing school or finding a career. They start to find a new meaning in life and are able to see the benefits of recovery. For many in recovery, estranged relationships with loved ones start to be repaired and new relationships develop. The recovering individual once again feels that others can rely on them and that they are contributing to the greater good. They may want to share their strength and hope in recovery with others or give back to their community. This can also be a vulnerable time for overconfidence and denial about the severity of their addictive illness can reappear. Some people in recovery relapse when things are going well or when they achieve a recovery milestone like 1 year clean and sober. It is important that healthcare providers continue to check in with their patients in recovery about how things are going to cheer the successes and support the more difficult times.

Recovery is a process, not a final destination, and the journey may be bumpy at times. We all tend to be hardest on ourselves and this is true for people trying to get clean and sober. Letting someone know that a relapse or a lapse is an opportunity, not a failure, can provide encouragement to try again. It often takes people multiple tries before they succeed in any new skill and this includes recovery. Relapses can provide information about previously unrealized risk factors and what additional support might be needed. Ask your patients how things are going for them with regard to their recovery goals. If reducing their use or abstinent, ask them how it feels to not be using their drug of choice and are they having any cravings to use. Cravings can be brief thoughts about using, wishful longing to use, fantasies about using, or even dreams about using. If they are having cravings, ask about how they are managing their cravings. Several options include changing your thoughts, purposefully stop thinking about drugs and think about something else, or following the thought through to the negative consequences that using the drug will bring. Sometimes cravings can lead to relapse. It may be helpful to increase recovery support and consider using MAT options discussed earlier.

As a professional working with patients who are seeking recovery from substance use disorders, one might ask what can I ask or say that might be helpful. Ask your patients or clients about their hopes or goals and what things get in the way of reaching those goals. Help your patients to break goals down into smaller, easier to attain goals so they can experience success. Ask your patients about how they are filling their time. Have they have discovered any new hobbies or do they have new goals for the future. Ask your patients where they get their support for recovery. Ask what meetings they have attended and whether they were helpful. There are many types of recovery meetings and supports, so if one meeting or support does not work, please try another. If they are attending 12-step meetings do they have a sponsor, a "home group," and what step are they working on? Inquire how their relationships have been going with friends and family and whether loved ones have noticed any changes. You can point out any positive changes that you are seeing. Ask whether their significant other is attending Al-Anon meetings. Al-Anon meetings can provide group support to loved ones, who may also be struggling by promoting self-care and limit setting with love. Family members who are getting their own support are better able to give their recovering loved ones space to work on their recovery. The recovering person can sometimes feel as if they are under the microscope when their loved ones are overly involved. Loved ones often lose themselves due to trying to protect or fix the addict. Al-Anon helps loved ones to focus on their own needs and feelings. These questions will provide an opportunity for exploration about goals, vulnerabilities, strengths, and successes. Depending on how your patient replies provide them with praise for the gains they have made, encouragement for future goals, and ask how you can support their recovery.

In summary, recovery is more than just abstinence. It is a process that unfolds with physical, psychological, psychosocial, and often spiritual changes for the individual. For many people seeking recovery, it is most easily supported when the individual is part of a recovering community. Behaviors associated with recovery are abstinence, getting to know oneself, finding passions in life again, reconnecting with one's values, and reintegrating into a community. People who are living a life suggestive of recovery are honest with themselves and others. They want to live a life that makes a difference and contributes to their communities. They want to be a person that others can rely on. They can enjoy life without drugs or alcohol. A common saying in recovery circles is, "My worst day in recovery is better than my best day using." Healthcare providers can play a large role in supporting patients' efforts towards finding recovery. Support and celebrate your patients' movements towards change. Continue to support progress even if variable. Most of all, never give up hope, because change is always possible.

References

1. Miller W, Rose G. Toward a theory of motivational interviewing. Am Psychol. 2009;64(6):527–37.
2. Rolnick S, et al. Negotiating behavior change in medical settings: the development of brief motivational interviewing. J Ment Health. 1992;1:25–37.
3. Reprinted by Permission of NA World Services, Inc. All rights reserved. The Twelve Steps of NA reprinted for adaptation by permission of AA World Services, Inc.
4. Jordi C, Farre M. Mechanisms of disease: drug addiction. N Engl J Med. 2003;349(10):975–86.
5. Kosten T, George T. The neurobiology of opioid dependence: implications for treatment. Sci Pract Perspect. 2002;1(1):13–20.

Part II
Ethical, Legal, Regulatory, and Policy Issues

Chapter 11
Commonly Used Interventions Intended to Limit Diversion and Abuse in Patients Receiving Opioid Therapy for Chronic Pain: Clinical Utility and Empirical Support

Steven D. Passik, Alicia Trigeiro, Kenneth L. Kirsh, and Stuart Gitlow

Whether a person has an obsessive or hysterical personality both are highly likely to stop their cars at a red light.

—Walter Mischel (1973)

11.1 Introduction

In a volume such as this one, devoted to those who have pain and comorbid addiction and dependence, it might be easy to view problems with adherence in opioid pain therapy as inevitable. There is a pervasive societal view inherent in the War on Drugs and in the scheduling of controlled substances maintaining that certain medications are inherently addictive and therefore almost anyone exposed to them will be vulnerable to loss of control and to engaging in a range of aberrant behaviors [1]. While we know this isn't the case over the population as a whole, that millions of Americans with chronic pain take these medications without developing problems of addiction

S.D. Passik, Ph.D.
Clinical Research and Advocacy, 16981 Via Tazon, San Diego, CA 92127, USA
e-mail: steven.passik@millenniumhealth.com

A. Trigeiro, M.S. (✉)
Millennium Health, 16981 Via Tazon, San Diego, CA 92127, USA
e-mail: Alicia.Trigeiro@millenniumhealth.com

K.L. Kirsh, Ph.D.
Clinical Research and Advocacy, 16981 Via Tazon, San Diego, CA 92127, USA

Clinical Affairs, Millennium Health, San Diego, CA 92127, USA
e-mail: Kenneth.kirsh@millenniumhealth.com

S. Gitlow, M.D., M.P.H., M.B.A.
Annenberg Physician Training Program in Addictive Disease,
153 Gaskill Street, Woonsocket, RI 02895, USA
e-mail: drgitlow@aol.com

© Springer International Publishing Switzerland 2016
A.M. Matthews, J.C. Fellers (eds.), *Treating Comorbid Opioid Use Disorder in Chronic Pain*, DOI 10.1007/978-3-319-29863-4_11

and/or abuse, when the focus is mainly the highest risk group one might think that all opioid pain treatment in such people is destined for disaster, but data is lacking to back up this assertion [2]. It is as if these drugs have a personality based upon their abuse liability; we all know that a major determinant of behavior is personality. But what if it isn't? What if Walter Mischel was right and regardless of personality variables, situational determinants are as likely or more likely to drive behavior. If that were the case, how to treat pain in a person at high risk of addiction or a person with a known history of addiction that develops into a serious painful illness and severe pain would become a question of creating the right situational conditions to help that person use their medications responsibly rather than keeping these medication options away from them entirely.

We know that it takes three factors to create addiction—an exposure to a potentially addictive substrate in a vulnerable person at a vulnerable time [3]. All people with chronic pain slated for an opioid trial are about to or have had such an exposure. And almost all of these people are at a vulnerable time; many will have had pain for months, will have started to withdraw from pleasurable activities, will have developed some measure of depression, and will have encountered financial and familial stressors related to their inability to function or work up to their baseline. Additionally, if we are evaluating the highest risk group of vulnerable patients, then we have also determined by their personal or family history of addiction, their comorbid psychiatric problems, their young age or their histories of trauma, that they are at high risk to loss of control, diversion, overuse, and abuse in being exposed to these agents.

One might be tempted to say that the way to manage pain in such people at high risk is to avoid the exposure entirely [4]. In certain pain syndromes in which opioids are proven to be or are viewed as ineffective or less effective than other interventions, this approach might be plausible in some patients at some points in their care. For example, if a person develops intractable migraines, a pain syndrome in which there is a community consensus that opioids are less effective than alternatives such as tryptans and that they may also be linked to rebound phenomena, then chronic opioids are low on the decision tree when thinking through potential treatments [5]. But if the patient in question also has a high risk of abuse or dependence, then opioids might fall off the decision tree entirely. But what if the patient has severe pain secondary to a disorder in which the literature supports opioid use and moreover has gone through many "safer" alternatives without benefit (safer is relative here; safer perhaps with regard to abuse potential though other medications might not be safer with regard to their potential for causing renal dysfunction, for example). What is the most humane thing to do if the high-risk person has severe pain from cancer or other life-limiting disease?

Rather than avoiding an exposure, the key questions become not whether opioids are to be used but which ones, how, and with what safeguards [6]. A discussion of which opioids might or might not be safer in this subgroup of patients is beyond the purview of this chapter. Sophisticated addiction practitioners might guess that set scheduling— rather than ad lib dosing—with long-acting medications (in abuse-deterrent formulations where possible) might be most reasonable, borrowing as it does from strategies used in medication-assisted addiction treatments such as methadone maintenance. In this chapter, we will discuss the commonly used behavioral and situational safeguards—or red lights to extend the Mischel metaphor—how they are applied clinically and, where applicable, supply what is known from empirical studies of such approaches.

11.2 Studies Combining Multiple Safeguards: Complex Interventions for a Complex Group of Patients

As one might imagine, clinically useful tools and safeguards have rarely been studied in isolation. More typically, investigators have conducted small, exploratory studies of programmatic interventions; often non-randomized and in the vein of demonstration projects. We will begin with a description of these and a brief discussion about why they might not have had as profound an impact on the standard of care as one might believe they deserve to have had. Despite this disappointment, the early success of such programs in limiting and containing aberrant drug-related behavior offers a glimmer of hope and a step towards eliminating the therapeutic nihilism many practitioners fall victim to when contemplating the management of pain in people with comorbid drug abuse.

In a 2010 study, Jamison and colleagues demonstrated that a complex intervention including education, monitoring (patient reported diaries of drug use, monthly urine drug testing), cognitive behavioral substance counseling both individually and in group formats led to a vast reduction in aberrant behaviors in a high-risk group of pain patients on opioid therapy as compared to a usual care high-risk group [7]. Additionally, they demonstrated that problematic use in the experimental group of patients was only as likely as in a low-risk control group. The histrionic personalities became similar to the obsessive personalities when the situational determinants were brought in line.

One might well ask why did this study virtually disappear into the literature and not have the type of impact a finding like this might ought to have had on the standard of care. For the past several years, the firestorm around opioids has continued to rage about whether they should be used at all, whether they work, or whether they have inherent risks that cannot be controlled outweighing any benefits likely to accrue from their use, when the dialogue might well have been refocused on what will it take to export interventions like this one to the healthcare system, teach them to prescribers (along with screening skills that are used to triage patients and guide the assignment of people into risk groups), and then reimburse/pay for them [8]? In truth, the Jamison study was funded by an R21 grant from the National Institute on Drug Abuse, a mechanism meant for developing and piloting interventions over a 2-year period on minimal budgets and the study included only 62 people (he did receive additional, though limited, funding from pharmaceutical companies) (Jamison, personal communication). There is no doubt that the intervention might have been in need of further study, refinement, and particularly to undergo a process in which its most potent components could be identified such that a more streamlined, cheaper, and more easily exportable product might have resulted. There also is little doubt that the intervention was labor-intensive and would have been expensive to export in its original form; and there was no data provided quantifying cost offsets that might have resulted from such an intervention and its potential to save the healthcare system vast amounts of money in myriad ways by limiting the overuse and abuse of opioids by pain patients which is now widely recognized as an amazingly costly expense.

Two other small studies have demonstrated similar results—a containment of aberrant behavior and/or drug misuse in people with pain and addiction or recent nonadherence by combining recovery support (frequent visits, limited supplies of medications) with accountability (opioid agreements, urine drug testing, pill counts) and psycho-education or psychotherapy. Wiedemer and Gallagher [9, 10] offered nonadherent veterans with problematic behavior in primary care-based opioid pain treatment a "second chance" with such a program showing a sharp increase in patients able to receive treatment uneventfully without further adherence issues with their opioids (and also, unfortunately a high rate of "self-discharge" with those unwilling to jump through hoops ostensibly seeking treatment in less restrictive settings even at their own peril). This particular result exemplifies why addressing drug abuse in pain management must be a community effort such that it is not so easy for people to ignore recommendations and seek refuge in practices unable or unwilling to apply the special safeguards needed. Bethea and colleagues [11] have similarly demonstrated that patients with recent histories of opioid abuse and chronic pain when treated with methadone-based regimens, accountability (urine drug testing), and an extensive menu of psychotherapies can not only avoid further opioid abuse, but even display trends toward less street drug use. Interestingly, the best predictor of a good response to this program was noted to be ratings of the therapeutic alliance made by the patients following therapy sessions. This observation begs the question of how the pain and addiction practitioner is to acquire the skills needed to administer treatment programs involving restrictions and safeguards that could be viewed negatively by patients if not introduced in an empathic fashion so as not to undermine the patient's ability to trust that the practitioner has their best interests at heart.

These studies inspire hope that the needs of this complex subgroup within the population of those with chronic pain might be able to be safely treated with opioids under the right conditions. It must be remembered though that the vast majority of opioid prescribing for chronic pain is done in overly taxed and busy treatment settings. One study suggested that, for example, primary care doctors use screening tools and perform risk assessments, even in high-risk patients, at a much lower rate than experts [12]. Primary care doctors are under pressure to see patients for short visits and cannot easily see patients with more frequent visits than once per month. While 8.8 million Americans are presently taking opioids for chronic pain, 5.5 million of them are being prescribed short-acting hydrocodone [13, 14]. If opioid therapy was being delivered in an individualized fashion, would greater than 60 % of patients be prescribed the same drug in the same low-risk model? Many have advocated for triaging patients into three levels of risk: low, medium and high [15]. Only the lowest risk patients (no history of addiction, no family history of addiction, no current psychiatric problems, older age) were ever intended for this once per month, minimally monitored, drug-only brand of opioid therapy; yet, there are indications that this is the predominant mode of delivering opioid therapy, driven largely by the reimbursement system. The system does not support payment for more expensive, potentially safer long-acting drugs, balks at more frequent visits, insist on charging co-pays for each prescription even if the prescriber doesn't feel the patient can safely manage a month's supply of medication, and won't pay for the psychological and rehabilitative treatments that patients require. There is even a recent trend balking at the cost of monitoring patients with urine drug testing at the recommended frequency suggested by expert consensus. The reimbursement system is a major impediment in this situation, though rarely given its share of the blame for the current state of affairs [8].

The expansion of opioid prescribing, occurring as it did within a healthcare system that struggles to come to terms with chronic medical problems, has only highlighted what our system is bad at managing. Our healthcare system does a bad job when illnesses require complex and ongoing risk assessment, psychological support, and communication among a multidisciplinary team of providers, with continuous monitoring and time. When the illness also occurs in situations in which patients are less likely to deal with us in good faith (whether out of embarrassment or fear that they will be denied access to care, or as a behavioral component of addictive illness), poor outcomes are to be expected. Opioids served to highlight this in chronic pain treatment. The only way forward is through advocacy for the kind of individualized pain care that patients deserve.

11.3 Specific Clinical Safeguards

11.3.1 Role of Urine Drug Testing in Medication Monitoring of Patients with chronic pain

Monitoring the medications of patients receiving opioid therapy for pain should be expected as part of therapy. UDT is a useful tool for the evaluation of patient adherence and urine drug testing (UDT) results provide objective data related to all aspects of adherence at a given point in time (the patient is taking their prescribed opioid medication; is not taking any other nonprescribed licit opioid medications; and is not using illicit drugs). The monitoring is comparable to checking for the effects of medication to regulate diabetes, cardiovascular irregularities, and other chronic medical conditions [16]. High-risk patients are occasionally untruthful about their drug use and behavioral monitoring by clinicians is of limited value in helping to identify the patients who misuse or abuse drugs. One study demonstrated that urine drug testing in patients who had undergone clinical assessment by experts in which it was determined that the patient had no problematic behavior nevertheless found unexpected results 20 % of the time [17].

Several studies have shown that drug testing in pain management may improve patient adherence [12, 18, 19]. Drug testing is also recommended in several clinical guidelines, including those of the American Pain Society, the American Academy of Pain Medicine, the American Society of Interventional Pain Physicians, and the Federation of State Medical Boards, among others [20–24]. Despite the evidence that urine drug monitoring improves patient adherence, it is still underutilized in pain management. A study involving a large primary care system discovered that 8 % of patients with chronic opioid therapy and only 24 % of highest risk group had undergone urine drug monitoring [8]. Physicians who routinely use urine drug testing are all too often not proficient in interpreting the results [25].

The frequency of urine drug testing for patients with chronic opioid therapy should be based on each patient's risk level. Guidelines generally recommend quarterly testing for so-called "standard risk" patients with more frequent testing used randomly as needed for higher risk patients or when there have been sentinel events (i.e., it is not uncommon to see aberrant behavior surface after many months of adherence in the setting of stressful life events). Low-risk patients (generally older patients without histories of addiction and with minimal comorbid psychiatric problems and often long periods of adherent opioid use) can be tested even less frequently according to guidelines at once or twice per year.

There are two main testing methodologies that can be used in UDT, immunoassay (IA) and gas chromatography mass spectrometry or liquid chromatography tandem mass spectrometry (GC-MS or LC-MS/MS). Immunoassay tests, also called presumptive tests, are primarily used for on-site testing as screening tools, because they are inexpensive and fast. This testing method is very convenient for situational use. This method of testing generally exhibits adequate sensitivity; however, it often cannot identify a specific metabolite and many cannot distinguish between different drugs of the same class (e.g., opioids). Cross-reactivity with other substances is very common with IA presumptive tests and this can produce more false positives, such as quinolone antibiotics and/or poppy seeds and opiates. IA typically also has higher cut-off levels, which can produce more false negatives. Definitive urine drug testing is generally performed in laboratories that use GC-MS or LC-MS/MS technology, which is a more sensitive and highly specific method of testing than immunoassay tests. In many instances, this type of technology is used in confirmation testing as a second test that is used to positively identify a drug or metabolite from a positive specimen. However, this type of testing can also be used as the initial and/or sole test since it provides more accurate information and it measures the concentrations of all drugs, metabolites, and illicit substances [26]. Reflex of only positive IA presumptive screening results to the laboratory will miss many potentially dangerous instances of the use of nonprescribed or illicit use [27]. GC-MS, while having comparable specificity to LC-MS/MS, requires higher volumes of urine, so specimens can be volatized for further testing. This method, however, has become somewhat outdated of late as it leans too heavily on the unreliable IA result to guide subsequent "confirmation" (the specimen must be volatized for the testing of each specific analyte to be tested). An outgrowth of forensic rather than clinical applications of testing for medication monitoring, more flexible LC-MS/MS technology does not require the clinician to "guess" at what drugs they are looking for based on history or the IA result and can improve detection of clinical adherence problems and may ultimately improve the safety of opioid therapy, particularly in high-risk patients who might be less than fully truthful about their substance use.

11.3.2   Pill (Patch) Counts

Another intervention used to promote adherence to medication regimens is pill or patch counting. A systematic chart review conducted by Chou et al. in 2009 suggests that there is, however, little or no reliable evidence on how pill counting affects patient outcomes or clinical decision making [28]. Clinically, pill counts can be a useful tool for the clinician concerned about binge pattern of medication use on the part of their patients or diversion. Pill counts are probably best employed on a random basis with short notice for the patient to come to the office with all of their remaining medication (or come to their pharmacy when the patient lives at a distance from the clinician's office and the pharmacist agrees to play this role). However, pill counts can be experienced as infantilizing or being treated "like a drug addict or criminal" and worse still can be highly disruptive to a patient's routines when, indeed, the goal of pain management is to facilitate return to function. Clinicians should weigh these considerations — for example, is it worthwhile to have the patient leave work to conduct a pill count. We have successfully used patch counts in patients on transdermal therapies wherein we have asked patients who live at a distance from our center to safely store used patches and then bring them to their office visit with the understanding that a full month's supply will only be renewed when all patches are accounted for and furthermore appear to be intact and untampered with. Clinicians conducting pill or patch counts should optimally do so with other staff or family members present as witnesses and should have the patient only touch and count their medications. We have heard of cases wherein clinicians have been accused of stealing medications when pill counts come up short (often by disgruntled, former patients who have had opioids discontinued or who have been discharged for nonadherence).

Whether or not pill counts are used, many patients who might find it difficult to adhere to treatment plans could benefit from more frequent visits to their provider in which smaller amounts of medication are provided. This is especially important for patient with a history of substance use disorder (SUD). Clinicians, for example, could divide a month's supply of medication into three 10-day prescriptions for patients who cannot handle a month's worth of medication [29].

11.3.3   Substance Use Agreements

A common and popular method to promote patient compliance with their medication regimen is the use of substance use agreements, often erroneously termed "patient contracts" in the past. Most agreements contain attempts to improve care through dissemination of information, facilitate a mutually agreed-upon course, or enhance compliance [30]. The agreement often includes descriptions of what exactly the clinician means by medication use and abuse, as well as the penalties for violating the contract, and the process for discontinuing the prescribed opioid. Terms for routine, random substance testing as part of the treatment plan are often explicitly stated [31]. A study involving a retrospective chart review of patients receiving chronic opioid medications in a primary care setting had an adherence rate to the agreement for opioids of over 60 % with a median follow-up of 22.5 months [32]. They found that agreements were discontinued in 37 % of the subjects, with only 17 % canceled for noncompliance and substance abuse while the rest were voluntary. Unfortunately, it is not known exactly how effective these agreements are in reducing nonadherence with opioids.

The use of agreements can also pose some problems, however, such as the inaccurate assurance that the patient is compliant and, if not carefully constructed and presented, the patient could perceive it as punishment. There is also the potential for agreements to have a negative stigma attached to them, especially if the patients have a history of substance abuse [31]. Agreements should never be written in absolute terms that preclude the use of clinical judgment lest the clinician be at risk of violating their own agreement. For example, "early renewals will never be granted" is too restrictive, whereas a statement such as "early medication renewals will not be automatically provided but will be provided at the discretion of the medical team" allows for more clinical judgment and interpretation based on circumstances [33]. Finally, they should represent a living document that is often revisited in the context of interactions with the patient to remind all parties of the goals and proposed outcomes if controlled substances are to be maintained as part of treatment.

11.4   Conclusion

Clinicians have many potential maneuvers and interventions at their disposal to aid in the use of controlled substances for pain treatment for patients all across the risk spectrum, but especially for those patients with a history of drug abuse, addiction, or nonadherence. In today's climate, wherein these medications are highly abused leaving in their wake overdose and criminality, clinicians have a duty to not conduct "business as usual" when it comes to ferreting out and responding to aberrant behavior. The patient's safety and that of the community in which they live are both at stake and clinicians are obliged to be thoughtful, observant, and humane. Indeed, the art of employing many of these simple strategies lies in introducing them into the care of the high-risk patient in a compassionate and empathic way that clearly communicates "whose side the clinician is on." When applied in just the right way, a lot of good can be done to help even some very challenging patient groups.

References

1. Beauchamp GA, Winstanley EL, Ryan SA, Lyons MS. Moving beyond misuse and diversion: the urgent need to consider the role of iatrogenic addiction in the current opioid epidemic. Am J Public Health. 2014;104(11):2023–9.
2. Daum AM, Berkowitz O, Renner Jr JA. The evolution of chronic opioid therapy and recognizing addiction. JAAPA. 2015;28(5):23–7.
3. Heit HA. Addiction, physical dependence, and tolerance: precise definitions to help clinicians evaluate and treat chronic pain patients. J Pain Palliat Care Pharmacother. 2003;17(1):15–29.
4. Collins ED, Streltzer J. Should opioid analgesics be used in the management of chronic pain in opiate addicts? Am J Addict. 2003;12(2):93–100.
5. Levin M. Opioids in headache. Headache. 2014;54(1):12–21.
6. Katz NP, Birnbaum H, Brennan MJ, Freedman JD, Gilmore GP, Jay D, Kenna GA, Madras BK, McElhaney L, Weiss RD, White AG. Prescription opioid abuse: challenges and opportunities for payers. Am J Manag Care. 2013;19(4):295–302.
7. Jamison RN, Ross EL, Michna E, Chen LQ, Holcomb C, Wasan AD. Substance misuse treatment for high-risk chronic pain patients on opioid therapy: a randomized trial. Pain. 2010;150(3):390–400.
8. Passik SD, Heit H, Kirsh KL. Reality and responsibility: a commentary on the treatment of pain and suffering in a drug-using society. J Opioid Manag. 2006;2(3):123–7.
9. Wiedemer NL, Harden PS, Arndt IO, Gallagher RM. The opioid renewal clinic: a primary care, managed approach to opioid therapy in chronic pain patients at risk for substance abuse. Pain Med. 2007;8(7):573–84.
10. Becker WC, Meghani SH, Barth KS, Wiedemer N, Gallagher RM. Characteristics and outcomes of patients discharged from the Opioid Renewal Clinic at the Philadelphia VA Medical Center. Am J Addict. 2009;18(2):135–9.
11. Bethea AR, Acosta MC, Haller DL. Patient versus therapist alliance: whose perception matters? J Subst Abuse Treat. 2008;35(2):174–83.
12. Starrels JL, Becker WC, Weiner MG. Low use of opioid risk reduction strategies in primary care even for high risk patients with chronic pain. J Gen Intern Med. 2011;26(9):958–64.
13. Kenan K, Mack K, Paulozzi L. Trends in prescriptions for oxycodone and other commonly used opioids in the United States, 2000-2010. Open Med. 2012;6(2):e41–7.
14. Volkow ND. America's addiction to opioids: heroin and prescription drug abuse. Testimony to Congress, May 14, 2014. http://www.drugabuse.gov/about-nida/legislative-activities/testimony-to-congress/2015/americas-addiction-to-opioids-heroin-prescription-drug-abuse#_ftn5. Last accessed Aug 22, 2015.
15. Passik SD, Kirsh KL. The interface between pain and drug abuse and the evolution of strategies to optimize pain management while minimizing drug abuse. Exp Clin Psychopharmacol. 2008;16(5):400–4.
16. Webster LR. The role of urine drug testing in chronic pain management: 2013 update. Pain Medicine News. December 2013. http://painmedicinenews.com/download/UDT_PMNSE2013_WM.pdf. Last accessed Aug 22, 2015.
17. Katz NP, Sherburne S, Beach M, Rose RJ, Vielguth J, Bradley J, Fanciullo GJ. Behavioral monitoring and urine toxicology testing in patients receiving long-term opioid therapy. Anesth Analg. 2003;97(4):1097–102.
18. Manchikanti L, et al. Does random urine drug testing reduce illicit drug use in chronic pain patients receiving opioids? Pain Physician. 2006;9(2):123–9.
19. Pesce A, et al. Illicit drug use in the pain patient population decreases with continued drug testing. Pain Physician. 2011;14(2):189–93.
20. Owen GT, Burton AW, Schade CM, Passik SD. Urine drug testing: current recommendations and best practices. Pain Physician. 2012;15(3):ES119–33.

21. Chou R et al. for American Pain Society-American Academy of Pain Medicine Opioids Guidelines Panel. Clinical guidelines for the use of chronic opioid therapy in chronic noncancer pain. J Pain. 2009;10(2):113–30.
22. Trescot AM, et al. Opioids in the management of chronic non-cancer pain: an update of the American Society of the Interventional Pain Physicians' (ASIPP) guidelines. Pain Physician. 2008;11(2 Suppl):S5–62.
23. Federation of State Medical Boards of the United States, Inc. (FSMB). Model policy on the use of opioid analgesics in the treatment of chronic pain. Washington, DC: Federation of State Medical Boards. 2013; http://www.fsmb.org/pdf/pain_policy_july2013.pdf. Last accessed Aug 22, 2015.
24. Gourlay DL, Heit HA. The art and science of urine drug testing. Clin J Pain. 2009; 26(4):267–358.
25. Reisfield GM, Salazar E, Bertholf RL. Rational use and interpretation of urine drug testing in chronic opioid therapy. Ann Clin Lab Sci. 2007;37(4):301–14.
26. Lum G, Mushlin M. Urine drug testing: approaches to screening and confirmation testing. Lab Med. 2004;6(35):369–373. http://www.pcls.com/wp-content/uploads/2014/04/UDT-Approaches-to-Screening-and-Confirmation-Testing.pdf. Last accessed Aug 22, 2015.
27. Kirsh KL. Winegarden W, McCarberg B, Stein GA, Pesce A, Passik SD. An analysis of laboratory immunoassay screen with reflex of positives to quantitation versus definitive laboratory quantitation methodologies for medication monitoring. International Conference on Opioids (ICOO): Basic Science, Clinical Applications & Compliance, Annual Meeting, Boston, MA. June 8–10, 2014.
28. Chou R, Ballantyne J, Fanciullo GJ, Fine PG, Miaskowski C. Research gaps on use of opioids for chronic noncancer pain: findings from a review of the evidence for an American Pain Society and American Academy of Pain Medicine clinical practice guideline. J Pain. 2009; 10(2): 147-159. http://www.jpain.org/article/S1526-5900(08)00830-4/pdf. Last accessed Aug 22, 2015.
29. Center for Substance Abuse Treatment. Managing chronic pain in adults with or in recovery from substance use disorders. Rockville (MD): Substance Abuse and Mental Health Services Administration (US); 2012 (Treatment Improvement Protocol (TIP) Series, No. 54.) 4, Managing addiction risk in patients treated with opioids. http://www.ncbi.nlm.nih.gov/books/NBK92046/. Last accessed Aug 22, 2015.
30. Fishman SF, Bandman TB, Edwards A, Borsook B. The opioid contract in the management of chronic pain. J Pain Symptom Manage. 1999;18(1):27–37.
31. Fishman SM, Wilsey B, Yang J, Reisfield GM, Bandman TB, Borsook D. Adherence monitoring and drug surveillance in chronic opioid therapy. J Pain Symptom Manage. 2000; 20(4):293–307.
32. Hariharan J, Lamb GC, Neuner JM. Long-term opioid contract use for chronic pain management in primary care practice. A five year experience. J Gen Intern Med. 2007;22(4):485–90.
33. Passik SD, Kirsh KL. Clinical aspects of the use of opioid agreements for chronic noncancer pain. In: Pasero C, McCaffery M, editors. Pain assessment and pharmacologic management. St. Louis: Elsevier; 2010, Appendix B, pp. 827–836.

Chapter 12
Prescription Monitoring Programs

Jonathan C. Fellers

12.1 Introduction

Prescription opioids are the second most commonly used illicit drug after cannabis. Their misuse has remained relatively stable over the past decade (Fig. 12.1); in 2014, an estimated 4.3 million Americans (1.6% of the population) had recently used prescription pain medications for non-medical purposes. Mirroring this trend, the prevalence of prescription opioid use disorder in 2014 was an estimated 1.9 million (0.7%) [1].

Unlike the flat rate of misuse and use disorders, overdose fatalities attributed to prescription opioids have surged over the last decade-and-a-half [2]. The disconnection between addiction rates and unintentional overdoses suggests other factors are driving this aspect of the prescription opioid epidemic. One powerful determinant of the increase is the corresponding rise in filled opioid prescriptions [3].

Prescriptions for opioids have grown steadily nationwide since the turn of the twenty-first century, until an inflection point was reached in 2011 [4]. The correlation between the amount of prescription opioids in circulation and risk of prescription opioid overdose is striking (Fig. 12.2). Access to opioids appears critical for the observed increase in overdoses.

To further define factors, a cohort study evaluated patients receiving opioid therapy for chronic non-cancer pain in a health maintenance organization [5]. A significant dose effect was seen for opioid overdose; patients receiving >100 morphine-milligram-equivalents (MMEs) were nine-times as likely to overdose compared to patients receiving 1–20 mg MMEs. Another case-control study identified several important contributors to opioid overdose mortality risk [6]. Each opioid prescription increased risk (OR = 1.2), as did each pharmacy (OR = 2.3). Multiple

J.C. Fellers, M.D. (✉)
Department of Psychiatry, Maine Medical Center,
216 Vaughan Street, Portland, ME 04102, USA
e-mail: jfellers@mmc.org

© Springer International Publishing Switzerland 2016
A.M. Matthews, J.C. Fellers (eds.), *Treating Comorbid Opioid Use Disorder in Chronic Pain*, DOI 10.1007/978-3-319-29863-4_12

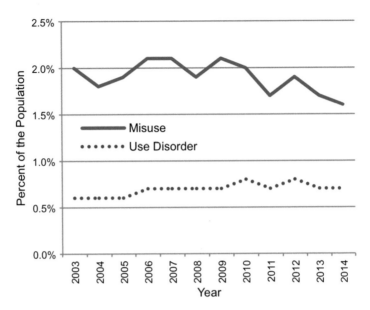

Fig. 12.1 National prevalence of prescription opioid misuse and use disorder. Misuse (non-medical use within the past 3 months) and use disorder (within the past year) have been relatively stable over the past 10+ years

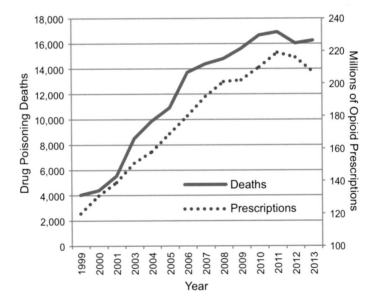

Fig. 12.2 National prescription opioid overdose deaths and prescriptions. *Primary axis*: From 1999 to 2013, overdose deaths from prescription opioids have increased 400%. *Secondary axis*: The number of prescriptions for opioids mirrors the overdose mortalities, with a 170% increase over the same period

prescriptions led to exponential risk (30 prescriptions, OR = 68.2). Other important factors included overlapping prescriptions for opioids (OR = 11.7) and high-dose opioid therapy (average >40 MMEs, OR 12.2). Taken together, these results suggest that a pattern of prescribing may be useful in identifying at-risk patients.

To this end, the government has focused on developing and implementing Prescription Drug Monitoring Programs (PDMPs) to warehouse controlled medication prescription data. It is hoped that through data analysis, profiles may emerge that can assist in identifying high-risk prescribing and intentional deception by patients [7]. This chapter will focus on PDMPs. We will begin with an overview of PDMPs. Then we will examine the information available in PDMPs, including constructs of risk based on PDMP data. Finally, we will review and synthesize research on the value of PDMPs in clinical practice.

12.2   What Are PDMPs?

PDMPs are centralized databases that collect information about the dispensing of controlled substances. States legislation establishes a PDMP as a repository for statewide data. The purpose of these programs is to reduce abuse, misuse, and diversion of prescription medications. Despite apparent utility for preventing opioid overdoses, no state includes this mission [8]. As of this writing, 49 states have implemented PDMPs while Missouri remains as the final holdout. A variety of departments may house the PDMP; state Departments of Health and Pharmacy Boards together administer PDMPs for two out of every three states.

State law defines reportable medications. All state PDMPs include schedule II medications like the opioids oxycodone, hydrocodone, and methadone. There is some variation in reporting schedule V medications (i.e., codeine containing cough medications) or other medications of concern (i.e., butalbital combination products) (Fig. 12.3).

When an entity (typically a pharmacy) dispenses a controlled substance, it must report the fill date, prescriber name, patient name, patient address, medication name, dose, and quantity dispensed; this is the source information for the PDMP. Some states require collection of the method of payment and/or identification of the person picking up the prescription.

It is important to recognize that while many controlled substance prescriptions are captured in a PDMP, there are some notable exceptions. First, Opiate Treatment Programs currently do not report methadone used for maintenance to PDMPs. Second, the Department of Veterans Affairs has limited reporting to state PDMPs (Fig. 12.4). Third, since PDMPs are run by individual states, information across state lines is not reported. There are many efforts underway to provide national connectivity between PDMPs. Finally, controlled medications dispensed while in the emergency room are not recorded.

States differ as per whom they recognize as authorized requestors for PDMP information, and whether training is required to receive access. All PDMPs allow

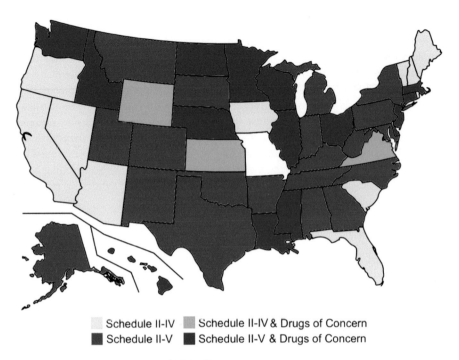

Schedule II-IV   Schedule II-IV & Drugs of Concern
Schedule II-V   Schedule II-V & Drugs of Concern

Fig. 12.3 Medications monitored by PDMPs

prescribers and pharmacists to access reports. Most also permit pharmacies, law enforcement, licensing boards, and patients. There are many interested parties including researchers, insurance companies, workers compensation insurance, and Medicaid fraud detection, and some states allow access. Access to PDMP information must be balanced with the need to protect its confidentiality.

Federal support has enabled the rapid expansion of PDMPs through two separate grant-funding mechanisms (Fig. 12.5). The US Department of Justice's Bureau of Justice Assistance administers the Harold Rogers Prescription Drug Monitoring Program (HRPDMP). It provides three types of grants for states targeting different phases of PDMP development: planning, implementation, and enhancement. Since funding began in 2003, grants have been awarded to over 47 states. The Bureau of Justice Assistance also funds the Brandeis PDMP Center of Excellence.

The 2005 National All Schedules Prescription Electronic Reporting Act (NASPER) created a grant program administered by the Substance Abuse and Mental Health Services Administration (SAMHSA). It provided states grant funding to implement or enhance prescription drug monitoring programs, with the goal of achieving consistent national standards for PDMPs. It was last funded in 2009 and 2010 when it supported 13 states. Grants are no longer available through NASPER.

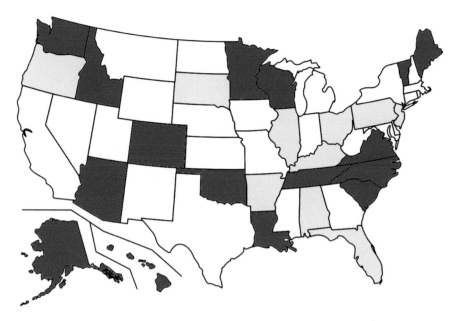

Fig. 12.4 States where US Veterans Affairs reports to PDMPs. States in *red* receive reports from all VA pharmacies in their PDMP. States in *yellow* obtain information from some VA pharmacies (color figure online)

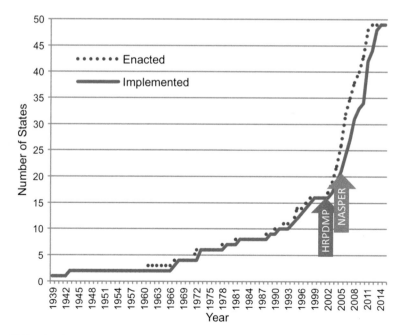

Fig. 12.5 Adoption of PDMPs in the United States. Federal support has accelerated expansion of PDMPs over the last decade

Table 12.1 Types of information available in PDMP reports

Information	Relevant questions
Compliance	•Were prescriptions filled?
	•Were prescriptions refilled early?
	•Were prescriptions refilled despite agreement to stop?
	•Was self-report accurate?
Medication reconciliation	•Were other providers prescribing medications?
	•What other medications were prescribed?
	•What is the dose and quantity of other medications?
Risk	•Are multiple controlled substances being prescribed?
	•How many total prescriptions are there?
	•Are large doses of medications being used?
	•Do prescriptions overlap such that available dose is higher?
	•How many prescribers are being used?
	•How many pharmacies are being used?
	•Is there evidence of deception? (i.e., discrepancy in amount prescribed vs. dispensed)
	•Is there evidence of diversion?

12.3 Information in PDMPs

Providers are faced with many challenges when deciding whether to prescribe controlled substances for pain. The diagnosis of a painful condition often requires patient cooperation and self-report, but completeness and accuracy are not assured. The inherent abuse liability of opioid medications poses a risk, and it is important that prescribers can trust their patients to handle the medication responsibly [9]. Therefore, the context of the encounter and collateral information are very important.

PDMPs offer an opportunity to independently verify prescription history. Since they capture every controlled prescription filled, many useful details can be extracted. Information about compliance, medications prescribed by other providers, and risk are contained in the PDMP report (Table 12.1). If a controlled substance was prescribed, the PDMP report will confirm whether the prescription was filled appropriately (suggesting starting and continuing the medication) and whether early refills occurred (possibly indicating increasing the dose). If a controlled substance was stopped, the report can identify if the prescription was refilled and therefore continued. Finally, if there was an agreement to notify the prescriber about any changes in prescriptions, the report can corroborate self-report.

Though obtaining information from and collaborating with other providers is important for patient care, a PDMP report provides a convenient substitute to aid medication reconciliation. The report can complete gaps from the patient self-report in regard to other providers, the names of other medications, and the dosing of those medications.

PDMP data can provide valuable information for risk-stratification. For overdose risk, several factors such as number of prescriptions, number of pharmacies, multiple controlled substances, overlapping prescriptions, and large doses of opioids are significant. Receiving prescriptions from five or more prescribers [10] and four or more pharmacies [11] have also been implicated in opioid-related death.

A PDMP report can inform the risk–benefit analysis when deciding to prescribe an opioid. If the report reveals other controlled substances, the risk is higher. In the case of concomitant benzodiazepines, overdose risk is tenfold higher [12]. Despite well-documented evidence to avoid sedative/hypnotics [13], the combination remains frequent in practice.

For suspected prescription fraud, a PDMP report can directly reconcile prescriptions. For example, if a prescriber writes a prescription for a certain quantity of an opioid, but the generated PDMP report deviates in amount dispensed, the discrepancy is a red flag for prescription alteration. Likewise, prescriptions found on a PDMP report that the prescriber did not write could indicate a stolen prescription pad or DEA registration number.

"Doctor shopping" describes the practice of seeing multiple different providers in order to find willing prescribers of controlled substances. A "doctor shopper" does not necessarily need to find one of the few prescribers who knowingly provide opioids to patients misusing and abusing them [14]. The patient can be successful by taking advantage of inter-provider differences in practice, feigning or exaggerating symptoms, and/or exploiting weaknesses in communication between providers. Such patients may also visit several pharmacies to evade suspicion. Patients may "doctor shop" in order to receive the treatment that they want, to feed an addiction, or to accumulate medications for diversion. The phenomenon of "doctor shopping" manifests on PDMP reports as multiple providers, multiple prescriptions, overlapping prescriptions, and multiple pharmacies.

One recent study attempted to estimate the number of "doctor shoppers" by statistically modeling prescription data [15]. An extreme subpopulation representing "doctor shoppers" was identified. They averaged seeing 10 prescribers for 32 prescriptions over the course of 10 months. With an estimated population of 135,000, the group consumed over 5.3 and 4 % of oxycodone and all opioids, respectively, dispensed nationwide. Since they are such a small sub-set of the population who receive an opioid prescription (0.7 %), screening every patient is impractical.

The high number of prescribers and prescriptions that define "doctor shoppers" make PDMPs uniquely positioned to identify them. PDMPs can isolate a similar population by identifying patients who receive prescriptions from a threshold number of prescribers, and from a threshold number of pharmacies, in a certain period of time. HRPDMP grantees used the metric of five or more prescribers, from five or more pharmacies, within a 3-month period ($5 \times 5 \times 3$). By varying the threshold, the sensitivity and specificity for detecting aberrant activity can be adjusted.

For the risk of substance use disorder, it is more challenging. A pattern of behaviors from a PDMP report, like deception, overlapping prescriptions, and "doctor shopping" are not diagnostic criteria for substance use disorders [16]. Addiction may lead to these behaviors, but it is better described as malingering.

12.4   Utility of PDMPs in Clinical Practice

Several studies have investigated whether the implementation of PDMPs has altered risks associated with controlled prescription medications. An ecological study looking at opioid misuse measures found that states with a PDMP showed a small mitigation in opioid overdoses, but no change in opioid treatment entrance [17]. This is an association and does not mean causation. Another study examining pre- and post-PDMP implementation found no difference in emergency room visits due to benzodiazepine misuse [18].

States quickly adopted PDMPs, but prescribers have been less enthusiastic. Prescribers largely know the programs exist, but they often do not use them [19]. Time constraints, inadequate training, and a lack of guidance on how to use the results appear responsible for the poor uptake [20]. It is difficult to justify the administrative burden when it is not clear how to apply information from the report.

Surveying a small sample of providers, one study identified a broad range in responses to how PDMPs were used [21]. The threshold for pulling a report and how a troublesome report was discussed with a patient varied widely. In a larger study, most providers would request a PDMP report if they suspected a problem, but only half would routinely check one on a new patient, and only one third would check prior to starting a controlled medication [22].

Some states have responded to the lackluster enrollment by mandating training (10 states), enrollment (21 states), and even access in certain situations (24 states) (Fig. 12.6). What is the effect of requiring prescribers to check a PDMP report prior to writing a scheduled prescription? A study of a dental practice in New York evaluated opioid prescribing pre- and post-implementation of New York's mandatory PDMP requirement [23]. A significant reduction in opioid prescriptions followed initial adoption and continued to decline thereafter (over 75 % reduction). Confounding this result was a significant change in patients within the clinic; prior to the PDMP requirement, surgical extraction was performed, but afterwards these cases were referred out. Despite this factor, the requirement clearly led to less opioid prescribing. It is highly likely that opioid prescribing was avoided due to the increased administrative burden of the PDMP mandate.

Several studies have looked at how PDMP reports can add to medical decision-making. In an emergency room setting, clinician judgment of drug-seeking behavior compared well with data from PDMP reports [24]. PDMP reports altered management in less than 10 % of cases (6.5 % giving opioid not planned, 3 % no longer giving opioids). In a general psychiatric clinic setting, again clinician judgment was able to identify prescription misuse accurately with about 70 % sensitivity [25]. PDMP reports only altered management in 2 % of cases, suggesting that pulling a report on every patient is not productive. Finally, a study in pain clinic patients suggests using an inconsistency scale, which includes checking a PDMP report, and assists in identifying patients at elevated risk for opioid misuse, abuse, or diversion [26].

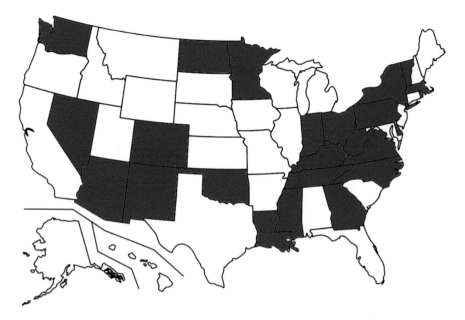

Fig. 12.6 States with regulations that require prescribers to access PDMP. States in *blue* oblige prescribers to check a PDMP on patients in certain circumstances. Criteria can range from narrow (patients prescribed opioids for workman's compensation claims — AZ) to broad (every controlled substance prescription with over 5 day supply — NY) (color figure online)

12.5 Conclusions

As prescription drug overdoses have reached epidemic proportions, government has responded by advancing PDMPs as a potential technological solution. Now widely implemented, PDMPs provide a valuable resource from a public health perspective. By consolidating controlled substance prescribing and dispensing records in one place, a PDMP enables identification of unusual activity in patients, prescribers, and pharmacies. Providers can use information in PDMPs to monitor compliance with prescribed treatment. Reports also provide valuable information for medication reconciliation, especially if patient report and collateral records are inadequate. Finally, PDMP reports provide a unique reference source when patient deception is suspected. Based on available data, the prevalence of "doctor shoppers" is very low. Consequently, having individual providers routinely screen PDMP reports is of low yield in detecting "doctor shopping." PDMP programs are better situated to identify such aberrant activity. In high-risk contexts (pain clinics, substance use treatment programs) and with high-risk patients (history of substance use disorder, on multiple controlled substances, on high-doses) yield improves. Some studies indicate that clinical judgment is quite good at predicting unusual activity on a PDMP report [24, 25]. Therefore, one approach might be to use clinical judgment, informed by the context of the encounter and the patient's history, to determine when a report is warranted. Despite the absence of best practice guidelines for using PDMPs in clinical practice, some states mandate providers to check reports in certain circumstances. Time will tell the consequence of such legislation.

References

1. Center for Behavioral Health Statistics and Quality. Behavioral health trends in the United States: Results from the 2014 National Survey on Drug Use and Health. 2015 (HHS Publication No. SMA 15-4927, NSDUH Series H-50).
2. United States Department of Health and Human Services (US DHHS). Underlying cause of death 1999-2013 on CDC WONDER Online Database. 2015.
3. Dart RC, Surratt HL, Cicero TJ, Parrino MW, Severtson SG, Bucher-Bartelson B, et al. Trends in opioid analgesic abuse and mortality in the United States. NEJM. 2015;372(3):241–8.
4. IMS Health. (1999-2013). National prescription audit.
5. Dunn KM, Saunders KW, Rutter CM, Banta-Green CJ, Merrill JO, Sullivan MD, et al. Opioid prescriptions for chronic pain and overdose: a cohort study. Ann Intern Med. 2010; 152(2):85–92.
6. Paulozzi LJ, Kilbourne EM, Shah NG, Nolte KB, Desai HA, Landen MG, et al. A history of being prescribed controlled substances and risk of drug overdose death. Pain Med. 2012; 13(1):87–95.
7. Clark T, Eadie J, Kreiner P, Strickler G. Prescription Drug Monitoring: An Assessment of the Evidence for Best Practices. Heller School for Social Policy and Management. The Prescription Drug Monitoring Program Center of Excellence: Brandeis University; 2012.
8. Davis CS, Johnston JE, Pierce MW. Overdose epidemic, prescription monitoring programs, and public health: a review of state laws. Am J Public Health. 2015;105(11):e9–11.
9. Miller J. The other side of trust in health care: prescribing drugs with the potential for abuse. Bioethics. 2007;21(1):51–60.
10. Hall AJ, Logan JE, Toblin RL, Kaplan JA, Kraner JC, Bixler D, et al. Patterns of abuse among unintentional pharmaceutical overdose fatalities. JAMA. 2008;300(22):2613–20.
11. Peirce GL, Smith MJ, Abate MA, Halverson J. Doctor and pharmacy shopping for controlled substances. Med Care. 2012;50(6):494–500.
12. Dasgupta N, Funk MJ, Proescholdbell S, Hirsch A, Ribisl KM, Marshall S. Cohort study of the impact of high-dose opioid analgesics on overdose mortality. Pain Med doi. 2015. doi:10.1111/pme.12907 [Epub ahead of print].
13. Webster LR, Reisfield GM, Dasgupta N. Eight principles for safer opioid prescribing and cautions with benzodiazepines. Postgrad Med. 2015;127(1):27–32.
14. Lembke A. Why doctors prescribe opioids to known opioid abusers. NEJM. 2012;367:1580–1.
15. McDonald DC, Carlson K. Estimating the prevalence of opioid diversion by "doctor shoppers" in the United States. PLoS One. 2014;8(7), e69241
16. Barrett SP, Meisner JR, Stewart SH. What constitutes prescription drug misuse? Problems and pitfalls of current conceptualizations. Curr Drug Abuse Rev. 2008;1(3):255–62.
17. Reifler LM, Droz D, Bailey JE, Schnol SH, Fant R. Do prescription monitoring programs impact state trends in opioid abuse/misuse? Pain Med. 2012;13(3):434–42.
18. Bachhuber MA, Maughan BC, Mitra N, Feingold J. Prescription monitoring programs and emergency department visits involving benzodiazepine misuse: early evidence from 11 United States metropolitan areas. Int J Drug Policy. 2016;28:120–3.
19. Feldman L, Williams KS, Coates J, Knox M. Awareness and utilization of a prescription monitoring program among physicians. J Pain Palliat Care Pharmacother. 2011;25(4):313–7.

20. Deyo RA, Irvine JM, Hallvik SE, Hildebran C, Beran T, Millet LM, et al. Leading a horse to water: facilitating registration and use of a prescription drug monitoring program. Clin J Pain. 2015;31(9):782–7.
21. Hildebran C, Cohen DJ, Irvine JM, Foley C, O'Kane N, Beran T, et al. How clinicians use prescription drug monitoring programs: a qualitative inquiry. Pain Med. 2014;15(7):1179–86.
22. Irvine JM, Hallvik SE, Hildebra C, Marino M, Beran T, Deyo RA. Who uses a prescription drug monitoring program and how? Insights from a statewide survey of Oregon clinicians. J Pain. 2014;15(7):747–55.
23. Rasubala L, Pernapati L, Velasquez X, Burk J, Ren YF. Impact of a mandatory prescription drug monitoring program on prescription of opioid analgesics by dentists. PLoS One. 2015;10(8), e0135957.
24. Weiner SG, Griggs CA, Mitchell PM, Langlois BK, Friedman FD, Moore RL, et al. Clinician impression versus prescription drug monitoring program criteria in the assessment of drug-seeking behavior in the emergency department. Ann Emerg Med. 2013;62(4):281–9.
25. Sowa EM, Fellers JC, Raisinghani RS, Santa Cruz MR, Hidalgo PC, Lee MS, et al. Prevalence of substance misuse in new patients in an outpatient psychiatry clinic using a prescription monitoring program. Prim Care Companion CNS Disord. 2014;16(1):pii: PCC.
26. Hamill-Ruth RJ, Larriviere K, McMasters MG. Addition of objective data to identify risk for medication misuse and abuse: the inconsistency score. Pain Med. 2013;14(12):1900–7.

Chapter 13
Federal Involvement in Pain Management Policy

H. Westley Clark

Vignette

The doctor's pain relief clinic was raided by federal agents. That raid was part of an ongoing investigation for possible over-prescribing for prescription painkillers to patients along with possible forgery and fraud. That warrant was served by the Drug Enforcement Administration's Indianapolis District Office, the County Drug Task Force, the local Police and the State Attorney General's Office's Medicaid Fraud Control Unit.

The warrant application noted eight drug overdose deaths of patients who received prescriptions from the doctor or one of his nurse practitioners. Subsequently, all the locations of the Pain Centers shut their doors, affecting an estimated 5000–10,000 patients in the state. Local officials called the influx of patients a community health crisis.[1]

The federal government has an extensive interest in pain management from multiple perspectives. This interest is magnified by the federal government's concern about the issues of misuse of prescription-controlled substances, especially prescription opioids. Through its multiple departments and agencies, the federal government has involvement that requires coordination and communication. That role ranges from regulatory, to research, to guidelines and education, to reimbursement and to enforcement. With the exception of such agencies such as the Department of Veterans Affairs (DVA), the Department of Defense (DoD), the Indian Health Services (IHS), and the Bureau of Prisons, the federal government's role is not to provide direct patient care, but it is concerned with appropriate pain management and the appropriate use of pain medication. Table 13.1. lists the acronyms of the various federal agencies actively involved in pain management policy.

---

[1] http://wane.com/2015/01/06/dea-arrests-fort-wayne-pain-doctor/ Accessed 2/5/2015.

H.W. Clark, M.D., J.D., M.P.H. (✉)
Public Health Program, Santa Clara University,
Kena 110, 500 El Camino Real, Santa Clara, CA 95053-0269, USA
e-mail: hclark@scu.edu

© Springer International Publishing Switzerland 2016
A.M. Matthews, J.C. Fellers (eds.), *Treating Comorbid Opioid Use Disorder in Chronic Pain*, DOI 10.1007/978-3-319-29863-4_13

Table 13.1 Federal agencies involved in pain management policy

Agency	Basic role in pain policy
FDA	Regulates the pharmaceutical industry, approves medications, recommends schedules
CMS	Pays for health services, concerned about waste, fraud, and abuse
SAMHSA	Collects data on misuse of prescription drugs, deals with substance use disorders, registers physicians for the use of buprenorphine, regulates opioid treatment programs, provides education
NIH	Funds research into the dimensions of pain, works with other federal agencies, provides education
CDC	Collects data on misuse of prescription drugs, fosters the use of PDMPS, provides education
AHRQ	Conducts research, provides education
HRSA	Provides education
ONDCP	Establishes policy about misuse of prescription drugs
DEA	Enforces the controlled substances act, schedules controlled substances, facilitates the arrest and prosecution of violators of the CSA, promotes awareness
IHS	Provides clinical pain care, provides education
DoD	Provides clinical pain care, provides pain care guidelines, provides education, conduct research
VA	Provides clinical pain care, provides pain care guidelines, provides education, conduct research

Most practitioners are aware of the increasing concern about the management and mis-management of pain. They are also aware of both the increase in overdose deaths and that several of the federal agencies in Table 13.1 have police powers that can be used to enforce criminal sanctions and penalties, including incarceration, for violating some of the more basic rules of prescribing controlled substances in the management of pain.

The vignette above was taken from an actual case. It demonstrates the collaboration and cooperation between state and federal officials when it comes to both prescription drug abuse and the often associated Medicaid fraud. Some Federal agencies have investigatory authority, in addition to police powers.

Good pain management should not be pursued under the threat of criminal sanctions, but it is important for clinicians who employ prescription opioids in the treatment of pain, particularly with patients with a history of prior substance misuse, to keep in mind that the use of controlled substances is regulated by both state and federal authorities and that the perceived misuse might carry criminal sanctions.

In addition, to investigatory and police powers, several federal agencies play an important role in establishing key principles associated with pain management.

The US Department of Health and Human Services (USDHHS) addresses the issue of prescription drug abuse within eight domains: (1) regulatory and oversight activities, (2) surveillance, (3) drug abuse prevention, (4) patient and public education, (5) provider education, (6) clinical practice tools, (7) drug abuse treatment, and (8) overdose prevention initiatives.[2] The following operating divisions within DHHS

[2] http://www.cdc.gov/HomeandRecreationalSafety/pdf/HHS_Prescription_Drug_Abuse_Report_09.2013.pdf, Addressing Prescription Drug Abuse in the United States. Accessed 2/10/2015.

play critical roles in prescription drug abuse policy: Food and Drug Administration (FDA), the Substance Abuse and Mental Health Services Administration (SAMHSA), the Centers for Disease Control and Prevention (CDC), the National Institutes of Health (NIH), the Centers for Medicare and Medicaid Service (CMS), the Health Resources Health and Services Administration (HRSA), and the IHS.

The US Department of Justice contains the Drug Enforcement Administration (DEA); The DEA is the entity that enforces the Controlled Substances Act and is responsible registering those clinicians who employ controlled substances in the treatment of pain and addiction.

The DoD and the DVA are also actively concerned about pain management policy and research. Both Departments, like DHHS's IHS, provide direct services. Therefore, they too are concerned about appropriate pain management policy and practice.

In its capacity as the lead federal agency for substance abuse policy, the Office of National Drug Control Policy (ONDCP) has addressed the issue of prescription drug abuse and overdose deaths.

13.1 Food and Drug Administration

Reviewing the role of the FDA in the management of pain and in pain policy is an excellent initial point of exploration. The FDA focuses on consumer protection, scientific credibility, regulatory activity as a part of its public health function. The FDA's modern era began in 1906 with the passage of the Pure Food and Drugs Act of 1906. The FDA has had a number of legislative enhancements in the over 100 years of its existence. It has grown to over 10,000 employees and a budget for fiscal year 2015 of over $4.4 billion dollars. The FDA's purpose, among many other things, is to provide Americans with safe and effective medications.

In 2007, the FDA Amendments Act permitted the FDA to require risk evaluation and mitigation strategies (REMS) from pharmaceutical companies to ensure that the benefits of prescription drugs outweigh their risks. The FDA can require a REMS before or after a drug is approved. The FDA told drug makers in 2011 that they must develop a REMS strategy for extended-release and long-acting opioid analgesics used to treat moderate-to-severe chronic pain. In doing so, the FDA acknowledged that other than opioids there were a limited number of options available for the treatment of pain. However, because of the complications associated with opioid use, e.g., misuse, abuse, overdose, and death, the FDA promulgated a risk management plan that affected more than 20 companies that made extended release/long-acting opioid medications. The cornerstone of this plan is to have the drug manufacturers make educational training available to prescribers on safe prescribing such medications.[3] The FDA expects companies to train at least 60 % of estimated 320,000 prescribers of extended release/long-acting opioids. In order to assist patients, the

---

[3] http://www.er-la-opioidrems.com/IwgUI/rems/home.action. Accessed 2/7/2015.

REMS includes a requirement for a Medication Guide that will be handed out by the pharmacist when the patient receives the medication covered by the REMS; this medication guide includes safety information.

REMS website contains information on Accredited Continuing Education for Healthcare Professionals and Materials for Healthcare Professionals. There are also Materials for Patients.[4]

The FDA's regulatory role allows it to encourage pharmaceutical companies to develop abuse-deterrent formulations of opioids.[5] The following prescription opioids are examples of medications with an abuse-deterrent capabilities: Zohyrdo ER, Hysingla ER[6], Embeda[7], and Targiniq ER[8] . While opioids with abuse-deterrent formulations may discourage the misuse of such medications, abuse is still a possibility by the oral route. In the post-marketing period, clinicians treating pain patients, especially those with co-occurring substance use disorders, can contribute to the knowledge about the impact of abuse deterrence by surveying those patients with prescription opioid use disorders who can report on the relative success of abuse deterrent formulations by using the FDA's Adverse Event Reporting System (FAER)[9] .

Beyond the issue of abuse deterrence, the traditional view is that the FDA does not regulate the practice of medicine, per se. The regulation of the practice of medicine has generally been viewed as a function of state authorities. To that end, when a medication that has been approved by the FDA for one purpose is used for another purpose with the intent to practice medicine, the FDA has been silent.[10] However, the FDA plays a major role in providing guidance and guidelines to clinicians and consumers about the appropriate use of medications; to this end, the FDA influences the practice of medicine, as well as regulating pharmaceuticals and pharmaceutical company practices.[11]

---

[4] Ibid.

[5] http://www.fda.gov/downloads/drugs/guidancecomplianceregulatoryinformation/guidances/ucm334743.pdf, Guidance for Industry Abuse-Deterrent Opioids-Evaluation and Labeling, FDA, January 2013. Accessed 2/7/2015.

[6] http://www.fda.gov/NewsEvents/Newsroom/PressAnnouncements/ucm423977.htm,   FDA approves extended-release, single-entity hydrocodone product with abuse-deterrent properties, November 20, 2014. Accessed 2/8/2015.

[7] http://www.fda.gov/NewsEvents/Newsroom/PressAnnouncements/ucm419288.htm,   FDA approves labeling with abuse-deterrent features for third extended-release opioid analgesic, October 17, 2014. Accessed 2/8/2015.

[8] http://www.fda.gov/NewsEvents/Newsroom/PressAnnouncements/ucm406407.htm,   FDA approves new extended-release oxycodone with abuse-deterrent properties, July 23, 2014. Accessed 2/8/2015.

[9] http://www.fda.gov/Drugs/GuidanceComplianceRegulatoryInformation/Surveillance/AdverseDrugEffects/, Accessed 2/15/2015, FDA Adverse Event Reporting System.

[10] http://www.fda.gov/RegulatoryInformation/Guidances/ucm126486.htm, Accessed 2/10/2015.

[11] http://www.fda.gov/ForConsumers/ConsumerUpdates/ucm220112.htm, "Combating Misuse and Abuse of Prescription Drugs: Q&A with Michael Klein, Ph.D. Accessed 2/19/2015.

Finally, the FDA's regulatory authority includes a cadre of special agents who work with federal, state, and local law enforcement agents to address violations of the Food, Drug, and Cosmetic Act.

Consequently, while the FDA does not regulate the "practice" of medicine, per se, it heavily influences both directly and indirectly pain policy. The FDA's influence is exercised through its responsibilities under the Food, Drug, and Cosmetics Act. The FDA is a member of the Interagency Pain Research Coordinating Committee (IPRCC) described below.

13.2 Centers for Medicare and Medicaid Services

CMS covers 100 million people through Medicare, Medicaid, the Children's Health Insurance Program, and the Health Insurance Marketplace. CMS concerns itself not just with the reimbursement for healthcare services, determining which procedures are reimbursable and which are not, but also with quality of care. Clearly, pain policies and pain management strategies extend beyond the use of prescription opioids for the treatment of pain. CMS uses payment policies to determine which pain management strategies are supportable.

In addition to the spectrum of reimbursement strategies, including intervention procedures that might be designed to avoid the use of prescription opioids in the treatment of pain, CMS has put together a number of education tools about drug diversion; these include: (1) Drug Diversion Toolkit,[12] (2) Drug Diversion in the Medicaid Program,[13] (3) Partners in Integrity: What Is a Prescriber's Role in Preventing the Diversion of Prescription Drugs?,[14] (4) Prescription Drug Diversion Resource Guide,[15] and (5) Analysis of Conditions Associated with High Opioid Use[16]: In addition, CMS developed prescriber education focused on FDA-approved dosage guidelines and promoted best practices.

---

[12] http://www.cms.gov/Medicare-Medicaid-Coordination/Fraud-Prevention/Medicaid-Integrity-Education/Provider-Education-Toolkits/Downloads/prescription-opioids-booklet0814.pdf, Drug Diversion Toolkit, Prescription Opioids-An Overview for Prescribers and Pharmacists. Accessed 2/10/2015.

[13] http://www.cms.gov/medicare-medicaid-coordination/fraud-prevention/medicaidintegrityprogram/downloads/drugdiversion.pdf, Drug Diversion in the Medicaid Program, State Strategies for Reducing Prescription Drug Diversion in Medicaid. Accessed 2/10/2015.

[14] http://www.cms.gov/medicare-medicaid-coordination/fraud-prevention/medicaid-integrity-education/provider-education-toolkits/downloads/prescriber-role-drugdiversion.pdf, Partners in Integrity, What is a Prescriber's Role in Preventing the Diversion of Prescription Drugs? Accessed 2/15/2015.

[15] http://www.cms.gov/Medicare-Medicaid-Coordination/Fraud-Prevention/Medicaid-Integrity-Education/Downloads/prescription-drugdiversion-resourceguide.pdf, Prescription Drug Diversion Resource Guide, accepted 2/15/2015.

[16] http://www.cms.gov/Medicare/Prescription-Drug-Coverage/PrescriptionDrugCovContra/Downloads/Analysis-of-Conditions-Associated-with-High-Opioid-Use.pdf, Analysis of Conditions Associated with High Opioid Use, Accessed 2/10/2015.

CMS, in conjunction with SAMHSA, CDC, National Institute on Drug Abuse (NIDA), and National Institute on Alcohol Abuse and Alcoholism (NIAAA), released an Information Bulletin in 2014 which focused on Medication Assisted Treatment for Substance Use Disorders[17]-outlined strategies for managing medication. Medicaid programs were reminded that they could use the following strategies: (1) Preferred Drug List (PDL) which indicated drugs that providers are permitted to use without prior authorization for payment, (2) Prior Authorization which requires a prescriber to obtain permission from Medicaid or the state agency vendor, (3) Quantity limits, where a state Medicaid agency may impose quantity limits on certain medications to prevent overprescription, (4) Duration Limits, where a state Medicaid agency may impose duration limits on certain medications to prevent overprescription, (5) Provider Selection and Credentialing, following state and federal regulations that establish guidance about who can provide certain prescription medications and in what setting. (6) Drug Utilization Reviews, a process applied either prospectively or retrospectively to a drug being dispensed, reviewing documentation of claims database to ascertain whether problems exist, and (7) Patient Review and Restriction Programs, which allows a state agency to restrict a beneficiary to obtain Medicaid services from designated providers only.

DHHS's Office of the Inspector General (IG) issued a report in 2013 entitled: "Prescribers with Questionable Patterns in Medicare Part D."[18] The IG recommended that CMS ensure the effective and systematic monitoring of prescribers to identify those with questionable patterns, provide guidance on how to effectively monitor prescribing patterns, provide education and training for prescribers, and follow-up on prescribers with questionable prescribing patterns.

In summary, CMS has substantially focused on drug diversion as its mission to address the prescription opioid problem; pain management is an inherent component of that discussion, but given the attention of prescription opioid diversion and abuse pain management threatens to be only a collateral issue.

13.3 Substance Abuse and Mental Health Services Administration

SAMHSA is the agency within DHHS that leads the public health efforts to advance the behavioral health of the nation. SAMHSA states that its mission is to reduce the impact of substance abuse and mental illness on America's communities. SAMHSA has a budget of $3.5 billion and over 600 employees; it is composed of the Center for Substance Abuse Treatment, the Center for Substance Abuse Prevention, the Center for Mental Health Services, the Center for Behavioral Health Statistics and

---

[17] http://medicaid.gov/Federal-Policy-Guidance/Downloads/CIB-07-11-2014.pdf,   Medication Assisted Treatment for Substance Use Disorders. Accessed 2/10/2015.

[18] http://oig.hhs.gov/oei/reports/oei-02-09-00603.pdf, Prescribers with Questionable Patterns in Medicare Part D. Accessed 2/19/2015.

Quality and four Offices. SAMHSA funds substance use prevention and treatment efforts in all 50 states and several territories, e.g., Puerto Rico and the US Virgin Islands. In addition, SAMHSA regulates Opioid Treatment Programs and registers physicians prescribing buprenorphine for the treatment of opioid use disorders. In addition to prevention and treatment efforts, SAMHSA collects surveillance data on patterns of substance use in the United States. It also collects information from facilities actively engaged in substance use treatment.

SAMHSA has sponsored training of clinicians in the use of pain medications and the misuse of pain medications for chronic pain.[19,20,21] One course, offered through Boston University, addresses: initiating opioid therapy, aberrant opioid taking behavior, lack of opioid benefit and excessive risk, high-dose opioids in an Inherited patient, illicit drug use in a patient on chronic opioid therapy, prescription drug monitoring programs (PDMP) questionable activity in an established patient, and PDMP's questionable activity in a new patient.[22]

In addition to promoting training, SAMHSA has published several documents that address the issue of managing pain. Pain Management Without Psychological Dependence, Substance Abuse In Brief Fact Sheet[23] is one. Managing Chronic Pain in Adults With or in Recovery From Substance Use Disorders, Tip 54[24] is a second one.

A third document is consumer-oriented, "You Can Manage Your Chronic Pain to Live a Good Life: A Guide for People in Recovery from Mental Illness or Addiction".[25] SAMHSA works closely with its HHS partners in the FDA, HRSA, CDC, NIH (particularly the NIDA and the NIAAA). In addition, SAMHSA collaborates with the Office of National Drug Policy and the DEA and with colleagues in the overall Department of Justice.

Furthermore, SAMHSA reaches out to various trade organizations such as the Association of State and Territorial Health Officials (ASTHO), the American Medical Association (AMA), the American Society of Addiction Medicine (ASAM), and the American Psychiatric Association (APA) to promote knowledge about pain management and the use of prescription opioids.

---

[19] http://www.medscape.com/viewarticle/712071, "Use of methadone in Chronic Pain Management—A Video Lecture from CSAT/SAMHSA. Accessed 2/19/2015.

[20] http://www.hawaii.edu/hivandaids/OxyContin%20%20%20%20%20Prescription%20Drug%20 Abuse.pdf. Accessed 2/15/2015.

[21] http://www.opioidprescribing.com/overview, "Safe and Effective Opioid Prescribing for Chronic Pain". Accessed 2/19/2015.

[22] Ibid.

[23] https://store.samhsa.gov/shin/content/MS993/MS993.pdf, Pain Management Without Psychological Dependence: A Guide for Healthcare Providers. Accessed 2/11/2015.

[24] http://store.samhsa.gov/product/TIP-54-Managing-Chronic-Pain-in-Adults-With-or-in-Recovery-From-Substance-Use-Disorders/SMA13-4671, TIP 54: Managing Chronic Pain in Adults With or in Recovery From Substance Use Disorders.

[25] http://store.samhsa.gov/product/You-Can-Manage-Your-Chronic-Pain-To-Live-a-Good-Life-A-Guide-for-People-in-Recovery-from-Mental-Illness-or-Addiction/SMA14-4783, You Can.

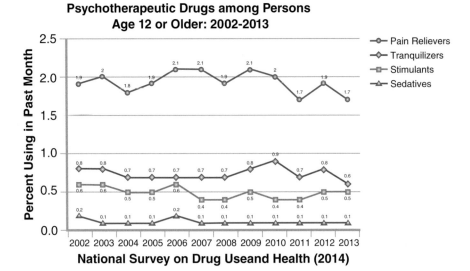

Fig. 13.1 Prevalence of the nonmedical use of prescription drugs during the past month

Another key activity of SAMHSA that should benefit clinicians concerned about pain and pain management is the collection of data. SAMHSA data has played a major role in influencing pain policy within the United States.

SAMHSA's National Survey on Drug Use and Health (NSDUH) is a primary source of statistical information on the use of illegal drugs, alcohol, and tobacco by the US civilian, noninstitutionalized population aged 12 and older in the United States. These data are collected annually, surveying over 67,000 people nationwide. The survey also collects data on mental disorders, including co-occurring substance use disorders. SAMHSA through NSDUH publishes both a summary of national findings for a quick review of general data and detailed tables. Figure 13.1 shows the prevalence of the nonmedical use of prescription drugs during the past month, with pain relievers, tranquilizers, stimulants, and sedatives separated out.

NSDUH collects prevalence data on the nonmedical use of pain relievers by geographic area, by county type, age, gender, race, and Hispanic ethnicity. NSDUH also collects prevalence data on specific pain relievers that are used nonmedically by age group. The following drugs are examples: codeine, hydrocodone, methadone, morphine, OxyContin®, tramadol, and Dilaudid®.

The data can also be used to determine the prevalence of substance use or mental illness among demographic or geographic subgroups, as well as to estimate the trends in these measures over time and to determine the need for substance abuse or mental health treatment services; as a result, SAMHSA publishes maps that are jurisdiction-specific capturing the prevalence of various drugs of abuse. Figure 13.2, for instance, represents the nonmedical use of pain relievers in the past year among individuals aged 12 or older by state in percentages based on the annual averages based on 2012 and 2013 data.

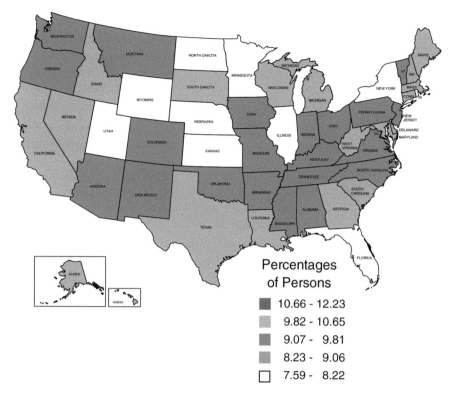

Fig. 13.2 Nonmedical use of pain relievers in the past year among individuals aged 12 or older by state in percentages based on the annual averages based on 2012 and 2013 data

These types of data can be used to promote prevention strategies, encourage treatment strategies, and educate consumers and clinicians. This type of information can aid clinicians in communicating with not only patients, but patient family members, state and tribal authorities, and professionals in the community.

In addition to NSDUH data, SAMHSA conducts a National Survey of Substance Abuse Treatment Services (N-SSATS), retrieving Information from 14,148 facilities throughout the United States. Detailing the types of services offered to those with substance use disorders allows for policy considerations for the treatment of those dependent on, among other things, prescription opioids.

SAMHSA also funds the Provider's Clinical Support System for Opioid Therapies (PCSS-O), which is a national training and mentoring project that focuses on the safe and effective use of opioid medication.[26] The PCSS-O offers no-cost CME programs on the use of opioids for the treatment of chronic pain.

---

[26] http://pcss-o.org/, PCSS-O. Accessed 2/20/2015.

13.4   National Institutes of Health

The NIH is made up of 27 Institutes and Centers, each with a specific research agenda. Of relevance to this chapter is that many of the NIH Institutes have come together to form the NIH Pain Consortium.[27] The goals of the NIH Pain Consortium are:

- To develop a comprehensive and forward-thinking pain research agenda for the NIH—one that builds on what we have learned from our past efforts.
- To identify key opportunities in pain research, particularly those that provide for multidisciplinary and trans-NIH participation.
- To increase visibility for pain research—both within the NIH intramural and extramural communities, as well as outside the NIH. The latter audiences include our various pain advocacy and patient groups who have expressed their interests through scientific and legislative channels.

While the focus of the NIH activity is research, that research encompasses a wide range of activities of interest. Such funding opportunities as Mechanistic Studies of Pain and Alcohol Dependence, Pharmacogenomics of Orofacial Pain Management, Clinical Evaluation of Adjuncts to Opioid Therapies for the Treatment of Chronic Pain, Chronic Overlapping Pain conditions, Pain in Aging, and the Neurobiology of Migraine encourage investigators working through public–private partnerships to increase knowledge about pain dynamics and pain management.

The NIH Pain Consortium has sponsored such meetings as: (1) Pathways to Prevention Workshop: The Role of Opioids in the Treatment of Chronic Pain,(2) Moving Molecules from Model systems to Medicine in Pain Research, and (3) Investigators Meeting on Chronic Overlapping Pain Conditions.

Furthermore, the NIH Pain Consortium sponsors an annual symposium on a topic relevant to pain; this meeting features NIH-supported researchers involved in pain research. Minutes of the meetings are posted on the Pain Consortium website. The first NIH Pain Consortium Symposium was held in 2006. The ninth symposium was held in 2014.[28]

The NIH has an Office of Pain Policy within the National Institute of Neurological Disorders and Stroke (NINDS), which works with the Pain Consortium.

In addition to the NIH Pain Consortium, the NIH participates in the IPRCC.[29] The IPRCC is a federal advisory committee facilitated by the Patient Protection and Affordable Care Act (PPACA) which prompted its creation by the Department of Health and Human Services.[30] The IPRCC consists of seven federal agencies and 12 non-federal members. The entities represented on the IPRCC include: Agency

---

[27] http://painconsortium.nih.gov/About/purpose.html. Accessed 2/19/2015.

[28] http://painconsortium.nih.gov/PC_Symposia_Meetings/symposiums/pc_symposia_index.html. Accessed 2/19/2015.

[29] http://iprcc.nih.gov/index.htm, The Interagency Pain Research Coordinating Committee. Accessed 2/19/2015.

[30] Public Law 111-148, Section 409J(b).

for Healthcare Research and Quality (AHRQ), the CDC, the FDA, the NIH, the DoD, and the DVA.
The mandate for the IPRCC as spelled out in the PPACA is to[31]:

- Develop a summary of advances in pain care research supported or conducted by the Federal agencies relevant to the diagnosis, prevention, and treatment of pain and diseases and disorders associated with pain.
- Identify critical gaps in basic and clinical research on the symptoms and causes of pain.
- Make recommendations to ensure that the activities of the NIH and other Federal agencies are free of unnecessary duplication of effort.
- Make recommendations on how best to disseminate information on pain care.
- Make recommendations on how to expand partnerships between public entities and private entities to expand collaborative, cross-cutting research.

Subsequently, the IPRCC moved to create a National Pain Strategy, which would be a comprehensive population level strategy for pain prevention, treatment, management, and research. The National Pain Strategy relied on key recommendations of the 2011 Institute of Medicine Report: Relieving Pain in America.[32] These were listed at the IPRCC website as[33]:

- Describe how efforts across government agencies, including public–private partnerships, can be established, coordinated, and integrated to encourage population-focused research, education, communication, and community-wide approaches that can help reduce pain and its consequences and remediate disparities in the experience of pain among subgroups of Americans.
- Include an agenda for developing physiological, clinical, behavioral, psychological, outcomes, and health services research and appropriate links across these domains.
- Improve pain assessment and management programs within the service delivery and financing programs of the federal government.
- Proceed in cooperation with the IPRCC and the NIH's Pain Consortium and reach out to private-sector participants as appropriate.
- Involve the appropriate agencies and entities.
- Include ongoing efforts to enhance public awareness about the nature of chronic pain and the role of self-care in its management.

The IPRCC recognized the need to create a National Pain Strategy Task Force in order to execute the elements of the National Pain Strategy, which was conceptualized as represented in Fig. 13.3.[34]

---

[31] Ibid.

[32] IOM (Institute of Medicine). Relieving pain in America: a blueprint for transforming prevention, care, education, and research. Washington, DC: The National Academies Press; 2011.

[33] http://iprcc.nih.gov/National_Pain_Strategy/NPS_Strategy_Description.htm.   Accessed 2/19/2015.

[34] http://iprcc.nih.gov/National_Pain_Strategy/oversight_panel.htm, National Pain Strategy Task Force. Accessed 2/19/205.

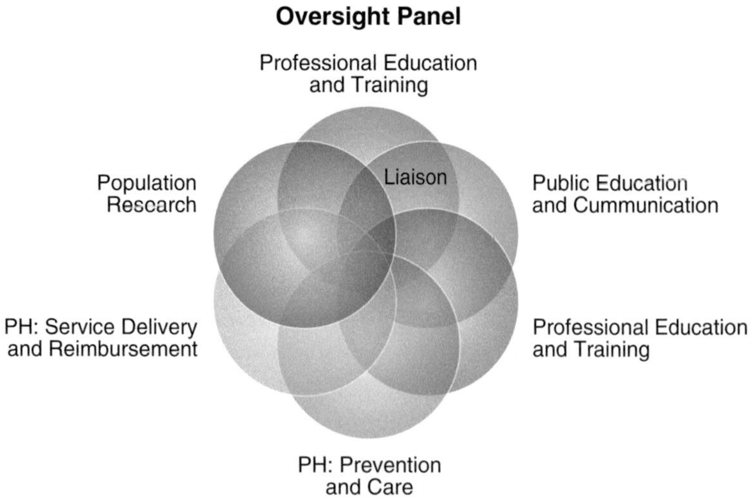

Oversight Panel

Professional Education
and Training

Population
Research

Liaison

Public Education
and Cummunication

PH: Service Delivery
and Reimbursement

Professional Education
and Training

PH: Prevention
and Care

Fig. 13.3 National Pain Strategy Task Force—Oversight Panel

IPRCC includes an oversight panel and working groups. The working groups include: (1) Professional Training, (2) Public Education and Communication, (3) Disparities, (4) Prevention and Care, (5) Service Delivery and Reimbursement, and (6) Population Research.

A Global Action Plan will derive from these activities. The issues will continue to be of concern to the various federal agencies actively involved in these discussions, with the NIH playing a major role in knowledge development. Clinicians concerned about pain management and pain medications whether for those with co-occurring disorders or otherwise will do well to check in at the NIH website from time to time.

In addition to the activities previously mentioned, the NIH also collects epidemiological data. The NIDA funds the Monitoring the Future (MTF) annual survey of 8th, 10th, and 12th graders to determine drug use patterns and activities of adolescents.[35]

Prescription drugs, including opioids, are a part of the MTF survey. OxyContin® and Vicodin® are two prescription opioids that are specifically addressed in the MTF survey. Figure 13.4 is an example of how trend data for OxyContin® could be charted using MTF data.

The National Institute of Drug Abuse offers an education course, "Opioid and Pain Management CMEs/CEs".[36] NIDA received funding from the White House ONDCP;

[35] Johnston LD, O'Malley PM, Miech RA, Bachman JG, Schulenberg J E. Monitoring the Future national survey results on drug use: 1975–2014: Overview, key findings on adolescent drug use. Ann Arbor: Institute for Social Research, the University of Michigan; 2015.

[36] http://www.drugabuse.gov/opioid-pain-management-cmesces, Opioid and Pain Management CMEs/CEs. Accessed 2/20/2015.

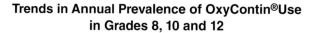

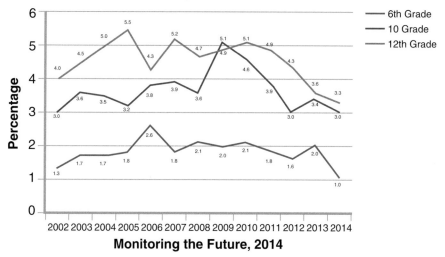

Fig. 13.4 How trend data for OxyContin® could be charted using MTF data

continuing education credits were provided by Medscape Education, the American Academy of Physician Assistants, the American Association of Nurse Practitioners, and the American Academy of Family Practitioners; both safe prescribing for pain and managing pain patients who abuse prescription drugs are covered.

13.5 The Centers for Disease Control and Prevention

The CDC is a major operating component of the Department of Health and Human Services and plays a major role in the federal activity around pain policy. Many clinicians are familiar with the CDC's role in addressing infectious diseases. However, the CDC maintains a broader role to protect America from health, safety, and security threats, both foreign and domestic.[37] Diseases that are chronic or acute, preventable or curable, or a product of human error or design fall within the area of concern of the CDC. The CDC's budget for fiscal year 2015 was $8.7 billion.[38] These funds are managed by over 20 Offices and Centers within the agency. The CDC is a member of the IPRCC of the federal government.

---

[37] http://www.cdc.gov/about/organization/mission.htm, Mission and Role of the CDC. Accessed 2/19/2015.

[38] http://www.cdc.gov/fmo/topic/Budget%20Information/FY2015-CDC-Operating-Plan-2-3-15. htm. Accessed 2/20/2015.

Of particular interest for those reading this book are the concerns of the CDC Office of Noncommunicable Diseases, Injury and Environmental Health, which includes the National Center for Injury Prevention and Control. In Fiscal Year 2015, CDC received from the Congress $20 million for prescription drug overdose prevention; this was targeted principally for prescription opioids and managed by the National Center for Injury Prevention and Control. The CDC sponsors the Youth Risk Behavior Surveillance (YRBS). The YRBS sampling consists of all regular public and private schools with students in at least one of grades 9–12 in the 50 states and the District of Columbia. The YRBS asks the following question about prescription drug use: "During your life, how many times have you taken a *prescription drug* (such as OxyContin, Percocet, Vicodin, codeine, Adderall, Ritalin, or Xanax) without a doctor's prescription?" While this question is not specific for prescription opioids, the data can be used to educate adolescents, parents, and professionals. In addition to the data, the CDC makes slides available for ready use.[39] Figure 13.5 is an example of the slides.

In addition to the YRBS data and accompanying slides, the CDC uses its Vital Signs mechanism to get the word out about opioid painkiller prescribing, providing infographics and recommendations to the public about the prescription opioid issue. Figure 13.6 is a screen shot of a recent CDC information effort.

CDC's National Center for Health Statistics collects data on severe headache or migraine, low back pain, and neck pain among adults aged 18 and over.[40] Additional data collected addresses the issue of drug poisoning deaths involving opioid analgesics.[41]

The CDC also offers a number of educational activities. These include information on arthritis pain,[42] primary care and opioid use, and balancing pain management and prescription opioid abuse.[43] CDC also published a policy impact document on prescription painkiller overdoses.[44]

In 2013, the CDC issued a Prescription Drug Overdose Status Report (PSR).[45] This report contained information about state pain clinic laws and the status of

---

[39] http://www.cdc.gov/healthyyouth/yrbs/slides/index.htm, Adolescent and School Health. Accessed 2/20/2015.

[40] http://www.cdc.gov/nchs/data/hus/2012/047.pdf, Severe headache or migraine, low back pain, and neck pain among adults aged 18 and over, by selected characteristics: United States, selected years 1997–2012. Accessed 2/20/2105.

[41] http://www.cdc.gov/nchs/data/hus/2012/032.pdf, Health, United States, 2012. Accessed 2/20/2015.

[42] http://www.cdc.gov/CDCTV/ArthritisPain/index.html. Accessed 2/20/2015.

[43] http://www.cdc.gov/primarycare/materials/opoidabuse/index.html. Accessed 2/20/2015.

[44] http://www.cdc.gov/homeandrecreationalsafety/rxbrief/, Policy Impact: Prescription Painkiller Overdoses. Accessed 2/22/2015.

[45] http://www.cdc.gov/psr/prescriptiondrug/index.html, Prescription Drug Overdose. Accessed 2/20/2015.

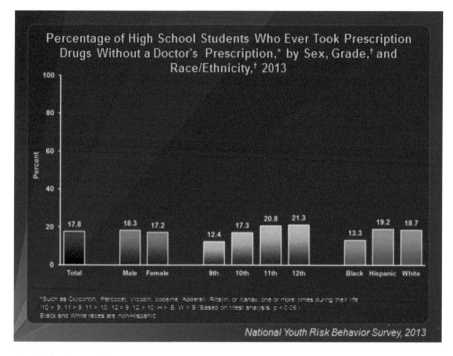

Fig. 13.5 Educational slides from the CDC

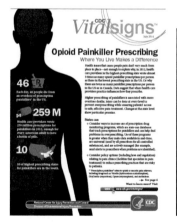
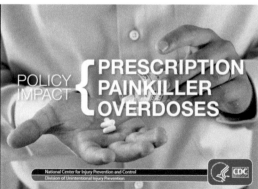

Fig. 13.6 Screen shot of a recent CDC information effort

PDMP following best practices. Of significance is the fact that the CDC website offered a state-by-state status report, permitting the public to assess their particular jurisdiction. In FY2016, the CDC requested $53.6 million to enhance its efforts to address drug overdose prevention with a focus on both illegal opioids and nonmedical use of legal opioids.[46] With the additional funds, CDC proposes to scale up existing state PDMP to improve clinical decision-making and to inform implementation of insurance innovations and evaluation of state-level policies. Should the Congress agree to it's FY2016 request, CDC also will scale up activities to improve patient safety by bringing together health systems and health departments to develop and track pain management and opioid prescribing quality measures in states with the highest prescribing rates.

13.6   Agency for Healthcare Research and Quality

The AHRQ's mission is to produce evidence to make healthcare safer, of higher quality, more accessible, equitable, and affordable. It works within the Department of Health and Human Services and with other partners. AHRQ's research priorities focus on: (1) improving healthcare quality and patient health outcomes; (2) producing evidence to make healthcare safer; (3) increasing accessibility by providing evidence on the effects of health insurance coverage expansions; and (4) improving healthcare affordability, efficiency, and cost transparency. AHRQ's FY2015 budget is $479 million and it has approximately 331 employees. AHRQ is a member of the IPRCC of the federal government.

AHRQ has created an Academy for Integrating Behavioral Health and Primary Care.[47] The Academy uses a web portal to organize critical subject matter, including information about pain, to identify the research to benefit those trying to change the healthcare system for the better. The Academy gathers research literature on integration and identifies opportunities for future research. The Academy maintains a searchable index to address critical issues. The pain literature compiled by the Academy addresses co-occurring disorders, such as pain and bipolar disorders, pain and depression, back pain and common mental disorders, and pain and substance use disorders in primary care.

In addition to the activities of the Academy, AHRQ released a report on the effectiveness and risks of long-term opioid treatment of chronic pain.[48] This report noted that evidence on long-term opioid therapy for chronic pain is very limited and suggests an increased risk of serious harms that appears to be dose-dependent. The report calls for more research to understand long-term benefits, risk of abuse and related outcomes, and effectiveness of different opioid-prescribing methods and risk mitigation strategies in the treatment of chronic pain.

---

[46] http://www.cdc.gov/fmo/topic/Budget%20Information/appropriations_budget_form_pdf/FY2016_CDC_CJ_FINAL.pdf. Accessed 2/15/2015.

[47] http://integrationacademy.ahrq.gov/aboutus.

[48] http://www.effectivehealthcare.ahrq.gov/ehc/products/557/1971/chronic-pain-opioid-treatment-report-141205.pdf. Accessed 2/20/2015.

13.7 Health Resources and Services Administration

The HRSA, another agency of the US Department of Health and Human Services, is the primary Federal agency for improving access to healthcare by strengthening the healthcare workforce, building healthy communities, and achieving health equity.[49] HRSA's programs provide healthcare to people who are geographically isolated and economically or medically vulnerable. This includes people living with HIV/AIDS, pregnant women, mothers, and their families and those in need of high-quality primary healthcare. HRSA also manages a drug-pricing program that requires drug manufacturers.

HRSA also supports the training of health professionals, the distribution of providers to areas where they are needed most, and improvements in healthcare delivery. HRSA has a budget of about $9 billion and has 1860 employees.

In addition to its funding for people living with HIV/AIDS and their medication need, HRSA supports nearly 1300 health centers that serve over 21 million people nationwide. Consequently, it has a substantial interest in pain management. HRSA also manages a drug-pricing discount program and is thus interested in formularies available to eligible healthcare organization/covered entities.[50]

HRSA has joined SAMHSA in sponsoring the Center for Integrated Health Solutions (CIHS).[51] CIHS focuses on the integration of primary and behavioral health services in order to address the needs of people with mental health and substance use disorders. CIHS offers a number of clinical practice activities, one of which is pain management. CIHS offers links to resources on the treatment of pain.[52] This includes education material.

13.8 Office of the National Drug Control Policy

The ONDCP advises the President on drug-control issues, coordinates drug-control activities and related funding across the federal government, and produces an annual National Drug Control Strategy. The 2014 National Drug Control Strategy includes a policy focus, "Preventing and addressing Prescription Drug Abuse."[53] This policy focus builds on ONDCP's 2011 Prescription Drug Abuse Prevention Plan, which created a framework for reducing prescription drug diversion and abuse.[54]

---

[49] http://www.hrsa.gov/about/index.html, About HRSA. Accessed 2/22/2015.

[50] http://www.hrsa.gov/opa/index.html, 340B Drug Pricing Program. Accessed 2/22/2015.

[51] http://www.integration.samhsa.gov/, SAMHSA-HRSA Center for Integrated Health Solutions. Accessed 2/22/2015.

[52] http://www.integration.samhsa.gov/clinical-practice/pain-management Accessed 2/22/2015.

[53] http://www.whitehouse.gov/sites/default/files/ondcp/policy-and-research/ndcs_2014.pdf, National Drug Control Strategy, 2014. Accessed 2/22/215.

[54] http://www.whitehouse.gov/sites/default/files/ondcp/issues-content/prescription-drugs/rx_abuse_plan.pdf, Epidemic: Responding to America's Prescription Drug Abuse Crisis. Accessed

ONDCP has the authority to convene federal agencies to develop policies around the misuse of controlled substances. There are four basic areas of policy that are incorporated in ONDCP's efforts: (1) Education of healthcare providers about opioid painkiller prescribing, (2) Expanding prescription drug-monitoring programs and promoting links among state systems and to electronic health records, (3) Increasing prescription return/take-back and disposal programs, and (4) Enforcement.

The education component of the National Strategy focuses less on appropriate pain management and more on the management of prescription of opioid, prescribing with the objective of reducing abuse and diversion. ONDCP has worked with the FDA, NIDA, SAMHSA, and education community to promote accessible educational opportunities toward that end.

The enforcement policy focus has four components: (1) Assisting States to Address Diversion and Pill Mills, (2) Driving Illegal Internet Pharmacies Out of Business, (3) Cracking Down on Rogue Pain Clinics that do not follow appropriate prescription practices, and (4) Overdose prevention and intervention. On the fourth point of the enforcement policy focus, ONDCP joined SAMHSA in the release of an opioid overdose toolkit.[55]

Despite the primary focus on the misuse of prescription opioid analgesics, it is clear that the ONDCP considers appropriate pain management an important goal. The use and misuse of opioid medications are intertwined, and the ability to appropriately use opioids for the treatment of pain from the federal perspective is tied to the ability to recognize when such medications are no longer being used in a clinically responsible manner.

13.9   Drug Enforcement Administration

The DEA's mission is to enforce the controlled substance laws and regulations of the United States as they apply to illegal and legal substances.[56] In the context of this chapter, the DEA's authority pertains to the manufacture, distribution, and dispensing of legally produced controlled substances. Clinicians who prescribe controlled substances for the treatment of pain are well aware that they must be registered with the DEA and that violations of the controlled substances act (CSA) may result in criminal penalties. In addition, those who treat opioid-dependent individuals with buprenorphine know that they must have an x-number in order to prescribe. The DEA has police powers which are used to investigate suspected violations of the CSA. Individuals who meet criteria for probable cause of violating the CSA may be arrested.

The DEA does not on its own determine that the use of a particular opioid is clinically appropriate; that is left to state authorities and to the medical community norms

---

2/22/2015.

[55] http://store.samhsa.gov/product/Opioid-Overdose-Prevention-Toolkit-Updated-2014/SMA14-4742. Accessed 2/22/2015.

[56] http://www.dea.gov/about/mission.shtml, DEA Mission Statement. Accessed 2/22/2015.

in the jurisdiction in which the medical standards are possibly being violated. The DEA's Office of Diversion Control plays a critical role registering clinicians and working with federal agencies about the appropriate use of controlled substances.

The DEA publishes lists of controlled substances schedules. DEA also publishes a list of doctors in which the DEA was involved in investigations that resulted in the arrest and prosecution of a physician registrant. The DEA works with the FDA and the NIH to determine the appropriate schedule of a drug.

The DEA works with ONDCP, the FDA, the NIH, SAMHSA, the VA, the DoD, HRSA, and CMS, in various capacities. The DEA also works with state and tribal authorities. It also conducts annual National Prescription Drug Take-Back Day.

The vignette at the beginning of this Chapter captures the close collaboration between federal authorities and state and local authorities in addressing questionable practices of licensed practitioners in the community. Clinicians should be aware that appropriate behavior in the treatment of pain requires good record keeping and informed clinical strategies.

In summary, the DEA's role in the management of pain is to make sure that any controlled substances being used for pain are being used in a medically necessary manner. When it becomes apparent that the CSA is being violated or that controlled substances are being used gratuitously, the DEA investigates and prosecutes.

13.10   Indian Health Services, Department of Veterans Affairs, and Department of Defense

These three federal entities provide direct patient care to their targeted populations, maintain formularies that include prescription opioids for analgesia, and employ direct service providers who decide when, where, and how much pain medications are to be prescribed and dispensed. Consequently, they have a vested interest in monitoring and influencing federal policies regarding pain management, both acute and chronic.

These entities operate and maintain clinics and hospitals, allow for services to be provided outside of their networks, and function within a broad array of state and federal laws and regulations.

13.11   Indian Health Services

The IHS is a system of healthcare within the USDHHS for individuals who are members of the 566 federally recognized American Indian and Alaska Natives in the United States. [57] The Department of the Interior's Bureau of Indian Affairs maintains the list of eligible Indian entities.[58]

---

[57] http://www.ihs.gov/, Indian Health Service. Accessed 2/22/2015.

[58] http://www.bia.gov/cs/groups/webteam/documents/document/idc1-029026.pdf, Department of the Interior, Bureau of Indian Affairs, Indian Entities Recognized and Eligible to Receive Services from the United States Bureau of Indian Affairs, Federal Register, Vol. 80, No. 9, January 14, 2015, pp. 1942–1948.

The IHS maintains a strategy for Pain Management that includes (1) proper patient assessment, (2) substance screening, (3) treatment planning, (4) monitoring, (5) informed consent, (6) safe storage of medications, (7) disposal, and (8) legal considerations for prescribers.[59] On the IHS website, providers are offered a range of resources to be taken into consideration for the management of pain.

13.12 Department of Defense and the Department of Veterans Affairs

While they are separate Departments, the DoD and the Department of Veterans Affairs (VA) have been working closely together on the matter of pain management. Following that work, they have developed websites, guidelines, and other resources to benefit patients and professionals functioning within the umbrella of their respective administrative authority.

In March of 2011, the DoD issued a memorandum for a Policy for Comprehensive Pain Management to the Assistant Secretaries of the Army, Navy, and Air Force.[60] The memorandum outlined policies for (1) comprehensive pain management, (2) pain assessment, (3) pain treatment and management, and (4) pain research. This memorandum followed the activities of a joint taskforce involving the DoD and the VA.[61]

In addition, the DoD and the Department of Veterans Affairs (VA) benefit from the activities of the Defense and Veterans Center for Integrative Pain Management which works to develop consensus recommendations for the military and the VA for the improvement in pain management, practice, education, and research.[62]

DoD and the VA working with professional organizations developed clinical practice guidelines for a number of medical conditions including pain.[63] They developed guidelines for (1) opioid therapy for chronic pain, (2) lower back pain, and (3) postoperative pain. They developed fact sheets for such phenomenon as managing the side effects of opioid therapy.[64]

---

[59] http://www.ihs.gov/painmanagement/, Pain Management. Accessed 2/23/2015.

[60] Policy for Comprehensive Pain Management from the Assistant Secretary of Defense, March 30, 2011. Accessed 2/23/2015 via google.

[61] http://www.regenesisbio.com/pdfs/journal/pain_management_task_force_report.pdf, Pain Management Task Force, Final Report May 2010. Accessed 2/23/2015.

[62] http://www.dvcipm.org/, Defense & Veterans Center for Integrative Pain Management. Accessed 2/23/2015.

[63] http://www.healthquality.va.gov/, VA/DoD Clinical Practice Guidelines. Accessed 2/23/2015.

[64] http://www.healthquality.va.gov/guidelines/Pain/cot/OpiodManagingSideEffectsFactSheet 23May2013v1HiResPrint.pdf, Managing Side Effects and Complications of Opioid Therapy for Chronic Pain. Accessed 2/23/2015.

13.13   Conclusion

The federal government has a substantial interest in pain management policy. That interest spans a broad spectrum of policy concerns from deciding what medications can be on the market through the FDA's activities, to regulating who can prescribe controlled substances through the DEA's activities, to pursuing research into the best approaches to pain management through the activities of NIH Pain Consortium, to promulgating guidelines and offering educational opportunities such as SAMHSA, HRSA, and the VA/DoD.

Anyone interested in pain management from either a clinical perspective or a policy perspective can find resources, often free of charge, on a number of the websites sponsored by agencies of the federal government.

Part III
Best Practices and Practice Models

Chapter 14
Multidisciplinary Pain Clinics

Andrea R. Diulio, Michael I. Demidenko, and Travis I. Lovejoy

14.1 Introduction

In the United States, 100 million adults suffer from chronic pain [1] and approximately one third of primary care patients are diagnosed with chronic non-cancer pain [2]. In recent years, opioid therapy has been a common treatment modality for chronic pain [3] and the rates of opioid prescribing nearly doubled between 2000 and 2010 [4]. Yet overreliance on these medications may led to pharmacologic tolerance, opioid-induced hyperalgesia [5], and in some cases abuse of opioids [6]. Additionally, a significant proportion of people with opioid use disorder experience chronic pain. Within opioid substitution programs, as many as 60 % of patients are diagnosed with chronic pain [7]. Considering the potential iatrogenic consequences of long-term opioid regimens for chronic pain, opioid therapy may be inappropriate for many individuals with opioid use disorder, necessitating alternative analgesic pharmacotherapies and other non-pharmacologic pain treatment approaches.

A.R. Diulio, Ph.D.
Mental Health & Clinical Neurosciences, VA Portland Health Care System,
3710 SW U.S. Veterans Hospital Road, Mail Code: P3MHDC, Portland, OR 97239, USA
e-mail: andrea.diulio1@va.gov

M.I. Demidenko, B.S. • T.I. Lovejoy, Ph.D., M.P.H. (✉)
Center to Improve Veteran Involvement in Care, VA Portland Health Care System,
3710 SW U.S. Veterans Hospital Road, Mail Code: R&D 66, Portland, OR 97239, USA
e-mail: travis.lovejoy@va.gov

© Springer International Publishing Switzerland 2016   177
A.M. Matthews, J.C. Fellers (eds.), *Treating Comorbid Opioid Use Disorder in Chronic Pain*, DOI 10.1007/978-3-319-29863-4_14

14.2 Comorbid Chronic Pain and Opioid Use Disorders

Chronic pain is associated with psychological distress, decreased mobility, obesity, limited physical function, social isolation, financial strain, and chronic disability [8]. Many of the factors that exacerbate chronic pain are also related to increased vulnerability to abuse opioids [9]. This has been supported by studies suggesting that the majority of patients involved in opioid replacement therapy have also been diagnosed with chronic pain [7], and in some instances, patients first developed an opioid use disorder after being prescribed opioid medication for the treatment of pain [10]. Additionally, inadequately managed pain in patients with an opioid use disorder has been associated with increased risk for continued opioid misuse [11]. Tailored treatment plans for comorbid chronic pain and opioid use disorder may thus need to simultaneously address the entire sequelae of chronic pain and addiction.

14.3 Challenges to Managing Chronic Pain in Patients with Comorbid Opioid Use Disorders

Management of chronic pain often includes the use of opioid medication. Precautions for the use of chronic opioid therapy should be employed with any patient with a history of an opioid use disorder due to the heightened risk for abuse. Patients who meet criteria for an opioid use disorder are at heightened risk for chronic pain relative to patients without a history of opioid use disorder (e.g. [7]). Among individuals receiving methadone maintenance treatment, up to 60 % are diagnosed with a chronic pain condition (e.g. [12,13]) and those who report abuse of prescription opioids in the past month are more likely to endorse chronic pain [14]. Unfortunately, few patients receiving opioid substitution therapy receive concurrent non-opioid pain management interventions [15]. Thus, some patients who over-medicate with opioids to manage pain may not be addressing a root cause of their opioid addiction. These patients may also be poor responders to singular pain treatment approaches. Studies indicate that individuals with concurrent chronic pain and opioid use disorders are at a heightened risk for poor pain treatment response, including continued functional impairment, maintenance of illicit substance use, and fatality (e.g. [12,16–18]).

The poor outcomes for this population may be due to the unique challenge of simultaneously treating two potentially debilitating disorders. This challenge is further complicated by the seemingly discrepant treatment objectives for each disorder. Historically, treatment for opioid use disorder intends to restore functioning by reducing drug use, while pain management attempts to restore functioning through analgesia [19]. When multiple providers, without an agreed upon treatment plan and objectives, treat the same patient for comorbid opioid use disorder and chronic pain, tension might arise due to the differing treatment approaches for each condition. Similarly, evidence suggests that if the burden of pain treatment falls upon a single provider, concern regarding the potential abuse of prescribed opioids and the lack of definitive clinical guidelines may lead to the under-treatment of pain in this population [20]. Although hesitation by providers to employ pain management interventions with this population has been documented, evidence suggests that patients with opioid use disorders who receive pain treatment endorse significant pain-related improvements [15].

14.4 Clinical Guidelines for the Management of Chronic Pain in Patients with Co-occurring Opioid Use Disorder

The American Pain Society and the American Academy of Pain Medicine developed a Pain Medicine Opioids Guidelines Panel to formulate recommendations regarding the long-term use of opioids to manage chronic pain. Due to the risk of aberrant drug-related behaviors, they propose intense monitoring be conducted for patients with a comorbid substance use disorder, in conjunction with behavioral therapies, and that chronic opioid therapy be discontinued if there is evidence of diversion or medication noncompliance [21]. The guidelines specify that although opioid medication may be risky for some patients with a history of substance abuse, it is not presumed that opioid medication is inappropriate treatment for all patients with a past history of a substance use disorder. Specific recommendations include frequent and intense pain reassessment to further improve pain-related outcomes, regular monitoring, including urine drug screens, limited prescription quantities, consultation or co-management with a mental health or substance use disorder provider, and use of prescription monitoring programs, if available, to identify when an individual is acquiring opioid medication from multiple providers (e.g. [22,23]). In addition, motivational counseling may be indicated to regularly reinforce a patient's motivation to adhere to the prescribed treatment plan, despite ongoing triggers to misuse or abuse substances [24]. These guidelines highlight the importance of a multidisciplinary approach to pain management in patients with opioid and other substance use disorders, as it may be unmanageable for a single provider or discipline to adequately address all aspects of chronic pain in patients with comorbid opioid use disorder.

14.5 Models of Pain Treatment

The growing demand for pain management has resulted in greater awareness to treating chronic pain and a variety of treatment models. Pain treatment approaches fall along a continuum from least to most comprehensive. Typically, a patient is initially prescribed analgesic pharmacotherapy through primary care, and if unresponsive to this treatment, is referred to one or more specialty services. The most basic treatment model is that of a single service clinic or modality-oriented clinic. This type of outpatient clinic provides a single treatment for pain, but often lacks the personnel and clinical expertise to provide a comprehensive pain assessment or pain treatment plan. Services within these clinics vary greatly, but examples include an acupuncture, biofeedback, physical therapy, or occupational therapy clinic. A single service clinic may be appropriate and most valuable for individuals living with mild forms of chronic pain, who have yet to develop significant pain-related disability. For patients whose pain is not adequately managed through a single treatment modality, more comprehensive pain treatment approaches may be required.

A more complex model of care is that of a pain clinic, which provides pain interventions that often target one pain condition, such as headache or back pain. Pain clinics may employ individuals from more than one discipline and can provide more comprehensive assessment and management of chronic pain than what is available in single service clinics. Nevertheless, pain clinics are often limited in the variety of services provided. Pain clinics commonly refer patients to outside providers for services that are not available within the clinic. This can result in fragmented patient care due to inconsistent communication and conflicting treatment orientations between providers in different clinics or healthcare systems. Patients also face the burden of keeping appointments across multiple clinics that can sometimes be geographically distant.

Multidisciplinary Pain Clinics (MPCs) are comprehensive, specialized inpatient or outpatient clinics composed of multiple pain-related disciplines. Clinical services often include physical therapy, occupational therapy, physical medicine and rehabilitation, pain education, and psychological/behavioral pain interventions. By providing global and intensive assessment and treatment interventions, MPCs are equipped to treat moderate-to-severe chronic pain that has resulted in diminished psychosocial functioning. The Commission on Accreditation of Rehabilitation Facilities (CARF) is the international accrediting body for MPCs. At the time of this writing, according to the CARF website (http://www.carf.org/home/), there are currently 69 accredited MPCs in the United States [25]. MPCs strive to improve psychosocial functioning and global life satisfaction by targeting the various factors that are maintaining or exacerbating the impairments one experiences as a result of chronic pain.

14.6   Disciplines Represented Within Multidisciplinary Pain Clinics

Significant variability exists across MPCs in the combination of pain treatments used for individual patients. This may partly be due to the notion that MPCs do not follow a single protocol to be used for all patients. Rather providers from various disciplines collaborate to identify what interventions may be most effective in addressing the unique impairments for each patient [26]. MPC staff typically comprise Physical Medicine and Rehabilitation Physicians, Nurses, Psychologists, Physical and Recreational Therapists, Social Workers, and Pharmacists. Some MPCs also include a Neurosurgeon, Orthospine Surgeon, Interventional Pain Specialist, and a Patient Advocate [27].

14.7 Advantages of Multidisciplinary Pain Clinics

The diversity of staff within an MPC naturally lends itself to a biopsychosocial conceptualization, assessment, and treatment of chronic pain. A biopsychosocial model of care assumes that a disorder is impacted by dynamic physiological, psychological, and social factors that interact to perpetuate, or worsen, symptoms [28]. This approach has widely replaced that of the dated biomedical model for chronic pain [29], which conceptualizes pain as solely affected by physical processes and does not consider the impact of social or psychological factors on the pain experience.

Potential contributions to a patient's pain that should be assessed include pain and general medical history, functional impairments, current and prior medications, past treatment compliance, previously tried procedures and interventions, legal history, social development, psychiatric history, and substance use history [30]. Due to the complexity of forming such a holistic conceptualization, the use of a multidisciplinary team is paramount. Involving experts from various disciplines in the assessment process helps to ensure that all relevant information is obtained. An MPC also ameliorates the burden of a single provider conducting the complete evaluation and ensures that clinicians only assess areas in which they have expertise.

Treatment within MPCs also applies a biopsychosocial approach. The application of multimodal evidence-based interventions to simultaneously target pain reduction and functional restoration aids in addressing the multiple contributors to a patient's pain. Effective interventions for comorbid opioid use disorder and chronic pain may include medication, substance use treatment, behavioral interventions, psychotherapy, weight loss, physical mobility, and conditioning [31]. Bearing in mind the assorted interventions necessary to improve functioning, it is vital that the various providers regularly collaborate to determine when modifications to the treatment plan should be implemented. Additionally, MPCs facilitate careful monitoring of the treatment regimen. This allows for input to be received from all disciplines, and modifications to be coordinated, before changes to the treatment plan are made.

14.8 Treatment Efficacy and Cost-Effectiveness

Considering the large number of patients who seek pain management and the rates of comorbidity between chronic pain and opioid use disorder, efficient and economical pain rehabilitation is needed. Unfortunately, conventional single service medical treatments have not demonstrated consistent efficacy or cost-effectiveness [32]. MPCs, on the other hand, have demonstrated superior outcomes across a number of studies and may produce long-term systemic cost benefits by reducing disability, lost work productivity, and the frequency with which high-cost services (e.g., emergency department visits and inpatient hospitalizations) are utilized by patients [32]. A review of evidence-based treatments for chronic pain demonstrated the efficacy of MPCs and identified that annual medical costs following treatment by an MPC were reduced by over 68% [32]. Further, the review found that more than two thirds of individuals treated by an MPC returned to work, compared to a little over one quarter of patients treated by single service models. These findings suggest that MPCs have a smaller economical cost in regard to lifetime disability and healthcare utilization, despite the increased cost at the onset of treatment.

14.9   Challenges/Considerations of Multidisciplinary Pain Clinics

Despite research to suggest the superiority and long-term cost-effectiveness of MPCs, there are unique challenges facing patients and providers who wish to utilize a multidisciplinary team. There are multiple stakeholders who impact healthcare access and barriers. For chronic pain, these stakeholders include, but are not limited to, the patient who is most likely interested in symptom management, third-party payers who may be interested in reducing future treatment utilization, and employers and worker compensation boards that are interested in closing claims by returning workers back to meaningful employment. The diverse players impacting the assessment and treatment of chronic pain can create a complex and politicized dimension to treatment.

Unfortunately, due to common cost-containment policies of third-party payers [32], many patients are unable to initiate treatment with an MPC. Moreover, the number of MPCs appears to be decreasing. The number of CARF-accredited MPCs in the United States is steadily decreasing from 210 in 1998, 84 in 2005 [33], to currently 69. The conflict between what has been found to be most effective for treating pain, the constraints of third-party payers, and the limitations of individual providers may prevent many patients from receiving the gold standard of evidence-based pain treatment and patients may, as a result, experience suffering from either untreated or undertreated pain. This in turn may lead to or perpetuate existing patterns of opioid misuse or abuse.

14.10   Conclusion

There is growing concern regarding the treatment of chronic pain and the associated risks of long-term opioid therapy, due to the threat of opioid misuse and abuse. The risk of iatrogenic effects of opioid therapy is greater for patients with a comorbid substance use disorder. Various treatment modalities exist for managing chronic pain, but considering the complex presentation of patients with comorbid chronic pain and opioid use disorder, MPCs may be the most appropriate pain treatment modality to address the complex and multifaceted needs of this patient population. Advantages of utilizing an MPC for this population include a comprehensive conceptualization of the biopsychosocial factors that influence pain and illicit opioid use behaviors, as well as coordinating various interventions to simultaneously target those factors. However, given the initial upfront cost associated with MPC treatment and reimbursement challenges in a third-party payer healthcare system, MPCs may not be available to many patients who could benefit from these services.

References

1. Institute of Medicine. Relieving pain in America: a blueprint for transforming prevention, care, education, and research. Washington, DC: The National Academies Press; 2011.
2. Johannes CB, Le TK, Zhou X, Johnston JA, Dworkin RH. The prevalence of chronic pain in United States adults: results of an Internet-based survey. J Pain. 2010;11(11):1230–9.
3. Mosher HJ, Krebs EE, Carrel M, Kaboli PJ, Vander Weg MW, Lund BC. Trends in prevalent and incident opioid receipt: an observational study in Veterans Health Administration 2004–2012. J Gen Intern Med. 2014;1–8.
4. Daubresse M, Chang HY, Yu Y, Viswanathan S, Shah ND, Stafford RS, Kruszewski SP, Alexander GC. Ambulatory diagnosis and treatment of nonmalignant pain in the United States, 2000-2010. Med Care. 2013;51(10):870–8.
5. Mao J. Opioid-induced abnormal pain sensitivity: implications in clinical opioid therapy. Pain. 2002;100(3):213–7.
6. Sullivan MD, Howe CQ. Opioid therapy for chronic pain in the United States: promises and perils. Pain. 2013;154:S94 S100.
7. Jamison RN, Kauffman J, Katz NP. Characteristics of methadone maintenance patients with chronic pain. J Pain Symptom Manage. 2000;19(1):53–62.
8. Stewart WF, Ricci JA, Chee E, Morganstein D, Lipton R. Lost productive time and cost due to common pain conditions in the US workforce. JAMA. 2003;290(18):2443–54.
9. Pud D, Cohen D, Lawental E, Eisenberg E. Opioids and abnormal pain perception: New evidence from a study of chronic opioid addicts and healthy subjects. Drug Alcohol Depend. 2006;82(3):218–23.
10. Tsui JI, Herman DS, Kettavong M, Alford D, Anderson BJ, Stein MD. Physician introduction to opioids for pain among patients with opioid dependence and depressive symptoms. J Subst Abuse Treat. 2010;39(4):378–83.
11. Tsui JI, Cheng DM, Coleman SM, Blokhina E, Bridden C, Krupitsky E, Samet JH. Pain is associated with heroin use over time in HIV-infected Russian drinkers. Addiction. 2013;108(10):1779–87.
12. Barry DT, Beitel M, Garnet B, Joshi D, Rosenblum A, Schottenfeld RS. Relations among psychopathology, substance use, and physical pain experiences in methadone-maintained patients. J Clin Psychiatry. 2009;70(9):1213.
13. Dhingra L, Masson C, Perlman DC, Seewald RM, Katz J, McKnight C, Homel P, Wald E, Jordan AE, Young C, Portenoy RK. Epidemiology of pain among outpatients in methadone maintenance treatment programs. Drug Alcohol Depend. 2013;128(1):161–5.
14. Rosenblum A, Parrino M, Schnoll SH, Fong C, Maxwell C, Cleland CM, Magura S, Haddox JD. Prescription opioid abuse among enrollees into methadone maintenance treatment. Drug Alcohol Depend. 2007;90(1):64–71.
15. Dunn KE, Brooner RK, Clark MR. Severity and interference of chronic pain in methadone-maintained outpatients. Pain Med. 2014;15(9):1540–8.
16. Bohnert AS, Ilgen MA, Trafton JA, Kerns RD, Eisenberg A, Ganoczy D, Blow FC. Trends and regional variation in opioid overdose mortality among Veterans Health Administration patients, fiscal year 2001 to 2009. Clin J Pain. 2014;30(7):605–12.
17. Trafton JA, Oliva EM, Horst DA, Minkel JD, Humphreys K. Treatment needs associated with pain in substance use disorder patients: implications for concurrent treatment. Drug Alcohol Depend. 2004;73(1):23–31.

18. Xiaobin C, Zunyou W, Li L, Lin P, Keming R, Changhe W, Wei L, Wenyuan Y, Jianhua L, McGoogan JM, and for the National Methadone Maintenance Treatment Program Working Group. Mortality among methadone maintenance clients in China: a six-year cohort study. PLoS One. 2013;8(12):e82476.
19. Berg KM, Arnsten JH, Sacajiu G, Karasz A. Providers' experiences treating chronic pain among opioid-dependent drug users. J Gen Intern Med. 2009;24(4):482–8.
20. Eyler EC. Chronic and acute pain and pain management for patients in methadone maintenance treatment. Am J Addict. 2013;22(1):75–83.
21. Chou R, Fanciullo GJ, Fine PG, Adler JA, Ballantyne JC, Davies P, Donovan MI, Fishbain DA, Foley KM, Fudin J, Gilson AM, Kelter A, Mauskop A, O'Connor PG, Passik SD, Pasternak GW, Portenoy RK, Rich BA, Roberts RG, Todd KH, Miaskowski C, and the American Pain Society-American Academy of Pain Medicine Opioids Guidelines Panel. Clinical guidelines for the use of chronic opioid therapy in chronic noncancer pain. J Pain. 2009;10(2):113–30.
22. Joranson DE, Carrow GM, Ryan KM, Schaefer L, Gilson AM, Good P, Eadie J, Peine S, Dahl JL. Pain management and prescription monitoring. J Pain Symptom Manage. 2002;23(3): 231–8.
23. Wu SM, Compton P, Bolus R, Schieffer B, Pham Q, Baria A, Van Vort W, Davis F, Shekelle P, Naliboff BD. The addiction behaviors checklist: validation of a new clinician-based measure of inappropriate opioid use in chronic pain. J Pain Symptom Manage. 2006;32(4):342–51.
24. Jamison RN, Edwards RR. Risk factor assessment for problematic use of opioids for chronic pain. Clin Neuropsychol. 2013;27(1):60–80.
25. CARF Provider search (n.d.). Retrieved on April 10, 2015 from: http://www.carf.org/advancedProviderSearch.aspx
26. Jeffery MM, Butler M, Stark A, Kane RL. Multidisciplinary pain programs for chronic noncancer pain. Technical Brief No. 8. (Prepared by Minnesota Evidence-based Practice Center under Contract No. 290-07-10064-I.) AHRQ Publication No. 11-EHC064-EF. Rockville: Agency for Healthcare Research and Quality; 2011.
27. Pain Clinic Guidelines (n.d.). Retrieved March 13, 2015 from http://www.iasp-pain.org/education/content.aspx?itemnumber=1471
28. Engel GL. The clinical application of the biopsychosocial model. J Med Philos. 1981;6(2):101–24.
29. Gatchel RJ, Peng YB, Peters ML, Fuchs PN, Turk DC. The biopsychosocial approach to chronic pain: scientific advances and future directions. Psychol Bull. 2007;133(4):581.
30. Malaty A, Sabharwal J, Lirette LS, Chaiban G, Eissa H, Tolba R. How to assess a new patient for a multidisciplinary chronic pain rehabilitation program: a review article. Ochsner J. 2014;14(1):96–100.
31. Liebschutz J, Beers D, Lange A. Managing chronic pain in patients with opioid dependence. Curr Treat Options Psychiatry. 2014;1(2):204–23.
32. Gatchel RJ, Okifuji A. Evidence-based scientific data documenting the treatment and cost-effectiveness of comprehensive pain programs for chronic nonmalignant pain. J Pain. 2006;7(11):779–93.
33. Schatman ME (2006). The demise of multidisciplinary pain management clinics? A potential strategy for addressing the conflicting ethos of business-oriented insurance and corporate healthcare versus the ends and means of right and morally sound patient care. January 1. Retrieved from http://www.practicalpainmanagement.com/resources/practice-management/demise-multidisciplinary-pain-management-clinics?page=0,4

Chapter 15
The Role of the Emergency Department in Chronic Pain Treatment

Sean W. Moore and Jeffrey Freeman

15.1 Introduction

Emergency physicians are presented with a unique opportunity when dealing with patients presenting with chronic pain. In emergency departments (EDs), up to 70 % of patients have pain as part of their presenting symptom [1, 2], and it has been estimated that about 11 % of all visits have an exacerbation of chronic pain as a chief complaint [3]. Up to 33 % of the American population will experience chronic pain each year.

There are many barriers to the effective management of patients with acute exacerbations of chronic pain (AECP). While patients often present when they are no longer responding to their usual medication regimen, many physicians are hesitant to prescribe opioids. This reluctance may be due to fears of causing, perpetuating, or worsening addiction, lack of knowledge about pain and its treatment, or having negative views about patients with chronic pain [4]. This, coupled with the lack of rapport or knowledge of prior treatment efforts, makes clinical care difficult in many interactions. Indeed, many patients in chronic pain who have been on a long-standing opioid regimen may be addicted or have developed tolerance or maladaptive behaviors. To further complicate matters, patients whose pain is undertreated can exhibit the phenomenon of pseudoaddiction, a condition where the patient is

S.W. Moore, M.D., C.M., F.R.C.P.C., F.A.C.E.P. (✉)
University of Ottawa, Ottawa, ON, Canada, K1N 6N5

Northern Ontario School of Medicine, Emergency Department, Lake of the Woods District Hospital, 21 Sylvan Street, Kenora, ON, Canada, P9N3W7
e-mail: seanwmoore@mac.com

J. Freeman, M.D. (✉)
Department of Emergency Medicine, University of Ottawa, Faculty of Medicine, 451 Smyth Road, Kenora, ON, Canada, P9N3W7
e-mail: Jfreeman@toh.on.ca

© Springer International Publishing Switzerland 2016   185
A.M. Matthews, J.C. Fellers (eds.), *Treating Comorbid Opioid Use Disorder in Chronic Pain*, DOI 10.1007/978-3-319-29863-4_15

exhibiting all the classic drug-seeking behaviors, such as increased frequency of ED usage and aggressively pursuing opioids. These behaviors occur because the patient is still in pain and they cease after the patient's pain is adequately controlled [5].

Chronic nonmalignant pain syndromes can have acute exacerbations of discomfort above and beyond their normal pain levels or may not have adequate pain control at baseline. These patients may be on chronic opioids and present to the ED for relief of their exacerbation because either they do not have access to their usual primary care provider or pain specialist or they simply do not have any continuity of care. Despite the widespread prevalence of this problem, there is a scarcity of studies about the treatment of AECP in EDs, with few guidelines or protocols about how to treat these patients humanely and effectively, and there is usually no established method for ensuring provider accountability for appropriate care [6].

The first task of the emergency physician often focuses on determining whether an acute medical condition has developed. Pain from chronic stable conditions may fluctuate or flare, or the chronic condition may be progressing. In addition, acute pain may be superimposed on the setting of a chronic painful condition. Consider the example of a patient with chronic non-cancer neck pain who, after receiving local trigger point injection, develops increased pain. The differential diagnosis of the new pain includes the possibility of spinal epidural abscess, postinjection pain, skeletal muscle injury, or simply failure of the procedure [7]. It is the complexity of differentiating an AECP from a new complication that makes the management of patients with chronic pain so challenging. Nonetheless, a careful history and physical examination will usually guide need for further diagnostic testing.

Many patients with chronic pain have clearly identified underlying etiology for their pain including progressive conditions such as cancer, multiple sclerosis, and sickle cell disease. It is often possible to decide *with the patient* whether extensive or invasive diagnostic tests are warranted. The emergency physician must decide how to treat symptoms until diagnostic testing is complete, as well as make management decisions once established that this is an AECP. Medications used for chronic pain include opioids, non-steroidal anti-inflammatory drugs (NSAIDS) as well as diverse agents including antidepressants, anticonvulsants, local anesthetics, NMDA receptor antagonists, steroids, and numerous other adjunctive therapies, which may help during an AECP [8].

15.2   What Is an Acute Exacerbation of Chronic Pain?

Chronic pain is difficult to define, but all chronic pain starts as acute pain. Despite the link to acute episodes, the pathways by which acute pain results in chronic pain remain elusive. The etiology of acute pain is often physical damage to nerve endings or an active inflammatory process sending pain signals to the central nervous system. These signals are an adaptive response; they give the patient an immediate motivation to remove the noxious stimuli. But, depending on the insult or injury, it is possible for acute pain to continue for months, and in many cases, there is no evidence to describe how much time it will take to heal. It is becoming more common to define chronic pain as pain that lasts beyond that which is normally expected for a particular injury [9]. When there is no longer a readily apparent etiology, chronic pain has set in and this no longer appears to serve any adaptive response. The experience of pain is certainly a physiologically complex phenomenon with multiple positive and negative feedback systems to modulate the signals. Chronic pain is now believed to be a result of remodeling or maladaptive changes to nociceptive pathways.

Breakthrough pain in patients with cancer has been more extensively studied and has been defined as a "transitory increase in pain in a patient to greater than moderate intensity which occurred on a baseline pain of moderate intensity or less" [10]. Cancer patients frequently have continuity of care with a multidisciplinary approach to their analgesia and a team composed of physicians (oncologists, pain specialists, and generalists), nurses, therapists, and psychosocial support. The team manages the patient's baseline pain with modifications in analgesia doses and dosing intervals; breakthrough pain is frequently treated with short-acting opioids to supplement daily doses of long-acting opioids. In general, the approach to patients with cancer should actively involve their specialists. In this text, we will focus on the AECP in chronic non-cancer pain, which may have a prevalence as high as 75 % [11].

Visits to the ED may occur due to multiple precipitants. Patients with AECP frequently present to the ED with multiple medical issues. The patient may simply not be receiving enough pain medication and is therefore undertreated, also known as oligoanalgesia. Perhaps the patient may have run out of their medications early, maybe due to taking more than prescribed because their pain is not well-controlled and is unable to get another prescription. These are prescribing and access to health-care issues. There is often the fear that the patient may be misusing their medications or distributing them for monetary gain. Finally, there is the possibility that this is a new medical issue, unrelated to their usual chronic pain. The best way to distinguish between all of these various reasons is taking a detailed history. It is important to ask the patient about what they believe is the cause of this visit and then to work with them to find a solution that will solve the problem at least until they can get back to their primary care physician or pain specialist.

15.3 Treatment of AECP Patients

15.3.1 Managing Patient Expectations

The patient's goals for their current emergency department visit must be addressed. It is important to help set realistic expectations for these patients. Most patients who have chronic pain have dealt with physicians frequently and have been frustrated by aspects of their care. One should ask specific questions to understand the reason for the immediate triggering event that led to the emergency visit. Visits may be precipitated by worsening pain, but can also be generated by suggestions from friends or physicians. In general, their goals are usually clear though often idealistic, and it is worth the time and effort to explore their expectations in an open discussion prior to aggressive treatment or diagnostic interventions. The goals for many patients fall into only a few categories: finding medications that are more effective for their pain (which may include stopping ineffective medications), having explanations for the cause of their pain, being referred to specialists or pain services, or referrals for physical therapies or special tests. In some cases, expectations may be unrealistic, include having immediate surgery, being admitted to discover the etiology of their pain, or achieving complete pain relief. Many patients with chronic pain have primary care physicians, but may report inadequate availability or dissatisfaction with responsiveness or sensitivity. It is well worth exploring the goals of the emergency visit with the patient before defining mutually the terms of success.

15.3.2   Diagnosis

Patients with chronic pain present to emergency departments with worsening of their pain (breakthrough pain), new painful conditions, or separate acute medical conditions. It is beyond the scope of this text to explore the diagnostic options for new pain or other acute medical conditions—simply be aware that there is often an interplay between the comorbid conditions. Consider having cautious periods of observation prior to exploring costly or potentially dangerous treatments or diagnostic testing—these patients are often over-imaged and exposed to unnecessary tests and radiation. Discuss with the patient the diagnostic rationale and explore options, benefits, and risks before assuming that exhaustive testing must be done to achieve diagnostic certainty (which is rarely feasible or even critical). Documentation of these discussions will minimize legal risk and help colleagues in understanding these plans of care.

On the other hand, the *diagnosis* of breakthrough pain in patients with chronic pain is rarely valuable to the management of the patient. Breakthrough pain is frequently incident-related (due to activity, position, or movement) and may be exacerbated by physical states (constipation, insomnia, vomiting). Pain is often increased due to variation in the patient's baseline tolerance, fatigue, dysphoria, frustration, or recent stressors. Medication factors are common and include non-compliance, end-of-dose failure, and tolerance. Occasionally, the breakthrough pain is due to disease progression, new processes, or may simply be idiopathic. Again, it is often prudent to embark on a process of shared decision-making prior to diagnostic ventures, which are rarely fruitful. As in other conditions, red flags should include immunocompromised states, new or unusual pain or symptoms, parenteral drug abuse, fever, objective neurological findings, altered mental status, and difficulty in communicating.

15.4   Opioids in the Management of AECP

The American Pain Society has published guidelines for using opioid therapy in chronic noncancer pain [12]. In their recommendations, chronic opioid use should be considered after carefully weighing the benefits versus the risk. Compared to the treatment of acute pain, there appear to be very few ED studies that compare treatment modalities for AECP. An AECP has different physiologic mechanisms than classical acute pain; the standard treatments used by emergency physicians might not be the most effective. There is also evidence that long-term opioid treatment activates some of the neuronal remodeling pathways that are implicated in the development of chronic pain, so adding short-acting opioids onto the chronic opioid therapy could actually reinforce the negative neurological effects [13].

Despite physician efforts to avoid opioids in chronic noncancer pain, this is the most frequently used drug class for managing AECP patients. Most patients with AECP have pain in the moderate-to-severe intensity range, which is frequently stated to be a reasonable range in which to prescribe an opioid analgesic. Short-acting opioids like codeine, oxycodone, morphine, hydrocodone, hydromorphone, and fentanyl may be considered depending on the clinical presentation. There is little evidence of superiority of one opioid over another, and choice of opioid is most often a regional preference. Mixed agonist–antagonist agents are not an effective treatment for an AECP. Drugs like buprenorphine have a ceiling effect, which may limit the amount of analgesia provided, and in opioid-dependent patients, may lead to an uncommon but distinctly unpleasant episode of precipitated withdrawal [14]. This class of drug is best used in a long-term treatment setting. Extended release preparations also have a slow onset and are less desirable in the acute care setting, whereas they are excellent agents for the long-term treatment of chronic pain. Nonetheless, if the patient is on a chronic opioid preparation, and has missed or vomited doses, attempts should be made to reintroduce this baseline analgesic and diminish withdrawal as a source of discomfort.

The route of administration of opioids is an important consideration. For an AECP, intravenous dosing is one of the best options as this route has a rapid onset regardless of the specific medication used. Doses may be quickly titrated to achieve immediate effect—most intravenous opioids have their maximal respiratory depressant effect within 3–15 min and small additional doses can be given safely at this time point with monitoring. Intramuscular injections have a slightly longer onset, are more painful, and do not provide as effective analgesia as intravenous treatment [15]. Other routes include intranasal and sublingual, both of which have a rapid onset and can be considered options [16]. Unfortunately, the peak effect of parenteral opioids wears off quickly. While patients may appreciate and want the euphoric or sedative effects of parenteral opioids, the goals of an ED visit are not often to simply induce sedation. Accordingly, following the initial prior discussions on treatment goals, parenteral and particularly IV dosing should be quickly supplanted by other routes if discharge plans are expected. Oral medications are frequently used both in the acute care setting and limited prescriptions may also be written in order to provide analgesia until the patient is able to reconnect with their long-term pain management provider.

Opioid medications carry significant risks of side effects and risks. Respiratory depression, constipation, and sedation are some of the well-known negative side effects of these drugs and their euphoric side effects may also contribute abuse potential. Normal physiologic response to long-term opioid use will result in physical dependency, and frequently psychological dependency as well. Opioid receptor tolerance is becoming better understood and likely results from decreased cell surface expression of receptors, with reduced coupling efficacy of receptor activation that occurs with chronic opioid use [17].

15.5   Non-opioid and Combination Analgesia

Acetaminophen is an excellent drug on its own and one that is frequently overlooked in treatments of AECP. Oral acetaminophen is widely available and intravenous acetaminophen is now available in some jurisdictions. In moderate-to-severe pain, even when previously ineffective, acetaminophen should be reconsidered as a first-line additive agent. Combined with an opioid, by using separate mechanisms, acetaminophen synergistically provides higher levels of analgesia than either agent alone [18]. By using a combination, patients need take less opioid, which may reduce the incidence of adverse events. Caution should be used when ordering drug combinations in conjunction with acetaminophen, as patients are often unaware that multiple sources of acetaminophen, including over-the-counter preparations, may result in inadvertent overdosage [19]. Hepatotoxicity is the major toxicity, and therefore, it is vital to ask specifically about any over-the-counter medications the patient may be using.

NSAIDS also have a role in the control of chronic pain and are widely prescribed alone or in combination for their analgesic effects. Most oral NSAIDs have similar analgesic effects, with a therapeutic dose ceiling for analgesia. There is little evidence that one class of NSAID is better or stronger than another, though there are occasionally advantages of trying agents from different classes. While true physical tolerance to the analgesic effects of NSAIDS probably is minimal, patients often react positively though transiently to a change in NSAID. The dose ceiling for analgesia is notably lower than the dose required to treat inflammation. Ketarolac is available for use in patients unable to tolerate oral NSAIDS, but its analgesia effect when given IM or IV is not superior to oral NSAIDS, and it has a higher risk of GI bleeding and other side effects than other NSAIDS [20]. NSAIDs also have numerous adverse effects including cardiovascular toxicity, renal impairment, and peripheral edema. They should be prescribed with caution in patients with allergies or potential drug interactions.

There is evidence that NMDA receptor blockers such as ketamine are effective treatments for AECPs without the adverse effects of reinforcing the chronic pain pathways, though there is little evidence that this agent works as a long-term solution [21]. Similarly, studies have explored the potential for short ED courses of sedatives (propofol) and lidocaine as alternatives in acute pain crises. While there are roles for many other classes of drugs in managing chronic pain, the initiation of most of these within the emergency department is difficult and prone to later complications if not under-supervised care.

Many chronic pain patients need long-term solutions that require more time than is available in the acute care setting. However, this does not mean that the EM physician should neglect suggesting some of these strategies. Some bedside education about the benefits of exercise, behavioral therapy, physical therapy, and holistic methods such as acupuncture or meditation can help patients cope with AECP without utilizing the ED. If the patient is not currently under the care of a multidisciplinary pain clinic, an ER visit may be an ideal opportunity to arrange for this. It has been shown that multidisciplinary approaches to pain management result in significantly improved pain ratings, decreased use of analgesia, and improved functionality [22]. The multidisciplinary approach of many pain clinics may reduce visits to other acute care settings. It has been also shown that in the Medicaid population, a population with significant prevalence of chronic noncancer pain, improved provider continuity is associated with lower ED usage [23].

Some institutions are experimenting with implementing non-opioid treatment protocols in an effort to cut down on the number of repeat visits that chronic pain patients will make to the emergency department. In a study at the University of Wisconsin [24], researchers identified patients who had presented to the ED more than 10 times in the past 12 months. They were able to show that instituting non-opioid treatment protocols resulted in a significant decrease in the number of ED visits in their subjects. Other institutions have tried limiting the doses of parenteral opioids, and when the patients became accustomed to the policy, they seemed to be willing to be discharged upon reaching their limit. Another study showed that when patients who had been frequenting emergency departments for chronic conditions were placed into a multidisciplinary program to encourage following care plans, the investigators were able to show a significant decrease in visits [25]. It should be pointed out that the emergency department is often the only point of contact where patients are able to find appropriate care for acute exacerbation of chronic pain, and it would not be humane to deny patients this care during an exacerbation given the fragmentation of our healthcare system.

15.6 Barriers to Treating Patients with AECP

There are many challenges to providing adequate analgesia to patients presenting with AECP. Preconceived notions about opioids and substandard analgesic practice patterns are important roadblocks to optimal care. Adequate treatment of pain is frequently an "afterthought" [26] and many physicians are concerned about potentially enabling addiction and adverse drug-related behaviors. Inability to properly treat patients requiring analgesia may result in exacerbation of mental health issues, as well as increasing chronic pain severity.

There is controversy over which analgesic modalities should be entertained in the acute care setting as well as the appropriateness of the ED as the optimal venue for chronic pain patients. Many patients' pain complaints are not effectively addressed during their ED visits. Explanations for this from ED physicians include fear of creating or perpetuating addiction, encouraging substance abuse, or fear that the drugs will be diverted to be sold on the street. The reluctance to prescribe opioids is fairly common and is inculcated at the very beginning of a medical student's education [27]. Pain control is often inadequately addressed in medical school curricula and opiophobic behaviors are modeled during clinical training. In fact, studies have demonstrated that as physicians gain experience in their practice, many show an increased discordance between their estimation of the patient's pain versus the patient's own report [28].

Patient expectations may also present specific barriers. Of patients presenting to the ED, one study reported that patients believe that about 75 % of their pain should be relieved and nearly one in five expect total pain relief [29]. This degree of pain relief is often an unattainable goal, especially in patients with chronic pain. Many patients become frustrated with treatment if they have unrealistic expectations and this issue should be discussed frankly at the onset of establishing goals together with patients.

Many of the behaviors displayed by patients with AECP predispose them to being labeled as "difficult patients." These behaviors include frequent visits to the ED, the subjective nature of pain symptoms, multiple prior investigations, multiple providers, frustration and anger, impatience, noncompliance, unclear goals, and counterproductive coping mechanisms. Since there are frequently no objective findings for a physician to treat, physicians are confronted with the dilemma of evaluating the legitimacy of pain presentations. This often sends confusing messages to patients who may interpret the interactions as confrontational rather than therapeutic.

Fear of the risk of addiction is a common concern for both the prescribing physicians as well as their patients. Although perhaps not as frequently cited as other problems limiting treatment of chronic pain, it remains an issue that must be addressed [2]. A survey of physicians found that fear of addiction represented a barrier to assessment and treatment of chronic pain patients [30]. Patients with chronic noncancer pain may also have comorbid substance abuse issues, as well as chemical dependence [31]. There is a wide distribution of addiction estimates reported in ED studies. It has been found that 10–16 % of outpatients and 25–40 % of hospitalized patients have problems with addiction [32]. However, other studies have shown that chronic pain patients have rates of addiction and dependence similar to that of the general population [33]. Variability in these prevalence estimates is in part due to failure to properly define terms like dependence, addiction, and abuse. It is reasonable to assume that there is a subset of patients who will develop addiction and adverse drug-related behaviors while taking opioids for legitimate pain [34]. Central to determining the risk is establishing the baseline addiction risk by routinely employing a stratification tool such as the Opioid Risk Tool [35].

Toxicology testing, including urine drug testing, has almost no part in the management of the patient with AECP. These tests have poor sensitivity and frequently do not test for certain many drugs, such as fentanyl, clonazepam, and several other drugs of abuse. They also have poor specificity in some cases, and the presence of drugs of abuse is neither helpful nor discriminating. However, urine drug testing may reveal the presence of other drugs of abuse, such as cocaine, which may indicate serious addiction and flag the need for addiction treatment or different medication approaches.

While difficult at times, patients suffering from addiction issues should be treated with dignity and respect. Many patients suffering from addiction have histories of abuse, sexual and physical trauma, and caregiver neglect that often contributed to their premorbid personalities long before they became addicted to opioids. It is helpful to give options rather than limiting choices, allowing patients as much autonomy of decision within whatever limits the physician deems reasonable. Escalation of emotions and confrontational approaches these patients often encounter within emergency departments are usually counterproductive, and sometimes simply stating your limitations clearly will be enough to clarify treatment decisions.

Patients with a known history of addiction and substance abuse may still be candidates for opioid analgesia. If pain is managed during the emergency encounter, short courses of outpatient opioids are an option that must be carefully considered. Negotiate with the patient on the expected time course of the exacerbation and the time to resolution or next follow-up. Rarely will scripts need to extend beyond 3 days or 20 pills. Consider writing prescriptions as 'daily dispense' and faxing the prescription directly to the pharmacy when permitted by local practices. Both these measures can decrease diversion and abuse.

Due to the large time commitment, follow-up, need for monitoring, and the multidisciplinary approaches, which are known to be more effective, the ED is not a practical place to begin long-term therapy. In acute settings, an emergency physician should take a careful history, especially focusing on the current and past use of analgesic medication and assess risk before prescribing an opioid. Even for experienced addiction physicians working in the ED, it can be difficult to identify drug-seeking patients and some contend that the only time it is necessary to distinguish drug-seeking patients from those truly in need of analgesia is if it changes the patients' management [36]. The evaluation of the patient should also include confirming that the patient is under the care of an appropriate primary care practitioner or pain clinic and communicating any changes in pharmacotherapy with them.

For patients in acute opioid withdrawal and a clear history of addiction, referral to appropriate opioid replacement therapy addiction services is recommended. Methadone and buprenorphine programs are effective strategies for opioid addiction that are cost-effective and reduce mortality and morbidity. Initiation of buprenorphine is an option in the emergency department in some jurisdictions, but should only be undertaken by those with a clear understanding of the mechanisms and pathway to ongoing care [37]. Despite being non-life threatening, help with symptom relief with clonidine, NSAIDS, and antiemetics may be useful in helping the patient endure the episode of withdrawal until addiction treatment can take place.

15.7 Clinical Approach to Acute Exacerbation of Chronic Pain

While there has been little focused research on best practices in the ED for AECP, it is important to have a consistent approach and be humane with patients seeking care in the ED. Strategies employing guidelines and protocols can reduce patient uncertainty and improve time and success to effective analgesia. Reduction of suffering and relief of pain are essential elements of emergency physician responsibility. Implementing departmental strategies measures may provide the ED physician increased confidence and aid in mitigating some of the barriers that may be encountered during these visits. Many of the issues central to treating patients with chronic noncancer pain, such as distinguishing between pseudoaddiction, regional pain disorders, or malingering, are not practical in the time-limited setting of the emergency department. These limitations should not be barriers to providing expeditious relief and subsequently working with the patient to address these issues in the longer term [38].

It is reasonable to first determine whether a patient is opioid-dependent and ensure that they are not currently in withdrawal. Physical dependency is a fundamental property of opioid treatment and is distinct from the chronic issue of addiction, which is characterized by maladaptive behaviors and use despite harm. It is difficult to evaluate a patient when they are suffering from opioid withdrawal, and it may be necessary to account for the patient's "opioid debt" before arriving at a reasonable dose adjustment. Secondly, a conversation with the patient to determine what the patient hopes to get out of the encounter must occur. If this patient's expectations are unrealistic, the achievable outcomes should be discussed, which often aids in improving patient satisfaction. Efforts should usually be made to confirm actual prescription medications and, if an opioid or prescription monitoring database is available, it should be checked. If primary care providers are easily available, attempts should be made to involve them in the management if appropriate.

Symptom control will often include more than just analgesia. Nausea should be aggressively treated and often responds to low-dose haloperidol when other antiemetics have failed. Vomiting is often complicated by dehydration and ketosis and responds best to aggressive saline fluid boluses followed by intravenous dextrose or refeeding. Constipation frequently requires education, and provision of a preprinted handout is often useful. Daily maintenance or bolus dosing of polyethylene-glycol powder solutions may be needed for severe constipation. Benzodiazepines should rarely be used in AECP patients, but may be carefully considered when anxiety or benzodiazepine withdrawal are critical components of the presentation.

After initiating symptom control, the focus should be on determination of further evaluation with lab tests or imaging. Differentiating between an AECP secondary to a known condition and pain arising from a new acute process may pose significant challenges. Careful history and physical examination should also elicit the patient's expectations and previous experience. Chronic pain patients frequently understand their pain origins and may be familiar with the exacerbations as well. If the character or location of the pain is significantly different, further investigation may be necessary.

After addressing the patient's current exacerbation, it is important to discuss with the management about future potential episodes. Significant time and resources are expended in managing AECP in the ED, largely because emergency physicians are not familiar with the prior management issues and have no established rapport with patients they are often meeting for the first time. Discussion should take place with the patient around linking with a chronic pain specialist or primary care physician whenever possible. If they have a primary care physician, planning should take place to deal with future pain exacerbations. Other resources, including social work, psychiatry, acute pain services, and addiction services may be consulted prior to discharging the patient or arranged following the ED visit. At the time of discharge, write out for the patient all the multiple venues you have discussed, both pharmacological and other, that may help in their management. These lists are often essential in the understanding that AECP is rarely just a matter of more opioids.

Every emergency department should consider developing systemic policies and procedures that help with the management of the patient presenting with an AECP. These include having education sessions for physicians and staff on the approach to this common but challenging patient group. Protocols should be in place for the quick approach to analgesia, with consideration to developing nurse-driven, physician-approved preorder sets. Analgesic protocols can also be developed for frequent diagnostic groups, such as patients with renal colic, migraine, or sickle-cell crisis that may be frequently initiated in a uniform manner. Patients who are well-known to ED staff will almost always require individualized care plans including the patient and their caregivers; neglecting these care plans in patients with AECP and frequent ED visits will often lead to escalation of visits, higher costs, and iatrogenic complications. Finally, since the patient with AECP will often require referrals and multidisciplinary follow-up, work with your specialists to develop quicker consultation and coordination of care.

15.8 Conclusions

Oligoanalgesia has long been recognized as an important problem, and efforts to improve appropriate ED analgesia have, for the most part, failed [39]. Many studies have examined reported pain levels on admission and compared it to levels on discharge. One study by Ducharme and Barber showed 69 % of patients presented to EDs with pain rated as moderate to severe [40]. Upon discharge, they reported 58 % of patients were still complaining of the same pain levels. Another study by Guru and Dubinsky revealed similarly poor response by physicians to patients in significant pain [41]. Studies by Stahmer [42] and Todd [43] have shown that providing adequate analgesia is a significant predictor of patient satisfaction. Pain intensity and adequate analgesia affect the patients' perception of their visits [13].

It is clear that emergency physicians need to focus on providing better analgesia and reduce the suffering of patients. In the past, treatment of pain was primarily symptomatic with little attention given to improving functional status or quality of life [44]. Research has made significant progress in elucidating the neurobiology of pain and we are now able to apply a mechanistic approach to target specific receptors and mediators [1]. It has been predicted that individualized genomic data can someday help choose the analgesic that is best suited to the patient [45]. At least 15 different μ-receptors for opioids have been identified. As we learn more about the neurophysiology of pain, we can hope for better agents to induce analgesia without the adverse effects that make opioid use so problematic. As the mechanisms of neuronal remodeling, reward behavior, and addiction are unlocked, new adjuvant drugs will be discovered that could act to alleviate some of the concerns about psychological opioid dependence.

Additionally, as we develop better metrics for measuring pain, we can deliver more appropriate levels of analgesia. Our current method of a one-dimensional pain measure is likely more indicative of the emotional component of the discomfort than the actual sensory aspect [46]. As the "fifth vital sign," it would certainly be helpful to have a more reliable system for quantifying pain, but the most humane and simple approach is simply to ask patients "would you like something to treat your pain" and provide them with further opportunities for reassessment and repeat doses.

Treatment of AECP with the aid of protocols for analgesia and implementing best practice guidelines will result in better care of our patients. Managing acute breakthroughs of pain episodes represents a central aspect in overall chronic pain management and has significant impacts on patient satisfaction and well-being. Ensuring safe, effective, and adequate analgesia to our patients remains one of the most important roles for the emergency physician, and we must continue to increase our efforts and strive to vastly improve upon the current practices, which do not meet patient needs.

References

1. Ducharme J. Acute pain and pain control: state of the art. Ann Emerg Med. 2000;35: 592–603.
2. Cordell WH, et al. The high prevalence of pain in emergency medical care. Am J Emerg Med. 2002;20:165–9.
3. Wilsey BL, Fishman SM, Ogden C, Tsodikov A, Bertakis KD. Chronic pain management in the emergency department: a survey of attitudes and beliefs. Pain Med. 2008;9(8):1073–80.
4. Weinstein SM, Laux LF. Physicians' attitudes toward pain and the use of opioid analgesics: results of a survey from the Texas cancer pain initiative. South Med J. 2000;93(5):479–87.
5. Rupp T, Delaney KA. Inadequate analgesia in emergency medicine. Ann Emerg Med. 2004;43:494–503.
6. Todd KH. Emergency medicine and pain: a topography of influence. Ann Emerg Med. 2004;43(4):504–6.

7. Cheng J, Abdi S. Complications of joint, tendon, and muscle injections. Tech Reg Anesth Pain Manag. 2007;11(3):141–7.
8. Todd KH. Defining acute versus chronic pain. In: Mace SE, Ducharme J, Murphy MF, editors. Pain management and sedation: emergency department management. 1st ed. New York: McGraw-Hill; 2006. p. 221.
9. Hansen GR. Management of chronic pain in the acute care setting. Emerg Med Clin North Am. 2005;23:307–38.
10. Portenoy RK, Hagen NA. Breakthrough pain: definition, prevalence and characteristics. Pain. 1990;41:273–81.
11. Portenoy RK, Bennett DS, Rauck R, Simon S, Taylor D, Brennan M, Shoemaker S. Prevalence and characteristics of breakthrough pain in opioid-treated patients with chronic noncancer pain. J Pain. 2006;7(8):583–91.
12. Chou R, Fanciullo GJ, Fine PG, et al. Clinical guidelines for the use of chronic opioid therapy in chronic noncancer pain. J Pain. 2008;10(2):113–30.
13. Chu LF, Angst MS, Clark D. Opioid induced hyperalgesia in humans: molecular mechanisms and clinical considerations. Clin J Pain. 2008;24(6):479–96.
14. Ferris FD, von Gunten CF, Emanuel LL. Ensuring competency in end-of-life care: controlling symptoms. BMC Palliat Care. 2002;1:5.
15. Tveita T, Thoner J, Klepstad P, Dale O, Jystad A, Borchgrevink PC. A controlled comparison between single doses of intravenous and intramuscular morphine with respect to analgesic effects and patient safety. Acta Anaesthesiol Scand. 2008;52(7):920–5.
16. Portenoy RK, Messina J, Xie F, Peppin J. Fentanyl buccal tablet (FBT) for relief of break-through pain in opioid treated patients with chronic low back pain: a randomized, placebo-controlled study. Curr Med Res Opin. 2007;23(1):223–33.
17. Christie MJ. Cellular neuroadaptations to chronic opioids: tolerance, withdrawal and addiction. Br J Pharmacol. 2008;154(2):384–96.
18. Beaver WT, McMillan D. Methodological considerations in the evaluation of analgesic combinations: acetaminophen (paracetamol) and hydrocodone in postpartum pain. Br J Clin Pharmacol. 1980;10(Supp2):215S–23S.
19. Wolf MS, et al. Risk of unintentional overdose with Non-prescription acetaminophen products. J Gen Intern Med. 2012;27(12):1587–93.
20. Turturro MA, et al. Intramuscular ketorolac versus oral ibuprofen in acute musculoskeletal pain. Ann Emerg Med. 1995;26:117–20.
21. Bell RF. Ketamine for chronic non-cancer pain. Pain. 2009;141:210–4.
22. Kitahara M, Kojima KK, Ohmura A. Efficacy of interdisciplinary treatment for chronic non-malignant pain patients in Japan. Clin J Pain. 2006;22(7):647–55.
23. Gill JM, Mainous AG, Nsereko M. The effect of continuity of care on emergency department use. Arch Fam Med. 2000;9:333–8.
24. Svenson JE, Meyer TD. Effectiveness of nonnarcotic protocol for the treatment of acute exacerbations of chronic nonmalignant pain. Am J Emerg Med. 2007;25:445–9.
25. Pope D, Fernandes CMB, Bouthillette F, Etherington J. Frequent users of the emergency department: a program to improve care and reduce visits. Can Med Assoc J. 2000;162(7):1017–20.
26. Fosnocht DE, Swanson ER, Barton ED. Changing attitudes about pain and pain control in emergency medicine. Emerg Med Clin North Am. 2005;23:297–306.
27. Weinstein SM, Laux LF, Thornby JI, et al. Medical students' attitudes toward pain and the use of opioid analgesics: implications for changing medical school curriculum. South Med J. 2000;93(5):472–8.
28. Marquié L, Raufaste E, Lauque D, Mariné C, et al. Pain rating by patients and physicians: evidence of systemic pain miscalibration. Pain. 2003;102(3):289–96.
29. Fosnocht DE, Heaps ND, Swanson ER. Patient expectations for pain relief in the ED. Am J Emerg Med. 2004;22(4):286–8.

30. Wilsey BL, Fishman SM, Crandall M, Casamalhuapa C, Bertakis KD. A qualitative study of the barriers to chronic pain management in the ED. Am J Emerg Med. 2008;26:255–63.
31. Gourlay DL, Heit HA. Pain and addiction: managing risk through comprehensive care. J Addict Dis. 2008;27(3):23–30.
32. Kissen B. Medical management of alcoholic patients. In: Kissen B, Begleiter H, editors. Treatment and rehabilitation of the chronic alcoholic. New York: Plenum; 1997.
33. Regier DA, Meyers JK, Kramer M, et al. The NIMH epidemiologic catchment area program. Arch Gen Psychiatry. 1984;41:934–58.
34. Weaver MF, Schnoll SH. Opioid treatment of chronic pain in patients with addiction. J Pain Palliat Care Pharmacother. 2002;26(3):5–26.
35. Webster LR, Webster RM. Predicting aberrant behaviors in opioid-treated patients: preliminary validation of the Opioid Risk Tool. Pain Med. 2005;6(6):432–42.
36. Hansen GR. The drug-seeking patient in the emergency room. Emerg Med Clin North Am. 2005;23:349–65.
37. D'Onofrio G, O'Connor PG, Pantalon MV, et al. Emergency department–initiated buprenorphine/naloxone treatment for opioid dependence. A randomized clinical trial. JAMA. 2015;313(16):1636–44.
38. Baker K. Chronic pain syndromes in the emergency department: identifying guidelines for management. Emerg Med Australas. 2005;17:57–64.
39. Marks RM, Sachar EJ. Undertreatment of medical inpatients with narcotic analgesics. Ann Intern Med. 1973;78:173–81.
40. Ducharme J, Barber C. A prospective blinded study on emergency pain assessment and therapy. J Emerg Med. 1995;13:571–5.
41. Guru V, Dubinsky I. The patient vs. caregiver perception of acute pain in the emergency department. J Emerg Med. 2000;18:7–12.
42. Stahmer SA, Shofer FS, Marino A, Shepherd S, Abbuhl S. Do quantative changes in pain intensity correlate with pain relief and satisfaction? Acad Emerg Med. 1998;5:851–7.
43. Todd KH, Sloan EP, Chen C, Eder S, Wamstad K. Survey of pain etiology, management practices and patient satisfaction in two urban emergency departments. CJEM. 2002;4(4):252–6.
44. Listed NA. Management of chronic pain syndromes: issues and interventions. Pain Med. 2005;6(S1):S1–S20.
45. Ducharme J. The future of pain management in emergency medicine. Emerg Med Clin North Am. 2005;23:467–75.
46. Clark WC, Yang JC, Tsui SL, et al. Unidimensional pain rating scales: a multidimensional affect and pain survey (MAPS) analysis of what they really measure. Pain. 2002;98(3):241–7.

Chapter 16
Assessing and Treating Co-occurring Mental Illness

Monique M. Jones and Marian Fireman

16.1 Introduction

In 2013, approximately 7.6 million adults in the United States endorsed symptoms of co-occurring substance use disorder (SUD) and mental illness [1]. Within that population, it is estimated that 2.3 million had a serious mental illness, which resulted in significant functional impairment in major interpersonal, social, and/or occupational life activities [1].

There have been several major studies conducted to quantify the prevalence of psychiatric disorders and SUDs among community populations particularly the Epidemiologic Catchment Area (ECA) Study [2], the National Comorbidity Survey (NCS) [3, 4], the National Comorbidity Survey Replication (NCS-R) [5], and the National Epidemiologic Survey on Alcohol and Related Conditions (NESARC) [6]. Individuals with a mental disorder have increased risk of also having a SUD; greater than twice the risk in comparison to those without a history of mental illness [2]. In those who have been diagnosed with either a psychiatric disorder or SUD, the majority have comorbid disorders [3]. Many studies combine nonmedical prescription opioid use (NMPOU) disorders with illicit opioid use disorders under the umbrella term, opioid use disorder. Therefore, the term opioid use disorder is used predominantly in this chapter. The term nonmedical prescription opioid use disorder will also be used in this chapter. It is defined as using an opioid in a nonmedical manner, without a prescription, or taking in larger doses than prescribed, or taking more frequently than prescribed [7]. In this text, the terms co-occurring and comorbidity shall be used interchangeably.

M.M. Jones, M.D. (✉) • M. Fireman, M.D.
Department of Psychiatry, Oregon Health & Science University,
3181 SW Sam Jackson, UHN80, Portland, OR 97239, USA
e-mail: jonemo@ohsu.edu; firemanm@ohsu.edu

© Springer International Publishing Switzerland 2016
A.M. Matthews, J.C. Fellers (eds.), *Treating Comorbid Opioid Use Disorder in Chronic Pain*, DOI 10.1007/978-3-319-29863-4_16

The term comorbidity is generally used to describe two or more diseases or disorders that are simultaneously present in an individual. However, researchers have begun to characterize two types of comorbidity. Depending on the disorders involved, there are concepts of homotypic comorbidity and heterotypic comorbidity [8]. Homotypic comorbidity is defined as concurring disorders within the same diagnostic group such as two or more SUDs (e.g., opioid use disorder and alcohol use disorder) [9]. Heterotypic comorbidity is defined as concurring disorders from different diagnostic groups such as SUD and a mental disorder (e.g., opioid use disorder and major depressive disorder) [9]. There is a paucity of research investigating the general population prevalence of two or more substances used simultaneously. This is especially true when looking at SUDs other than alcohol use disorder (AUD); few studies separate the drug disorders into specific types (e.g., opioids, cannabis, cocaine, amphetamines, etc.). Additionally, many epidemiological studies addressed SUDs by analyzing lifetime prevalence rather than current use (within the most recent 12-month period) which inflates comorbidity estimates. When using lifetime prevalence, instances where disorders may not have occurred simultaneously are included.

16.2   Overview of Chapter

This chapter is not intended as a comprehensive text of heterotypic comorbid mental health disorders. Rather, it is hoped that this chapter will provide concise information about epidemiology, diagnosis, screening, and treatment of co-occurring heterotypic disorders in the context of opioid use disorders and/or chronic pain. In brief, potential etiologic relationships between psychiatric syndromes and substance use have implications on diagnosis and treatment options. Four general models for comorbidity have been formulated [10, 11]. One model suggests that SUDs develop secondary to psychiatric syndromes. This includes the self-medication model which postulates that individuals seek substances to alleviate unpleasant symptoms. [10, 11] A second model is that SUDs precipitate secondary mental illness [10, 11]. Common factor models propose that shared vulnerabilities such as genetic factors or trauma increase the risk of having both disorders [10, 11]. The bidirectional theory hypothesizes that disorders become related over time due to interactional effects [10]. There is evidence supporting each model.

16.2.1   Assessment

Several approaches may be utilized for assessment which are summarized in Table 16.1.
    Though screening tools should not replace a full diagnostic assessment, they are helpful in providing a preliminary indication of whether a patient has mental health problems and/or substance use issues. Synopses of several validated screening tools are included in Table 16.2.

Table 16.1 Synopsis of validated diagnostic assessment tools

Name	Comment
Structured Clinical Interview for DSM-IV (SCID)[1]	• SCID-I: Determines Axis I disorders (e.g., mood disorders, and anxiety disorders, etc.)
	• SCID-II: Determines Axis II disorders (e.g., personality disorders)
	• SCID-5: Uses DSM-5 diagnostic criteria
	• Takes approximately ½–2 h to administer
Mini-International Neuropsychiatric Interview (M.I.N.I.)[2]	• Determines major DSM-IV Axis I disorders
	• Short and structured
	• Takes approximately 15 min to administer
Psychiatric Research Interview for Substance and Mental Disorders (PRISM)[3]	• Determines DSM-IV Axis I, Axis II, and comorbid substance use
	• Discerns substance-induced disorders and primary psychiatric disorders
	• Takes approximately 1–3 h to administer

1. First MB, Spitzer RL, Gibbon M, Williams JBW. *Structured Clinical Interview for DSM-IV-TR Axis I Disorders, Patient Edition. (SCID-I/P)*. New York, NY; 2002
2. Sheehan D V., Lecrubier Y, Sheehan KH, et al. The Mini-International Neuropsychiatric Interview (M.I.N.I.): the development and validation of a structured diagnostic psychiatric interview for DSM IV and ICD-10. *J Clin Psychiatry*. 1998;59(Suppl 20):22–33
3. Hasin D, Samet S, Nunes E, Meydan J, Matseoane K, Waxman R. Diagnosis of comorbid psychiatric disorders in substance users assessed with the psychiatric research interview for substance and mental disorders for DSM-IV. *Am J Psychiatry*. 2006;163(4):689–696. doi:10.1176/appi.ajp.163.4.689

16.3   Mood Disorders

16.3.1   Epidemiology

Various epidemiological studies have demonstrated that SUDs and affective disorders are often comorbid. Studies from the more recent past have extracted data from the NESARC, a large nationally representative survey of over 40,000 participants. In one study, NMPOU disorders were associated with 2.4 times risk of lifetime Major Depressive Disorder (MDD), 4.9 times risk of lifetime Bipolar I Disorder (BPI), and 4.3 times the risk of bipolar II disorder (BPII) [7]. Another study investigated gender differences in lifetime prevalence associations between mood disorders and SUDs; women with opioid use disorder tended to have higher associations with mood disorders in comparison to men [12]. Individuals who were heroin and nonmedical prescription opioid users appeared to be at increased risk of mood disorders in comparison to heroin-only or nonmedical prescription opioid-only users [13]. One study of data extracted from the NESARC specifically examined individuals with lifetime opioid use disorder and comorbid lifetime prevalence of an Axis I or Axis II disorder revealed that 51 % had MDD, 20.1 % had BPI, and 9.6 % had BPII [14].

202   M.M. Jones and M. Fireman

Table 16.2 Synopsis of validated screening tools

Name	Assesses	Comment
Beck Depression Inventory (BDI)[1]	Depression	21-items, self-administered
Montgomery-Asberg Depression Rating Scale (MADRS)[2]	Depression	10-items, clinician administered
Hamilton Depression Rating Scale (HAM-D)[3]	Depression	21-items, clinician administered
Patient Health Questionnaire (PHQ-9)[4]	Depression	9-items, clinician or self-administered
Young Mania Rating Scale (YMRS)[5]	Mania	11-items, clinician administered
Bech-Rafaelson Mania Scale (MAS)[3]	Mania	11-items, clinician administered
Hamilton Anxiety Rating Scale (HAM-A)[6]	Anxiety	14-items, clinician administered
Four-Dimensional Symptom Questionnaire (4DSQ)[7]	Distinguish general distress from anxiety, depression, and somatization	50-items, self-administered
Yale-Brown Obsessive Compulsive Scale (Y-BOC)[8]	OCD	10-items, clinician administered
Clinician-Administered PTSD Scale (CAPS)[9]	PTSD	17-items, clinician administered
Short Form of PTSD Checklist-Civilian Version (PCL-C)[10]	PTSD	6-items, clinician administered
PTSD Symptom Scale—Self-Report Version (PSS-SR)[11]	PTSD	17-items, self-administered
Brief Psychiatric Rating Scale (BPRS)[12]	Depression, anxiety, hallucinations, and unusual behaviors	16-items, clinician administered
Positive and Negative Syndrome Scale (PANSS)[13]	Schizophrenia symptom severity	30-items, clinician administered
Adult ADHD Self-Report Scale (ASRS) Symptom Checklist[14]	ADHD	18-items, self-administered

1. Beck A, Steer R, Ball R, Ranieri W. Comparison Of Beck Depression Inventories-IA And-II In Psychiatric Outpatients. *J Pers Assess.* 1996;67(3):588–597
2. Montgomery S, Asberg M. A new depression scale designed to be sensitive to change. *Br J Psychiatry.* 1979;134:382–389
3. Beck P, Bolwig T, Kramp P, Rafaelsen O. The Bech-Rafaelsen Mania Scale and the Hamilton Depression Scale. *Acta Psychiatr Scand.* 1979;59(4):420–430
4. Kroenke K, Spitzer RL, Williams JB. The PHQ-9: validity of a brief depression severity measure. *J Gen Intern Med.* 2001;9:606–613
5. Young RC, Biggs JT, Ziegler VE, Meyer DA. A rating scale for mania: reliability, validity and sensitivity. *Br J Psychiatry.* 1978;133:429–435
6. Hamilton M. The assessment of anxiety states by rating. *Br J Med Psychol.* 1959;32(1):50–55
7. Terluin B, van Marwijk HWJ, Adèr HJ, et al. The Four-Dimensional Symptom Questionnaire (4DSQ): a validation study of a multidimensional self-report questionnaire to assess distress, depression, anxiety and somatization. *BMC Psychiatry.* 2006;6:34. doi:10.1186/1471-244X-6-34
8. Goodman WK, Price LH, Rasmussen SA, et al. The Yale-Brown Obsessive Compulsive Scale: Development, use, and reliability. *Arch Gen Psychiatry.* 1989;46(11):1006–1011

(continued)

Table 16.2 (continued)
9. Blake DD, Weathers FW, Nagy LW, et al. A clinician rating scale for assessing current and life-time PTSD: the CAPS-1. *Behav Ther*. 1990;13:187–188
10. Lang AJ, Stein MB. An abbreviated PTSD checklist for use as a screening instrument in primary care. *Behav Res Ther*. 2005;43:585–594
11. Foa E, Cashman L, Jaycox L, Perry K. The validation of a self-report measure of PTSD: The Posttraumatic Diagnostic Scale. *Psychol Assess*. 1997;9:445–451
12. Overall JE, Gorham DR. The Brief Psychiatric Scale. *Psychol Rep*. 1962;10:799–812
13. Kay SR, Fiszbein A, Opler LA. The positive and negative syndrome scale (PANSS) for schizophrenia. *Schizophr Bull*. 1987;13(2):261–276
14. Kessler RC, Adler L, Ames M, et al. The World Health Organization Adult ADHD Self-Report Scale (ASRS): a short screening scale for use in the general population. *Psychol Med*. 2005;35(2): 245–256
15. Ewing JA. Detecting Alcoholism: The CAGE Questionnaire. *JAMA*. 1984;252(14):1905–1907
16. T. Babor, J. C. Higgins-Biddle, J. B. Saunders MGM. The Alcohol Use Disorders Identification Test: Guidelines for use in primary care. *Geneva World Heal Organ*. 2001:1–40
17. Skinner HA. The drug abuse screening test. *Addict Behav*. 1982;7:369–371
18. Humeniuk R, Ali R, Babor TF, et al. Validation of the Alcohol, Smoking And Substance Involvement Screening Test (ASSIST). *Addiction*. 2008;103(6):1039–1047

There have been a number of studies that demonstrated the strong association between pain and depression. One review noted that individuals with moderate to severe pain that impaired function, and/or was refractory to treatment, were likely to have more depressive symptoms and worse depression outcomes including increased healthcare utilization and lower quality of life [15].

16.3.2 Treatment

Though there are no definitive guidelines for treatment of co-occurring depressive disorders and opioid use disorder, there have been a number of studies investigating efficacy of various treatment modalities. One review highlighted that antidepressant medications combined with concurrent therapy exert modest beneficial effects with patients with comorbid depressive symptoms and SUDs [16]. In another study of methadone maintenance treatment (MMT) patients, psychotropic medication treatment was associated with reduction in depressive symptoms and decreased benzodiazepine abuse [17]. Two studies demonstrated reduction in depressive symptoms using imipramine, a tricyclic antidepressant (TCA) [18, 19]. There have also been a number of negative studies that showed no difference between MMT patients with depression who received a psychotropic medication or not. Two studies that compared fluoxetine, a selective re-uptake inhibitor (SSRI), to placebo demonstrated no effect differences between the groups [20, 21]. Desipramine, another TCA, was not shown to decrease depressive symptoms in MMT patients compared to placebo [22, 23]. Due to mixed results in studies evaluating opioid use disorder and comorbid depression, two reviews postulated the need for more studies that control for variables such as antidepressant class and psychosocial interventions in this population subset [24, 25]. Duloxetine, a dual re-uptake inhibitor of norepinephrine and serotonin (SNRI), has shown promise in effectively treating depressive and painful physical symptoms. [26] In patients with comorbid pain and depression, a review noted improvement of both measures simultaneously with antidepressant treatment; however, it also noted that many studies included in the review were of short duration, uncontrolled, and focused on measurement of pain response [15].

There is evidence that non-pharmacological modalities for comorbid depression and substance use can be efficacious. However, few studies have looked specifically at opioid use disorders and affective syndromes. In one study, active injection drug users were randomized to either assessment only or combined cognitive behavioral therapy (CBT) plus pharmacotherapy (citalopram (SSRI), venlafaxine (SNRI), or bupropion, a weak norepinephrine dopamine reuptake inhibitor (NDRI)) [27]. The group that received combined treatment had higher depression remission rates and decreased frequency of heroin use in comparison to the control group [27]. Behavior Therapy for Depression in Drug Dependence (BTDD) was developed to treat co-occurring substance use and depressive disorders in MMT patients; one study demonstrated a decrease in depressive symptoms from baseline, but no change in opioid and cocaine use [28]. A review of CBT in comparison to other psychotherapies for co-occurring depression and substance use supported treatment over no treatment, but showed little evidence that CBT was more effective than other psychotherapies in this population [29].

In general, data are lacking in investigations of comorbid bipolar disorder and SUDs; this is especially striking when evaluating opioid use disorders and bipolar disorder co-occurrence. Due to paucity of data, definitive guidelines are limited. Aripiprazole, an atypical psychotic with a novel mechanism of action as a dopamine-2 receptor partial agonist, was found to have associated symptomatic improvement when patients were switched to it from other medication regimens [30]. Integrated Group Therapy (IGT) is a group treatment specifically designed for patients with both substance dependence and bipolar disorder; studies have demonstrated decreased substance use days and mood episodes with this intervention [31–33]. Two reviews of the available data in patients with comorbid bipolar disorder and substance use suggested that an integrative approach that included pharmacological interventions (i.e., mood stabilizers [lithium, antiepileptic medications, and/or atypical antipsychotics]) combined with appropriate psychosocial interventions (e.g., 12-step groups, IGT, or individual psychotherapy) created best outcomes (e.g., reduced hospital admissions and improved life satisfaction) [34, 35].

16.4   Anxiety Disorders

16.4.1   Epidemiology

Many studies have demonstrated associations between anxiety disorders and comorbid SUD. A study that examined NMPOU patients found there was a high association with lifetime prevalence of various anxiety disorders [7]. The authors noted 4.3 times risk of panic disorder with agoraphobia, 4.0 times risk of panic disorder without agoraphobia, 2.4 times risk of social phobia, 2.3 times risk of a specific phobia, and 2.7

times risk of generalized anxiety disorder (GAD) [7]. Whereas women with opioid use disorder demonstrated higher associations with mood disorders in comparison to men, this trend appeared to be reversed with many anxiety disorders [12]. Individuals who are heroin and nonmedical prescription opioid users appear to be at increased risk of anxiety disorders in comparison to heroin-only or nonmedical prescriptions opioid-only users [13]. Studies of individuals with a lifetime opioid use disorder show significant comorbidity with anxiety disorders [14]. Approximately 14.9% had panic disorder without agoraphobia, 4.9% had panic disorder with agoraphobia, 12.7% had social phobia, 18.5% had specific phobia, and 12.3% had GAD [14].

16.4.2   Treatment

Various studies have investigated treatments and treatment outcome for comorbid anxiety disorders and SUDs. Patients on buprenorphine maintenance for opioid dependence were found to be at increased risk for relapse if they had co-occurring anxiety disorders, active alcohol abuse, or active nonmedical use of benzodiazepines [36]. Anxiety sensitivity, referring to the fear of anxiety-related sensations due to the belief that such sensations have harmful consequences, was linked to higher premature attrition rates from treatment in heroin and/or cocaine/crack-dependent patients [37]. Buspirone, a non-benzodiazepine anxiolytic medication, did not significantly reduce anxiety in opioid-dependent persons, but was associated with trends toward decreased depression scale scores and slower return to substance use [38]. A study that randomly assigned substance abusing OCD patients to 3 different treatment conditions: a) integrated OCD substance abuse treatment, b) substance abuse treatment, or c) progressive muscle relaxation control condition—indicated that individuals who received the combined intervention had greater reduction of OCD symptom severity, stayed in treatment longer, and had lower overall relapse rates at 1-year follow-up [39]. One review created a decisional flowchart for opioid-dependent patients who entered treatment. Those with severe anxiety symptoms should have specific management for the anxiety disorder [40]. This should include with consideration of SSRI therapy and psychotherapy along with treatment as usual (TAU), aimed at achieving long-term abstinence from opioids [40]. Finally, another review suggested that pharmacotherapeutic treatment for comorbid anxiety and substance use disorders should follow routine clinical practice guidelines and preferentially use agents with a low abuse potential [41].

16.5   Posttraumatic Stress Disorder

16.5.1   Epidemiology

Several large epidemiological studies examined PTSD and SUD co-occurrence. One study evaluated PTSD among substance users by extracting data from an arm of the ECA study [42]. Cocaine and heroin users were combined and were found more likely, in comparison to other groups, to report more PTSD-qualifying traumatic events and symptoms and to meet criteria for PTSD [42]. A retrospective study that involved over 140,000 Iraq and Afghanistan veterans with at least one pain diagnosis revealed that 32 % received a diagnosis of PTSD (with or without other psychiatric disorders) [43]. Those with a diagnosis of PTSD had higher-risk opioid use and increased risk for injuries and overdose [43]. Veterans with both a SUD and PTSD were over four times as likely to be prescribed opioids in comparison to veterans without a psychiatric disorder [43]. Over 18,000 active US military service members from 2001 to 2008 were examined in a 2014 study to determine whether opioid abuse/dependence diagnosed during service was associated with a prior PTSD diagnosis [44]. The study revealed that service members with an opioid abuse or dependence diagnosis were 28 times more likely than controls to have prior diagnosis of PTSD [44].

Pain syndromes and PTSD comorbidity are highly prevalent. Current PTSD diagnosis has been linked to increased subjective ratings of pain, increased pain-related impairment ratings, and higher likelihood of opioid analgesics used for pain control in civilian populations [45]. Individuals with a PTSD diagnosis have a greater likelihood of being prescribed opioid analgesics [46]. These individuals tend to have more severe PTSD symptoms and were more likely to be prescribed any type of analgesic pain medication [46].

16.5.2   Treatment

Treatment to address concurrent PTSD and SUDs has been evolving. In the past, the standard of care was to treat the SUD first. It was thought that attempts to focus on the trauma symptoms during the early stages of SUD treatment would exacerbate hyperarousal symptoms and negative affect which would lead to relapse. However, emerging data revealed that an integrated approach that addressed both PTSD and SUDs improved recovery rates. Seeking Safety (SS) is a manualized CBT group therapy designed to specifically treat PTSD and substance using patients. It uses cognitive, behavioral, and interpersonal coping skills over 24 structured sessions. In a small study, SS was combined with Exposure Therapy, a behavioral therapy that encourages systematic confrontation to a feared object or context in a safe space to attenuate a person's fear response [47]. Male PTSD and SUD patients demonstrated improved outcome results in 11 different measures including decreased drug use, decreased trauma symptoms, and decreased anxiety [47]. SS combined with another manualized CBT treatment, Relapse Prevention, demonstrated improvement in women's PTSD and psychiatric symptoms along with reductions in substance use [48]. Relapse Prevention is a behavioral approach that teaches individuals with SUDs how to anticipate and cope with the potential for relapse. In one study of individuals with comorbid PTSD and substance dependence, Concurrent Treatment of PTSD and SUDs Using Prolonged Exposure (COPE) along with TAU was compared with TAU alone. Those receiving the combined treatment showed improved

PTSD symptoms without worsening of substance dependence as compared with TAU for a substance dependence-only group [49]. Interestingly, most individuals within the COPE group continued to use substances during the study disputing the notion that abstinence is necessary to do trauma work and receive benefit [49]. Serotonin-reuptake inhibitors are U.S. Food and Drug Administration (FDA)-approved for PTSD treatment. Pharmacological studies of co-occurring PTSD and SUDs are lacking, and of the studies done, PTSD and AUD are the comorbid conditions investigated [50]. A 2013 literature review of comorbid PTSD and opioid addiction further noted the lack of studies evaluating integrated behavioral therapies and medication-assisted treatment for opioid dependence [51].

16.6 Psychotic Disorders

16.6.1 Epidemiology

Studies have shown that schizophrenia often co-occurs with SUDs. The ECA study reported that participants with a lifetime prevalence of Schizophrenia were 8.8 times more likely to have an opioid use disorder in their lifetime [2]. Individuals with a lifetime prevalence of self-reported psychotic disorder were approximately ten times more likely to have an opioid use disorder according to the NESARC study results [52].

16.6.2 Treatment

A number of studies have examined patients with comorbid psychotic disorders and SUDs. Schizophrenia with comorbid SUD has been associated with poor treatment outcome and poor treatment adherence. Behavioral Treatment for Substance Abuse in Severe and Persistent Mental Illness (BTSAS) is a social learning intervention that includes motivational interviewing, urinalysis contingency, and social skills training. BTSAS was more effective than Supportive Treatment for Addiction Recovery (STAR) in percentage of clean urine drug screens, attendance to sessions, and retention in treatment [53]. Specifically, within the schizophrenia spectrum, heroin addicts on combined opioid agonist therapy and olanzapine, an atypical antipsychotic, in comparison to those on combined therapy with haloperidol, a typical antipsychotic, had improved retention rates in treatment and increased negative urine drug screens [54]. A recent review of the literature indicated that clozapine, an atypical antipsychotic reserved for use in treatment-resistant schizophrenia because of the potential for serious side effects, demonstrated improved SUD treatment outcomes. Most studies with clozapine have been limited to psychotic patients with AUD; [55] use in co-occurring psychotic and opioid use disorders require further study.

16.7   Personality Disorders

16.7.1   Epidemiology

There is limited research investigating all personality disorders and co-occurring of substance use. More studies have examined antisocial personality disorder (ASPD) and comorbid substance use. The ECA study revealed that persons with lifetime ASPD had 24.3 times increased risk for opioid use disorder in their lifetime [2]. In persons with NMPOU disorders, there is an 8.1 risk of lifetime ASPD. [7] Another study extracted data from the NESARC and found that of individuals with lifetime opioid use disorder, 30.3 % had ASPD, 18.3 % had obsessive compulsive personality disorder, 15.9 % had paranoid personality disorder, 11.9 % had schizoid personality disorder, 10.4 % had avoidant personality disorder, and 9.4 % had histrionic personality disorder [14]. Synthesizing data from various studies, in treated addicts, ASPD lifetime prevalence ranged from 3.0 to 27.0 % and borderline personality disorder (BPD) lifetime prevalence ranged from 5.0 to 22.4 % [56].

16.7.2   Treatment

Few studies investigated the efficacy of integrated approaches to treat co-occurring personality disorders and SUDs. There are no medications FDA-approved for personality disorder treatment. A review that examined pharmacotherapeutic interventions for personality disorders demonstrated that none of the medications, regardless of class (e.g., antidepressants, mood stabilizers, and antipsychotics), produced a remission of BPD [57]. Additionally, there is a dearth of studies exploring pharmacological treatment for personality disorders other than BPD.

Nevertheless, there are some behavioral therapies that show benefit in personality disorders. Dialectical behavior therapy (DBT) is a specific form of CBT originally developed to help individuals change patterns of behavior that are harmful, such as self-injurious behaviors and suicidal thinking. DBT, in comparison to TAU, was associated with reduction in substance abuse and improved treatment retention in substance-dependent BPD patients [58]. Patients on MMT with personality disorders were found to have higher dropout rates from treatment; and BPD, ASPD, and histrionic personality disorder patients demonstrated poorest overall treatment outcomes [59].

16.8   Attention Deficit/Hyperactivity Disorder

16.8.1   Epidemiology

A number of studies have shown increased risk for substance use disorder in individuals with attention deficit/hyperactivity disorder (ADHD). Adults with ADHD are approximately 7.9 times more likely than controls to have comorbid drug dependence within the previous 12 months [60]. Roughly 19.4 to 27.2 % of patients with SUDs have comorbid ADHD [61]. In comparison to controls, individuals with ADHD were 2.5 times more likely to develop illicit substance abuse/dependence [62]. Persons with ADHD combined subtype were more elevated risk for opioid use disorders in comparison to ADHD inattentive subtype or ADHD hyperactive-impulsive subtype [63].

16.8.2   Treatment

Psychostimulants are first-line FDA-approved medications for ADHD treatment. However, medications often prescribed for ADHD have abuse potential [64] and medical users of psychostimulants are more likely to be approached to divert their medication [65]. In individuals with ADHD and comorbid opioid dependence and/ or cocaine dependence, age of first substance use was earlier, there were a greater number of co-occurring SUD and psychiatric disorder diagnoses, there were more suicide attempts, and there were greater number of hospitalizations due to either psychiatric or substance issues [66]. This underscores the need for interventions that address both ADHD and the co-occurring SUDs. Given the concerns for the higher abuse potential of prescribed stimulants, bupropion has been used as an alternative medication to reduce ADHD symptoms. A 12-week double-blind study that compared the efficacy of sustained-release methylphenidate, a psychostimulant, or sustained-release bupropion to placebo in MMT participants with ADHD demonstrated no significant differences between the groups in reducing ADHD symptoms. [67]

16.9   Eating Disorders

Although there is evidence that eating disorders are comorbid with SUDs, this association has not been seen for opioid use disorders.

16.10   Summary

The co-occurrence of opioid use disorders with psychiatric syndromes is common and highly prevalent. The negative impact that these conditions have on the individual patient, family, and community as a whole cannot be fully quantified. As health-care providers, it is important to screen, assess, and appropriately triage patients to the appropriate level of care to address their immediate needs. The philosophy in treating these comorbid conditions has shifted from one of sequential management of each disease process to an integrated approach to handle multiple disorders simultaneously and evidence continues to grow that this consolidated method leads to better outcomes for patients with reduced substance use and symptomatology for psychiatric conditions. An integrated approach generally includes pharmacotherapeutic and behavioral interventions. More research of opioid use disorder patients in the context of comorbid mental disorders is needed. In particular, studies to investigate specific psychotropic medications and psychosocial interventions are crucial so that integrated models of care and treatment algorithms may be created specifically for this population.

References

1. Substance Abuse and Mental Health Services Administration Centre for BHS and Quality. Results from the 2013 National survey on drug use and health: mental health detailed tables. Rockville; 2014.
2. Regier DA, Farmer ME, Rae DS, et al. Comorbidity of mental disorders with alcohol and other drug abuse: results from the Epidemiologic Catchment Area (ECA) study. JAMA. 1990;264:2511–8.
3. Kessler RC, Mcgonagle KA, Zhao S, et al. Lifetime and 12-month prevalence of DSM-III-R psychiatric disorders in the United States: Results From the National Comorbidity Survey. Arch Gen Psychiatry. 1994;51:8–19.
4. Warner LA, Kessler RC, Hughes M, Anthony JC, Nelson CB. Prevalence and correlates of drug use and dependence in the united states: results from the national comorbidity survey. Arch Gen Psychiatry. 1995;52:219–29.
5. Kessler RC, Chiu WT, Demler O, Merikangas KR, Walters EE. Prevalence, severity, and comorbidity of 12-month DSM-IV disorders in the National Comorbidity Survey Replication. Arch Gen Psychiatry. 2005;62(6):617–27. doi:10.1001/archpsyc.62.6.617.
6. Compton WM, Thomas YF, Stinson FS, Grant BF. Prevalence, correlates, disability, and comorbidity of DSM-IV drug abuse and dependence in the united states: results from the national epidemiologic survey on alcohol and related conditions. Arch Gen Psychiatry. 2007;64:566–76.
7. Huang B, Dawson DA, Stinson FS, et al. Prevalence, correlates, and comorbidity of nonmedical prescription drug use and drug use disorders in the United States: Results of the National Epidemiologic Survey on Alcohol and Related Conditions. J Clin Psychiatry. 2006;67(7):1062–73.
8. Angold A, Costello EJ, Erkanli A. Comorbidity. J Child Psychol Psychiatry. 1999;40(1):57–87. doi:10.1111/1469-7610.00424.
9. Falk D, Yi H, Hiller-Sturmhöfel S. An epidemiologic analysis of co-occurring alcohol and drug use and disorders. Alcohol Res Health. 2008;31(2):100–10.
10. Mueser KT, Drake RE, Wallach MA. Dual diagnosis: a review of etiological theories. Addict Behav. 1998;23(6):717–34. doi:10.1016/S0306-4603(98)00073-2.
11. Kessler RC. The epidemiology of dual diagnosis. Biol Psychiatry. 2004;56(10):730–7. doi:10.1016/j.biopsych.2004.06.034.
12. Conway KP, Compton WM, Stinson FS, Grant BF. Lifetime comorbidity of DSM-IV mood and anxiety disorders and specific drug use disorders: results from the National Epidemiologic Survey on Alcohol and Related Conditions. J Clin Psychiatry. 2006;67(2):247–57. http://www.scopus.com/inward/record.url?eid=2-s2.0-33644823142&partnerID=tZOtx3y1.
13. Wu L-T, Woody GE, Yang C, Blazer DG. How do prescription opioid users differ from users of heroin or other drugs in psychopathology: results from the National Epidemiologic Survey on Alcohol and Related Conditions. J Addict Med. 2011;5(1):28–35. doi:10.1097/ADM.0b013e3181e0364e.

14. Grella CE, Karno MP, Warda US, Niv N, Moore AA. Gender and comorbidity among individuals with opioid use disorders in the NESARC study. Addict Behav. 2009;34(6-7):498–504. doi:10.1016/j.addbeh.2009.01.002.
15. Bair MJ, Robinson RL, Katon W, Kroenke K. Depression and pain comorbidity: a literature review. Arch Intern Med. 2003;163:2433–45. doi:10.1097/ALN.0b013e31822ec185.
16. Nunes EV, Levin FR. Treatment of depression in patients with alcohol or other drug dependence: a meta-analysis. JAMA. 2014;291(15):1887–96.
17. Schreiber S, Peles E, Adelson M. Association between improvement in depression, reduced benzodiazepine (BDZ) abuse, and increased psychotropic medication use in methadone maintenance treatment (MMT) patients. Drug Alcohol Depend. 2008;92(1-3):79–85. doi:10.1016/j.drugalcdep.2007.06.016.
18. Kleber HD, Weissman MM, Rounsaville BJ, Wilber CH, Prusoff BA, Riordan CE. Imipramine as treatment for depression in addicts. Arch Gen Psychiatry. 1983;40(6):649–53. doi:10.1001/archpsyc.1983.04390010059007.
19. Nunes EV, Quitkin FM, Donovan SJ, et al. Imipramine treatment of opiate-dependent patients with depressive disorders. A placebo-controlled trial. Arch Gen Psychiatry. 1998;55(2):153–60. doi:10.1001/archpsyc.55.2.153.
20. Petrakis I, Carroll KM, Nich C, Gordon L, Kosten T, Rounsaville B. Fluoxetine treatment of depressive disorders in methadone-maintained opioid addicts. Drug Alcohol Depend. 1998;50(3):221–6. doi:10.1016/S0376-8716(98)00032-5.
21. Dean AJ, Bell J, Mascord DJ, Parker G, Christie MJ. A randomised, controlled trial of fluoxetine in methadone maintenance patients with depressive symptoms. J Affect Disord. 2002;72(1):85–90.
22. Gonzalez G, Feingold A, Oliveto A, Gonsai K, Kosten TR. Comorbid major depressive disorder as a prognostic factor in cocaine-abusing buprenorphine-maintained patients treated with desipramine and contingency management. Am J Drug Alcohol Abuse. 2003;29(3):497–514. doi:10.1081/ADA-120023455.
23. Kosten T, Falcioni J, Oliveto A, Feingold A. Depression predicts higher rates of heroin use on desipramine with buprenorphine than with methadone. Am J Addict. 2004;13(2):191–201. doi:10.1080/10550490490435966.
24. Nunes EV, Sullivan MA, Levin FR. Treatment of depression in patients with opiate dependence. Biol Psychiatry. 2004;56(10):793–802. doi:10.1016/j.biopsych.2004.06.037.
25. Pedrelli P, Iovieno N, Vitali M, Tedeschini E, Bentley KH, Papakostas GI. Treatment of major depressive disorder and dysthymic disorder with antidepressants in patients with comorbid opiate use disorders enrolled in methadone maintenance therapy: a meta-analysis. J Clin Psychopharmacol. 2011;31(5):582–6. doi:10.1097/JCP.0b013e31822c0adf.
26. Detke MJ, Lu Y, Goldstein DJ, Hayes JR, Demitrack MA. Duloxetine, 60 mg once daily, for major depressive disorder: a randomized double-blind placebo-controlled trial. J Clin Psychiatry. 2002;63(4):308–15.
27. Stein MD, Solomon DA, Herman DS, et al. Pharmacotherapy plus psychotherapy for treatment of depression in active injection drug users. Arch Gen Psychiatry. 2004;61(2):152–9. doi:10.1001/archpsyc.62.2.224.
28. Carpenter KM, Smith JL, Aharonovich E, Nunes EV. Developing therapies for depression in drug dependence: results of a stage 1 therapy study. Am J Drug Alcohol Abuse. 2008;34(5):642–52. doi:10.1080/00952990802308171.
29. Hides L, Samet S, Lubman DI. Cognitive behaviour therapy (CBT) for the treatment of co-occurring depression and substance use: current evidence and directions for future research. Drug Alcohol Rev. 2010;29(5):508–17. doi:10.1111/j.1465-3362.2010.00207.x.
30. Brown ES, Jeffress J, Liggin JDM, Garza M, Beard L. Switching outpatients with bipolar or schizoaffective disorders and substance abuse from their current antipsychotic to aripiprazole. J Clin Psychiatry. 2005;66(6):756–60. doi:10.4088/JCP.v66n0613.
31. Weiss RD, Griffin ML, Kolodziej ME, et al. A randomized trial of Integrated Group Therapy versus group drug counseling for patients with bipolar disorder and substance dependence. Am J Psychiatry. 2007;164(1):100–7. doi:10.1176/appi.ajp.164.1.100.

32. Weiss RD, Griffin ML, Jaffee WB, et al. A "community-friendly" version of integrated group therapy for patients with bipolar disorder and substance dependence: A randomized controlled trial. Drug Alcohol Depend. 2009;104(3):212–9. doi:10.1016/j.drugalcdep.2009.04.018.

33. Weiss RD. Treating patients with bipolar disorder and substance dependence: lessons learned. J Subst Abuse Treat. 2004;27(4):307–12. doi:10.1016/j.jsat.2004.10.001.

34. Levin FR, Hennessy G. Bipolar disorder and substance abuse. Biol Psychiatry. 2004;56(10):738–48. doi:10.1016/j.biopsych.2004.05.008.

35. Albanese MJ, Pies R. The bipolar patient with comorbid substance use disorder: recognition and management. CNS Drugs. 2004;18(9):585–96. doi:10.2165/00023210-200418090-00004.

36. Ferri M, Finlayson AJR, Wang L, Martin PR. Predictive factors for relapse in patients on buprenorphine maintenance. Am J Addict. 2014;23(1):62–7. doi:10.1111/j.1521-0391.2013.12074.x.

37. Lejuez CW, Zvolensky MJ, Daughters SB, et al. Anxiety sensitivity: a unique predictor of dropout among inner-city heroin and crack/cocaine users in residential substance use treatment. Behav Res Ther. 2008;46(7):811–8. doi:10.1016/j.brat.2008.03.010.

38. McRae AL, Sonne SC, Brady KT, Durkalski V, Palesch Y. A randomized, placebo-controlled trial of buspirone for the treatment of anxiety in opioid-dependent individuals. Am J Addict. 2004;13(1):53–63. doi:10.1080/10550490490265325.

39. Fals-Stewart W, Schafer J. The treatment of substance abusers diagnosed with obsessive-compulsive disorder: an outcome study. J Subst Abuse Treat. 1992;9(4):365–70. doi:10.1016/0740-5472(92)90032-J.

40. Fatséas M, Denis C, Lavie E, Auriacombe M. Relationship between anxiety disorders and opiate dependence—a systematic review of the literature. Implications for diagnosis and treatment. J Subst Abuse Treat. 2010;38(3):220–30. doi:10.1016/j.jsat.2009.12.003.

41. Back SE, Brady KT. Anxiety disorders with comorbid substance use disorders: diagnostic and treatment considerations. Psychiatr Ann. 2008;38(11):724–9. doi:10.3928/00485713-2008 1101-01.

42. Cottler LB, Comton WM, Mager D, Spitznagel EL, Janca A. Posttraumatic stress disorder among substance users from the general population. Am J Addict. 1992;149(5):664–70.

43. Seal KH, Ying S, Cohen G, et al. Association of Mental Health Disorders with Prescription Opioids and High-Risk Opioid Use in US Veterans of Iraq and Afghanistan. JAMA. 2012;307(9):940–7. doi:10.1001/jama.2012.234.

44. Dabbs C, Watkins EY, Fink DS, Eick-Cost A, Millikan AM. Opiate-related dependence/abuse and PTSD exposure among the active-component U.S. Military, 2001 to 2008. Mil Med. 2014;179(8):885–90. doi:10.7205/MILMED-D-14-00012.

45. Phifer J, Skelton K, Weiss T, et al. Pain symptomatology and pain medication use in civilian PTSD. Pain. 2011;152(10):2233–40. doi:10.1016/j.pain.2011.04.019.

46. Schwartz AC, Bradley R, Penza KM, et al. Pain medication use among patients with posttraumatic stress disorder. Psychosomatics. 2006;47(2):136–42. doi:10.1176/appi.psy.47.2.136.

47. Najavits LM, Schmitz M, Gotthardt S, Weiss RD. Seeking safety plus exposure therapy: an outcome study on dual diagnosis men. J Psychoactive Drugs. 2005;37(4):425–35. doi:10.108 0/02791072.2005.10399816.

48. Hien DA, Cohen LR, Miele GM, Litt LC, Capstick C. Promising treatments for women with comorbid PTSD and substance use disorders. Am J Psychiatry. 2004;161(8):1426–32. doi:10.1176/appi.ajp.161.8.1426.

49. Mills KL, Teesson M, Back SE, et al. Integrated exposure-based therapy for co-occurring posttraumatic stress disorder and substance dependence: a randomized controlled trial. JAMA. 2012;308(7):690–9.

50. McCauley J, Kileen T, Gros DF, Brady KT, Back SE. Posttraumatic stress disorder and co-occurring substance use disorders: advances in assessment and treatment. Clin Psychol (New York). 2012;19(3):1–27. doi:10.1111/cpsp.12006.Posttraumatic.

51. Fareed A, Eilender P, Haber M, Bremner J, Whitfield N, Drexler K. Comorbid posttraumatic stress disorder and opiate addiction: a literature review. J Addict Dis. 2013;32(2):168–79. doi:10.1080/10550887.2013.795467.

52. Lev-Ran S, Imtiaz S, Le Foll B. Self-reported psychotic disorders among Individuals with substance use disorders: findings from the National Epidemiologic Survey on Alcohol and Related Conditions. Am J Addict. 2012;21(6):531–5. doi:10.1111/j.1521-0391.2012.00283.x.

53. Bellack AS, Bennett ME, Gearon JS, Brown CH, Yang Y. A randomized clinical trial of a new behavioral treatment for drug abuse in people with severe and persistent mental illness. Arch Gen Psychiatry. 2006;63(4):426–32. doi:10.1001/archpsyc.63.4.426.

54. Gerra G, Di Petta G, D'Amore A, et al. Combination of olanzapine with opioid-agonists in the treatment of heroin-addicted patients affected by comorbid schizophrenia spectrum disorders. Clin Neuropharmacol. 2007;30(3):127–35. doi:10.1097/wnf.0b013e31803354f6.

55. Zhornitsky S, Rizkallah E, Pampoulova T, et al. Antipsychotic agents for the treatment of substance use disorders in patients with and without comorbid psychosis. J Clin Psychopharmacol. 2010;30(4):417–24. doi:10.1097/JCP.0b013e3181e7810a.

56. Verheul R. Co-morbidity of personality disorders in individuals with substance use disorders. Eur Psychiatry. 2001;16(5):274–82. doi:10.1016/S0924-9338(01)00578-8.

57. Paris J. Pharmacological treatments for personality disorders. Int Rev Psychiatry. 2011;23(3):303–9. doi:10.3109/09540261.2011.586993.

58. Linehan MM, Schmidt H, Dimeff LA, Craft JC, Kanter J, Comtois KA. Dialectical behavior therapy for patients with borderline personality disorder and drug-dependence. Am J Addict. 1999;8(4):279–92.

59. Cacciola JS, Alterman AI, Rutherford MJ, McKay JR, Mulvaney FD. The relationship of psychiatric comorbidity to treatment outcomes in methadone maintained patients. Drug Alcohol Depend. 2001;61(3):271–80. doi:10.1016/S0376-8716(00)00148-4.

60. Kessler RC, Adler L, Barkley R, et al. The prevalence and correlates of adult ADHD in the United States: results from the National Comorbidity Survey Replication. Am J Psychiatry. 2006;163(4):716–23. doi:10.1176/appi.ajp.163.4.716.

61. Van Emmerik-van Oortmerssen K, van de Glind G, van den Brink W, et al. Prevalence of attention-deficit hyperactivity disorder in substance use disorder patients: a meta-analysis and meta-regression analysis. Drug Alcohol Depend. 2012;122(1-2):11–9. doi:10.1016/j.drugalcdep.2011.12.007.

62. Lee SS, Humphreys KL, Flory K, Liu R, Glass K. Prospective association of childhood attention-deficit/hyperactivity disorder (ADHD) and substance use and abuse/dependence: A meta-analytic review. Clin Psychol Rev. 2011;31(3):328–41. doi:10.1016/j.cpr.2011.01.006.

63. De Alwis D, Lynskey MT, Reiersen AM, Agrawal A. Attention-deficit/hyperactivity disorder subtypes and substance use and use disorders in NESARC. Addict Behav. 2014;39(8):1278–85. doi:10.1016/j.addbeh.2014.04.003.

64. Mao AR, Babcock T, Brams M. ADHD in adults: current treatment trends with consideration of abuse potential of medications. J Psychiatr Pract. 2011;17(4):241–50. doi:10.1097/01.pra.0000400261.45290.bd.

65. McCabe SE, Boyd CJ, Teter CJ. Medical use, illicit use, and diversion of abusable prescription drugs. J Am Coll Health. 2006;54(5):269–78. doi:10.1016/j.biotechadv.2011.08.021.Secreted.

66. Arias AJ, Gelernter J, Chan G, et al. Correlates of co-occurring ADHD in drug-dependent subjects: prevalence and features of substance dependence and psychiatric disorders. Addict Behav. 2008;33(9):1199–207. doi:10.1016/j.addbeh.2008.05.003.

67. Levin FR, Evans SM, Brooks DJ, Kalbag AS, Garawi F, Nunes EV. Treatment of methadone-maintained patients with adult ADHD: double-blind comparison of methylphenidate, bupropion and placebo. Drug Alcohol Depend. 2006;81(2):137–48. doi:10.1016/j.drugalcdep.2005.06.012.

Chapter 17
Assessing and Treating Co-occurring Substance Abuse

Jyothsna Karlapalem and Monica L. Broderick

17.1 Non-opioid Substance Abuse, Chronic Pain, and Opioid Use Disorder: A Complex Interaction

In order to manage co-occurring substance abuse in patients with chronic pain and opioid use disorder effectively, we need to find out if such comorbidities exist, and if they do, we need to understand how these conditions relate to one another.

A review of current literature answers the former in the affirmative. However, consideration of the relationship between chronic pain, opioid use disorders, and non-opioid substance use leaves us with a truly complex web with several interconnections (Fig. 17.1).

1. There is evidence for prevalence of non-opioid substance use in patients with chronic pain.

   Estimates of co-occurring substance abuse in patients with chronic pain and opioid use disorder vary widely in literature. Nevertheless, there is a significant body of literature attesting to the fact that these comorbidities exist. A systematic review of 38 studies published between 1950 and 2010 found that 3–48 % of patients with chronic noncancer pain have a current substance use disorder [1, 2]. The wide variation in prevalence rates across studies is due to differences in study population as well as methods used to assess substance use disorders.

J. Karlapalem, M.B.B.S. (✉)
Department of Psychiatry, SUNY Downstate Medical Center,
450 Clarkson Avenue B5-495, Brooklyn, NY 11203, USA
e-mail: jyothsnawudali@gmail.com

M.L. Broderick, M.D.
Department of Psychiatry, Kings County Hospital Center/SUNY Downstate Medical Center,
451 Clarkson Avenue, Brooklyn, NY 11203, USA
e-mail: monica.broderick@nychhc.org

© Springer International Publishing Switzerland 2016   215
A.M. Matthews, J.C. Fellers (eds.), *Treating Comorbid Opioid Use Disorder
in Chronic Pain*, DOI 10.1007/978-3-319-29863-4_17

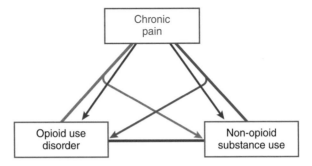

Fig. 17.1 Complex interaction: non-opioid substance use, chronic pain, and opioid use disorder

2. Non-opioid substance use is a risk factor for developing opioid use disorder in chronic pain patients.

   For example, a large study of 15,160 US veterans with chronic pain found that a diagnosis of non-opioid substance abuse is a strong predictor for opioid abuse and dependence with an odds ratio of 2.34. In the same study, a diagnosis of another mental health disorder was only a moderate predictor of opioid abuse or dependence in this population with an Odds ratio of 1.46 [3, 4]. In another study of 199 patients in a pain rehabilitation program, Huffman et al. found that patients with non-opioid substance abuse disorders have 28 times the odds of developing therapeutic opioid addiction [4].

3. Chronic pain itself may be an independent risk factor for substance use and may worsen treatment outcomes for non-opioid substance use.

   For instance, Larson et al. in their study of 397 patients admitted to a detoxification program found that persistent pain increased the risk of relapse for any substance use (adjusted odds ratio 4.2) at 24 months follow-up [5]. In another prospective study of 582 veterans receiving addiction treatment, veterans with chronic pain were less likely to be abstinent from alcohol or drugs and had worse Alcohol Severity Index (ASI) composite scores compared to those with no pain at 12 months follow-up [6].

4. The presence of pain in patients with opioid use disorders is associated with continued use of opioids and poor retention in substance abuse treatment [7]. In addition, chronic pain in patients with opioid use disorders is associated with increased severity of medical and psychiatric comorbidities [7].

   Even though the non-opioid substance abuse has been well-known as a risk factor for opioid misuse in chronic pain patients for at least a decade [8], recent studies in prescribing practices continue to find a large number of patients with a history of substance abuse who are still prescribed opioids for chronic pain. In a large scale study based on adult health plan enrollees, Weisner et al. (2009) found that 17 % of patients with prior substance abuse history were on prescription opioids compared to 2.9 % of those without substance abuse histories [4, 9].

The same study also found that patients with prior substance abuse history who are prescribed opioids are more likely to be on higher doses and long-acting formulations of opioids and are more likely to be prescribed sedative hypnotics as well. Given the complex interaction between these three conditions and continued practice of prescribing opioids to patients with known history of substance abuse, some knowledge about patterns of comorbid substance use in chronic pain patients is essential. This will help us to actively assess and treat these specific conditions.

17.1.1 Common Patterns of Co-occurring Substance Abuse

The Pain and Opioids IN Treatment (POINT) study was a 2-year prospective cohort study of about 1500 people prescribed with pharmaceutical opioids for their chronic pain, based in Australia [10]. In this study, over 75 % of these patients reported lifetime tobacco use and 30 % endorsed current daily use of tobacco. Thirty percent of the patients in this sample had a lifetime alcohol use disorder, 10 % had cannabis use disorder, and 5 % had lifetime amphetamine use disorder.

In terms of recent use, 12.9 % reported using cannabis and 1.6 % reported using amphetamines. Over 37.5 % patients had at least one item positive on Opioid-related Behaviors in Treatment (ORBIT) scale during the study period. About 34 % of the patients in this cohort were also prescribed benzodiazepines (Table 17.1).

In another study of patients entering a pain rehabilitation program, 59 % had a lifetime history of non-opioid substance abuse disorder and 14.9 % had active sedative hypnotic use disorder [4]. In patients with opioid dependence on methadone maintenance ($n=404$), Dhingra et al. found that about 104 patients had clinically significant pain (CSP). Among the CSP patients, 42.3 % endorsed cocaine use, 18.3 % endorsed nontherapeutic opioid use, and 1.9 % endorsed amphetamine use [11].

In summary, tobacco, alcohol, benzodiazepines, cannabis, amphetamines, and cocaine seem to be the common substances used by patients with chronic pain and opioid dependence listed in order from most common to least common in terms of prevalence. However, we need to review the risk for each substance of abuse to decide which ones we need to be most vigilant about.

Table 17.1 Non- opioid substance use in POINT cohort ($n=1514$)

Substance	Lifetime use	Lifetime use disorder	Used in last 12 months
Tobacco	75.9 %	31.1[a]	31.1[a]
Alcohol	92.8	30.7	60.5
Cannabis	43.2	11.7	10.9
Amphetamines	13.9	5.6	1.6

[a]This number reflects people who endorsed current daily smoking, lifetime use disorder was not reported for tobacco

17.2 Rationale for the Need to Actively Assess and Treat for Comorbid Substance Abuse

Why do we need to actively assess and treat for comorbid substance abuse? While specific interactions exist for different substances, increased risk of overdose and death seems to be common to many substances and is the most serious of them all.

17.2.1 Risk of Overdose and Death

Calcaterra et al. used death certificate data to analyze pharmaceutical opioid overdose deaths in the US between 1999 and 2009. Along with a fourfold increase in the overall death rate due to overdose in the study period, they found that opioid-related deaths commonly involved additional substances including alcohol, sedatives, or prescription drugs. They also found that the combination of pharmaceutical opioids and benzodiazepines was the most common cause of polysubstance overdose death [12].

Similarly, Madadi et al. used the coroner's records of Ontario to study opioid-related deaths in the city between 2006 and 2008. They found that accidental death related to opioids was significantly associated with a personal history of substance abuse. Of the 1359 opioid-related deaths in the study period, there was history of illicit substance abuse in over 44 % of cases, history of alcohol abuse in 21 %, and history of prescription opioid abuse in 43 %. Alcohol was detected during coroner's examination in over 32 % of cases; cocaine was found in over 29 % [13].

The above findings illustrate the role of comorbid substance abuse in opioid-related mortality. In addition, there is ample data to suggest that comorbid substance abuse affects multiple outcomes in patients with chronic pain and opioid dependence as discussed later in this chapter. In view of high prevalence of comorbid substance abuse, wide variation in comorbidity patterns, and possibility of multiple comorbid substance abuse concerns in the same individual, it is important to understand the interaction between opioids and specific substances of abuse. Knowledge of these specific interactions will help providers to educate patients about relative risks of various substances, as well as help tailor treatment based on individual comorbidity patterns.

17.2.2 Tobacco

Smoking is comorbid in over 80 % of patients in substance abuse population. There is evidence to support that smoking cessation does not impair outcomes for presenting substance abuse issue in any way and may actually enhance successful outcomes for the same [14]. Despite this, tobacco use is undertreated in this population. Given the high mortality and morbidity associated with smoking, it is vital to address tobacco use aggressively in treating chronic pain patients as well.

In a structured review of studies that dealt with smoking in pain patients published between 1966 and 2011, 100% of the studies reviewed supported the study hypotheses that chronic pain patients who smoke are more likely to be on opioids, are also more likely to be on a higher dose, have drug and alcohol dependence, and have aberrant drug-related behavior [15]. Another study of over 1200 patients entering a 3-week pain rehabilitation program found that smokers were less likely to complete the treatment compared to nonsmokers and past smokers [16].

While treatment outcomes for smoking cessation in substance-abusing population are modest, even modest results may help to decrease mortality and morbidity rates for these patients [14]. Additionally, chemicals in cigarette smoke are known to induce the metabolism of opioids. Hence, while advising smoking cessation in patients on opioid therapy, one needs to be mindful of the possibility of increased opioid drug levels with smoking cessation [17] and decrease the dose of opioids as needed to avoid toxicity. Further, patients need to be made aware that smoking decreases the analgesic effects of opioids at any given dose, in view of this interaction.

17.2.3 Alcohol

Alcohol abuse is concerning in patients with chronic pain who are on opioid therapy primarily due to risk of additive CNS and respiratory depressant effects contributing to psychomotor impairment and mortality. Even without significant pharmacokinetic interaction, co-administration of alcohol and opioids decreases the ventilatory response to hypercapnia [18].

However, the phenomenon of "dose dumping" is a major concern when alcohol and some formulations of long-acting opioid are taken together. This refers to unintended, rapid release of a large fraction of the opioid from a modified release opioid preparation and may increase the risk of overdose and abuse liability of these drugs [19]. Regardless of the formulation, consumption of opioids with alcohol may produce more euphoric effects than either substance alone [19, 20], possibly contributing to addictive potential of both substances. In view of this, we need to caution our patients regarding additive risk of overdose when combining opioids with alcohol, particularly if they are on a long-acting formulation. We should also educate patients and their families about this risk and provide them with naloxone rescue kits, in addition to aggressive treatment of alcohol use disorders in these patients.

17.2.4 Benzodiazepines

Patients who are prescribed high doses of opioids are significantly more likely to receive high doses of benzodiazepines [19]. Hence, it is important to consider interactions between these two classes of medications. Similar to alcohol, benzodiazepines carry the risk of additive CNS and respiratory depression when used along with opioids. Combined opioid and benzodiazepine use accounted for majority of polysubstance overdose deaths in the US between 1999 and 2009 [12].

Even during medical or surgical procedures, co-administration of benzodiazepines and opioids might result in hypoxemia, apnea, and respiratory depression [21, 22].

Conversely, a history of benzodiazepine use is a strong predictor of moderate-to-high opioid use at a later time. This persists even after adjusting for musculoskeletal pain, smoking, alcohol, and socioeconomic variables, suggesting that benzodiazepine use is a stronger predictor for future opioid use than even self-reported pain [23].

Patients who are on both opioids and benzodiazepines have more pain-related and behavioral management problems. Also, among patients with noncancer pain, benzodiazepine use is associated with more total months of prescribed opioids, higher mean daily doses, and a greater risk of a psychogenic chronic pain diagnosis and a diagnosis of alcohol abuse/dependence [19, 24]. Given these interactions, we need to review our patients' current medications carefully before prescribing benzodiazepines or opioids. In addition to education about risk of overdose and provision of naloxone rescue kits, we should also discuss possibility of poor outcomes when these medications are taken together and suggest alternative treatments when available.

17.2.5 Cannabis

A number of states in the US have enacted legislation decriminalizing or legalizing cannabis. So, it's becoming imperative to understand the ramifications in chronic pain patients who may be prescribed both medical marijuana and opioids concurrently. While recent literature shows that liberal marijuana laws in certain states are associated with decreased opioid-related mortality, further studies need to examine whether this is related to the effect of possible confounders like aggressive campaigns to prevent opioid overdose like distribution of naloxone rescue kits and aggressive patient education programs in these states [25].

Experts believe that analgesic effects of cannabis and opioids are additive in nature. For example, Abrams et al. conducted an interventional study of 21 patients receiving sustained-release morphine or oxycodone. They administered vaporized cannabis to these patients in the laboratory and found that cannabis augments analgesic effects of opioids even without significantly altering plasma opioid concentrations [26].

However, this does not seem to translate into better clinical outcomes in patients with chronic pain who use both cannabis and opioids. In a longitudinal analysis of POINT study population, patients who reported using cannabis had been prescribed opioids for longer, were on higher opioid doses, and were more likely to be nonadherent with their opioid use. Also, those who reported using cannabis specifically for pain reported greater pain severity, greater interference from and poorer coping with pain, and more days out of role in the past year [27]. While this points to clear association between cannabis abuse and worsened clinical pain in chronic pain population, causality or directionality is difficult to establish from this data.

However, Reisfield et al., in their 2009 review of literature, found that cannabis use in chronic opioid patients shows statistically significant associations with present and future aberrant opioid-related behaviors [28]. In a related commentary, the same authors highlighted the psychomotor impairments in cannabis use and association with motor vehicle crashes particularly when used with other CNS depressants like alcohol. They cautioned against prescribing opioids to patients who are also prescribed medical cannabis, particularly if there is suspicion of other substance abuse [29]. Hence, patients need to be warned about increased risk of opioid abuse, worsening pain outcomes in the long term, as well as additive impairments in complex tasks like driving or operating heavy machinery when they use opioids and cannabis together.

17.2.6   Cocaine

Risk of increased rates of opioid-related mortality is a major concern for cocaine abuse.

Cocaine was convincingly implicated in up to 29 % of opioid-related deaths in a large North American city in a span of 2 years [13]. This is probably related to QT prolongation with cocaine [30], which might be additive when given with opioids. A history of cocaine use increases the odds of failing to resolve aberrant drug-related behaviors in a pain rehabilitation program; odds ratio 4.97 [31]. Past cocaine use was also found to be an independent predictor of prescription opioid misuse in a large academic practice; odds ratio 4.3 [32].

Because of the serious consequences like death and overdose and also adverse outcomes for pain management as well as opioid use disorders listed above, it is imperative to actively assess for comorbid non-opioid substance abuse and treat them aggressively as discussed below.

17.3   Approach to Assessment of Co-occurring Substance Abuse

Guidelines for opioid therapy in patients with chronic noncancer pain recommend screening for substance abuse before initiation of opioid therapy [31]. There are a variety of screening instruments like Opioid Risk Tool (ORT) [8] (Fig. 17.2), Screener and Opioid Assessment for Patients with Pain (SOAPP) [33], and so on. Where indicated, more specific screening instruments such as the Alcohol Use Disorders Identification Test—Consumption (AUDIT-C) questionnaire or CAGE questionnaire to assess alcohol abuse or Drug Abuse Screening Test (DAST-10) for illicit substance abuse may be used. All patients will benefit from a thorough

Opioid Risk Tool (Adapted from Webster and Webster, 2005) Mark each that applies. Risk level based on total score values Low risk: 0-3 Moderate risk: 4-7 High risk > 8		
Item	Item score for Females	Item score for Males
1.Family history of substance abuse		
• Alcohol	( )1	( )3
• Illegal drugs	( )2	( )3
• Prescription drugs	( )4	( )4
2.Personal history of substance abuse		
• Alcohol	( )3	( )3
• Illegal drugs	( )4	( )4
• Prescription drugs	( )5	( )5
3.Age	( )1	( )1
4.History of preadolescent sexual abuse	( )3	( )0
5.Psychological disease		
• Attention Deficit disorder, Obsessive compulsive disorder, Bipolar disorder, Schizophrenia	( )2	( )2
• Depression	( )1	( )1

Fig. 17.2 Opioid risk tool. Modified from Webster LR, Webster RM. Predicting aberrant behaviors in opioid-treated patients: preliminary validation of the Opioid Risk Tool. Pain Med. 2005 Dec;6(6):432–42

assessment of smoking history given mortality and morbidity associated with tobacco regardless of other clinical issues. A good clinical interview is invaluable not only in assessing for substance abuse, but also to build a therapeutic alliance with the patient. At baseline, all patients should be assessed for current use of alcohol, cannabis, opioids, benzodiazepines, and sedating over-the-counter preparations; also, stimulants and their use should be quantified. Openness and nonjudgmental stance on the part of clinician are key to elicit this information. Also, family history of substance abuse should be assessed as there is some shared vulnerability for drug abuse that is inherited [34, 35].

The 6 As approach advocated by Baca et al. [14, 36] to address smoking cessation in substance abusers might be adapted to serve as a good framework to assess and treat comorbid substance abuse in this patient population (Fig. 17.3).

Fig. 17.3 Management of
co-occurring substance
use: 6 As

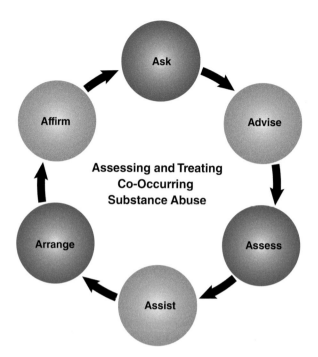

1. ASK: Ask about substance abuse to identify the risk factors. An open-ended question like "Can you tell me about your _____ (substance) use?" is likely to yield more information than a closed question like "Do you smoke marijuana?"
2. ADVISE: Clear, personalized advice about interaction between substance abuse and opioids, counseling about risk of overdose, poor clinical outcomes
3. ASSESS: Assess the patient's willingness by asking "How important on a scale of 0–10 is it for you to quit _____ (any substance)?" or "How willing or ready are you on a scale of 0–10 to quit_____ (any substance)?"
4. ASSIST: Assist in developing a quit plan. Ideally, this should involve presenting the patient with a menu of options and help patients come up with their own plan.
5. ARRANGE: Arrange for treatment and referrals as per the quit plan and arrange for follow-up with the patient later. Follow-up on these referrals is key to treatment success.
6. AFFIRM: Affirm past successes and acknowledge patient's strengths to improve treatment adherence [32].

While subjective reports by patients and clinical interviews are helpful, objective assessment of substance abuse is essential as many patients may not report substance abuse histories. This usually involves urine toxicology, blood alcohol levels, breathalyzer tests, reviewing prescription monitoring programs for other prescription medications like benzodiazepines and other controlled medications, obtaining prior records, and consultation with other specialties like psychiatry, pain management, and physical therapy.

17.3.1   Urine Toxicology

There is a fair amount of evidence to suggest that urine drug screens decrease illicit substance abuse as well as prescription drug abuse in patients receiving chronic pain management therapy [37, 38]. Routine point of care immunoassays can be administered in office-based settings and can help as a first step. However, it is essential to keep in mind some of their limitations [36, 38] (see Table 17.2).

Hence, in selective cases, chromatography is indicated, especially if urine is negative for prescribed opioid or there is suspicion of a false positive result on immunoassay. Any positive urine drug screen should prompt an assessment of detailed medication use and substance use in the past seven days and the results should be discussed with patients in a timely fashion. Referral to addiction treatment may be appropriate if there is a repeated pattern of positive urine drug screens. If clinical suspicion for substance abuse is high, but urine toxicology remains negative, adulteration or subversion of urine drug testing should be considered.

While observed urine collection is widely used in substance abuse settings, it is rarely implemented in family practice or pain management clinics [39]. An indirect method to assess urine dilution is to measure urine creatinine. A urine creatinine level of less than 2–3 mmol/L indicates urine dilution. Cold urine is another crude red flag to suspect dilution. Possible delays in handling samples make urine temperature hard to use clinically as an indicator of dilution as urine samples can cool within minutes.

How often should we get urine drug screens? A "universal" approach to urine toxicology reduces stigma associated with urine drug testing. All patients are treated in the same fashion, making urine drug screens a routine part of evaluation, same as measuring blood pressure or other vital signs [39]. While universal baseline urine toxicology screen is recommended by many guidelines, there are variations in frequency of urine toxicology testing thereafter. One approach is to stratify patients into low-, medium- and high-risk groups based on initial screening instrument used (e.g., ORT). Urine drug screens should be randomly administered every 3–6 months in high-risk group, 6–12 months in medium-risk group, and 1–2 years in low-risk group [2]. Another approach is to do a baseline toxicology screen and then follow-up test within 1-3 months, to monitor for compliance, and every 6 months after that to screen for substance abuse [35].

In case of alcohol, breathalyzer test and blood alcohol levels are affordable options, but can only detect acute alcohol consumption. But, use of newer tech-

Table 17.2 Limitations of immunoassays

1. Do not differentiate among various opioids, unless newer immune assays for specific opiates are used
2. Can show false positive results
3. May miss semisynthetic opioids like methadone, fentanyl, etc.
4. Do not distinguish among various benzodiazepines
5. May miss intermediate acting benzodiazepines like clonazepam

niques like measurement of EtG/EtS (Ethyl glucuronide and Ethyl sulphate) allows for alcohol to be detected up to 4 days even after it is completely eliminated. Given the interaction between alcohol and certain modified release preparations of opioids, testing for EtS/EtG might be relevant in selective cases [19, 40].

17.3.2 Prescription Monitoring Programs

Prescription monitoring programs help to reduce prescription drug abuse or "doctor shopping" and provide information on patterns of prescriptions used by individual patients [41]. While they are mostly limited to state boundaries, they have still been helpful to assess risk of interactions between various controlled medications prescribed to a patient. American Society of Interventional Pain Physicians (ASIPP) guidelines recommend utilizing prescription-monitoring programs at baseline for all patients and at intervals during opioid therapy, as per their risk level, to gather prescription data. When prescription-monitoring programs are not available, they recommend gathering data from all patient's previous physicians and pharmacies. Prescription-monitoring programs may be particularly helpful in case of intermediate acting benzodiazepines like clonazepam, which may not be detected in routine immunoassay-based urine toxicology screens.

17.3.3 Consultation with Other Specialties

In case of patients who show only partial response to opioids or may benefit from specific interventions, consultation with pain management and physical therapy may be helpful to decrease pain-related disability and improve patient outcomes. In addition, careful assessment and management of psychiatric comorbidities is needed to optimize pain management issues. There is evidence to support that patients with chronic noncancer pain who also have a psychiatric illness are more likely to be on opioids and are less likely to benefit from those [42]. In addition, they are frequently prescribed opioids with benzodiazepines, increasing the risk of opioid-related overdose and death. Particular caution is advised in case of patients with suicidal thoughts as a study of opioid-related overdose in Ontario classified 21 % of the deaths as suicide. Close monitoring by a psychiatrist is indicated in such cases [12, 35].

17.4 Approach to Treatment of Co-occurring Substance Abuse

A comprehensive biopsychosocial approach to patients with chronic pain and comorbid substance abuse should include thoughtful medication management along with psychotherapy and adjunctive social services to improve functioning [43]. While evidence on integrated approach to chronic pain and substance abuse is limited, there have been encouraging results for an integrated primary care-based treatment approach to address several comorbid conditions like mood and substance abuse disorders with cognitive behavioral therapy (CBT) and Motivational Interviewing (MI)-based interventions [44]. Careful attention should be paid to drug interactions when prescribing medications to decrease substance abuse in patients receiving opioid therapy. In addition, other psychiatric comorbidities should also be managed with appropriate medications.

17.4.1 Medication Management

There are limited number of studies that looked at specific pharmacotherapies for co-occurring substance abuse in chronic pain patients or those with opioid dependence.

Petrakis et al. found that Disulfiram was helpful to reduce frequency and quantity of cocaine use in opioid-dependent patients on methadone maintenance [45]. Nicotine replacement therapy has been shown to have modest benefit in terms of abstinence rates in substance abuse population [46]. Even if there is little specific literature for this patient population, evidence-based pharmacological approaches to treat comorbid substance abuse should be considered in this patient population, where no contraindications exist. In addition, thoughtful management of opioids and other adjunctive pain medications needs to be a priority. Considering the importance of treating co-occurring substance abuse and dearth of data to manage this condition in patients with chronic pain or opioid dependence, it is pertinent to review FDA-approved pharmacotherapy for substance abuse [46].

17.4.2 Tobacco

1. Nicotine replacement therapy (NRT): This includes products that allow smokers to obtain nicotine without other harmful products that are present in tobacco, like gum, nasal spray, oral spray, patches, or lozenges. They reduce cravings for tobacco and can be used for quitting as well as cutting down. More than one form of NRT like patch with gum/lozenges may be needed to optimize NRT.
2. Varenicline: This acts as a partial agonist of nicotinic receptor and reduces cravings as well as withdrawal symptoms. There is some evidence to suggest it is superior to NRT. Common side effects include nausea and other gastrointestinal side effects. Varenicline carries FDA warning for serious neuropsychiatric symptoms, and careful monitoring is needed in patients with comorbid psychiatric illness.
3. Bupropion SR: This acts by increasing dopamine and norepinephrine levels in the mesolimbic system and locus ceruleus simulate reward achieved by nicotine. Insomnia is the most common adverse effect. Bupropion SR increases risk for seizures and caution advised in Bulimia.

17.4.3 Alcohol

In addition to psychosocial treatments, most guidelines recommend pharmacotherapy as the default position for moderate-to-severe alcohol dependence or for mild alcohol dependence not responding to psychosocial interventions alone [47].

1. Naltrexone: Naltrexone is contraindicated in patients who are currently using opiates as this might result in precipitated opiate withdrawal. Further, patients on Naltrexone cannot take opiates even for legitimate pain concerns, limiting the scope of its use in chronic pain patients. This acts as a mu opioid antagonist and is thought to mitigate "high" associated with alcohol use and reduces cravings. It is available in oral preparation as well as once monthly injections. Naltrexone is useful for patients who are not yet ready to quit, but want to cut down on alcohol. When prescribed in patients abstaining from alcohol, naltrexone is thought to prevent "a lapse from becoming a relapse." Naltrexone has also been found to be effective in decreasing binges even when taken on as needed basis.
2. Acamprosate: This acts as a functional NMDA antagonist and has evidence base for maintaining abstinence or "preventing a lapse." It is more effective when started early in the period of abstinence as it mitigates the hyper-glutamergic state caused by alcohol withdrawal.
3. Disulfiram: This acts by inhibiting the enzyme aldehyde dehydrogenase. This causes accumulation of acetaldehyde when taken with alcohol which results in an aversive reaction with dizziness, nausea, vomiting, and even hypotension at times. Non-adherence is a major concern with Disulfiram, but it was found to be effective when adherence was ensured by witnessed administration.

Other medications that have some evidence base include Baclofen and Topiramate, but they are not approved by the FDA for this indication. They may be considered if patient does not respond to Naltrexone, Acamprosate, and Disulfiram. There are no FDA-approved medications for cannabis, cocaine, or amphetamine use disorders at this time, but psychosocial treatments are helpful.

17.4.4 Psychotherapy

Screening Brief Intervention and Referral to Treatment (SBIRT) is designed to routinely assess and treat patients at risk of substance abuse in primary care settings [48]. While screening is discussed in the section above, the brief interventions are usually MI-based methods to enhance patients' motivation for change. CBT and Contingency management (CM) are other evidence-based psychotherapeutic approaches that have been helpful in substance abuse population. In addition to referral to substance abuse treatment programs, 12 step-based programs like Twelve Step Facilitation (TSF) may also help to improve outcomes. Referral to quit lines is another referral option for smoking cessation [14]. Social interventions like work placement programs for disabled patients and peer support groups for certain chronic pain conditions might be useful adjuncts to improve quality of life and functional status.

In summary, co-occurring substance use disorders in chronic pain patients dependent on opioids need to be managed aggressively to reduce risk of overdose and death as well as improve pain outcomes and outcomes for opioid dependence. Tobacco, alcohol, benzodiazepines, cannabis, cocaine and amphetamine use disorders are common comorbidities in this patient population. Careful, aggressive screening and assessment of comorbid substance abuse, random urine toxicology screens with immediate discussion of any abnormal results with patient and providing brief interventions, pharmacotherapy, and referrals when appropriate are key to the management of comorbid substance abuse in patients with chronic pain who are dependent on opioids.

References

1. Morasco BJ, Gritzner S, Lewis L, Oldham R, Turk DC, Dobscha SK. Systematic review of prevalence, correlates, and treatment outcomes for chronic non-cancer pain in patients with comorbid substance use disorder. Pain. 2011;152(3):488–97.
2. Chang Y-P, Compton P. Management of chronic pain with chronic opioid therapy in patients with substance use disorders. Addict Sci Clin Pract. 2013;8:21.
3. Edlund MJ, Steffick D, Hudson T, Harris KM, Sullivan M. Risk factors for clinically recognized opioid abuse and dependence among veterans using opioids for chronic non-cancer pain. Pain. 2007;129(3):355–62.
4. Huffman KL, Shella ER, Sweis G, Griffith SD, Scheman J, Covington EC. Nonopioid substance use disorders and opioid dose predict therapeutic opioid addiction. J Pain. 2015; 16(2):126–34.
5. Larson MJ, Paasche-Orlow M, Cheng DM, Lloyd-Travaglini C, Saitz R, Samet JH. Persistent pain is associated with substance use after detoxification: a prospective cohort analysis. Addiction. 2007;102(5):752–60.
6. Caldeiro RM, Malte CA, Calsyn DA, Baer JS, Nichol P, Kivlahan DR, et al. The association of persistent pain with out-patient addiction treatment outcomes and service utilization. Addiction. 2008;103(12):1996–2005.
7. Dunn KE, Brooner RK, Clark MR. Severity and interference of chronic pain in methadone-maintained outpatients: pain in methadone-maintenance patients. Pain Med. 2014;15(9): 1540–8.
8. Webster LR, Webster RM. Predicting aberrant behaviors in opioid-treated patients: preliminary validation of the Opioid Risk Tool. Pain Med. 2005;6(6):432–42.
9. Weisner CM, Campbell CI, Ray GT, Saunders K, Merrill JO, Banta-Green C, et al. Trends in prescribed opioid therapy for non-cancer pain for individuals with prior substance use disorders. Pain. 2009;145(3):287–93.
10. Campbell G, Nielsen S, Bruno R, Lintzeris N, Cohen M, Hall W, et al. The Pain and Opioids IN Treatment study: characteristics of a cohort using opioids to manage chronic non-cancer pain. Pain. 2015;156(2):231–42.
11. Dhingra L, Perlman DC, Masson C, Chen J, McKnight C, Jordan AE, et al. Longitudinal analysis of pain and illicit drug use behaviors in outpatients on methadone maintenance. Drug Alcohol Depend. 2015;149:285–9.

12. Calcaterra S, Glanz J, Binswanger IA. National trends in pharmaceutical opioid related over-dose deaths compared to other substance related overdose deaths: 1999-2009. Drug Alcohol Depend. 2013;131(3):263–70.
13. Madadi P, Hildebrandt D, Lauwers AE, Koren G. Characteristics of opioid-users whose death was related to opioid-toxicity: a population-based study in Ontario, Canada. PLoS One. 2013; 8(4), e60600.
14. Baca CT, Yahne CE. Smoking cessation during substance abuse treatment: What you need to know. J Subst Abuse Treat. 2009;36(2):205–19.
15. Fishbain DA, Cole B, Lewis JE, Gao J. Is smoking associated with alcohol-drug dependence in patients with pain and chronic pain patients? An evidence-based structured review. Pain Med. 2012;13(9):1212–26.
16. Hooten WM, Townsend CO, Bruce BK, Warner DO. The effects of smoking status on opioid tapering among patients with chronic pain. Anesth Analg. 2009;108(1):308–15.
17. Wahawisan J, Kolluru S, Nguyen T, Molina C, Speake J. Methadone toxicity due to smoking cessation—a case report on the drug-drug interaction involving cytochrome P450 isoenzyme 1A2. Ann Pharmacother. 2011;45(6), e34.
18. Ali NA, Marshall RW, Allen EM, Graham DF, Richens A. Comparison of the effects of thera-peutic doses of meptazinol and a dextropropoxyphene/paracetamol mixture alone and in com-bination with ethanol on ventilatory function and saccadic eye movements. Br J Clin Pharmacol. 1985;20(6):631–7.
19. Gudin JA, Mogali S, Jones JD, Comer SD. Risks, management, and monitoring of combina-tion opioid, benzodiazepines, and/or alcohol use. Postgrad Med. 2013;125(4):115–30.
20. Zacny JP, Gutierrez S. Subjective, psychomotor, and physiological effects of oxycodone alone and in combination with ethanol in healthy volunteers. Psychopharmacology (Berl). 2011;218(3):471–81.
21. Bailey PL, Pace NL, Ashburn MA, Moll JW, East KA, Stanley TH. Frequent hypoxemia and apnea after sedation with midazolam and fentanyl. Anesthesiology. 1990;73(5):826–30.
22. Faroqui MH, Cole M, Curran J. Buprenorphine, benzodiazepines and respiratory depression. Anaesthesia. 1983;38(10):1002–3.
23. Skurtveit S, Furu K, Bramness J, Selmer R, Tverdal A. Benzodiazepines predict use of opi-oids—a follow-up study of 17,074 men and women. Pain Med. 2010;11(6):805–14.
24. Hermos JA, Young MM, Gagnon DR, Fiore LD. Characterizations of long-term oxycodone/acetaminophen prescriptions in veteran patients. Arch Intern Med. 2004;164(21):2361–6.
25. Bachhuber MA, Saloner B, Cunningham CO, Barry CL. Medical cannabis laws and opioid analgesic overdose mortality in the United States, 1999-2010. JAMA Intern Med. 2014; 174(10):1668–73.
26. Abrams DI, Couey P, Shade SB, Kelly ME, Benowitz NL. Cannabinoid-opioid interaction in chronic pain. Clin Pharmacol Ther. 2011;90(6):844–51.
27. Degenhardt L, Lintzeris N, Campbell G, Bruno R, Cohen M, Farrell M, et al. Experience of adjunctive cannabis use for chronic non-cancer pain: findings from the Pain and Opioids IN Treatment (POINT) study. Drug Alcohol Depend. 2015;147:144–50.
28. Reisfield GM, Wasan AD, Jamison RN. The prevalence and significance of cannabis use in patients prescribed chronic opioid therapy: a review of the extant literature. Pain Med. 2009;10(8):1434–41.
29. Reisfield GM. Medical cannabis and chronic opioid therapy. J Pain Palliat Care Pharmacother. 2010;24(4):356–61.
30. Magnano AR, Talathoti NB, Hallur R, Jurus DT, Dizon J, Holleran S, et al. Effect of Acute Cocaine Administration on the QTc Interval of Habitual Users. Am J Cardiol. 2006;97(8): 1244–6.
31. Meghani SH, Wiedemer NL, Becker WC, Gracely EJ, Gallagher RM. Predictors of resolution of aberrant drug behavior in chronic pain patients treated in a structured opioid risk manage-ment program. Pain Med. 2009;10(5):858–65.
32. Ives TJ, Chelminski PR, Hammett-Stabler CA, Malone RM, Perhac JS, Potisek NM, et al. Predictors of opioid misuse in patients with chronic pain: a prospective cohort study. BMC Health Serv Res. 2006;6:46.

33. Akbik H, Butler SF, Budman SH, Fernandez K, Katz NP, Jamison RN. Validation and clinical application of the Screener and Opioid Assessment for Patients with Pain (SOAPP). J Pain Symptom Manage. 2006;32(3):287–93.

34. Tsuang MT, Lyons MJ, Meyer JM, Doyle T, Eisen SA, Goldberg J, et al. Co-occurrence of abuse of different drugs in men: the role of drug-specific and shared vulnerabilities. Arch Gen Psychiatry. 1998;55(11):967–72.

35. Kahan M, Wilson L, Mailis-Gagnon A, Srivastava A. National Opioid Use Guideline Group. Canadian guideline for safe and effective use of opioids for chronic noncancer pain: clinical summary for family physicians. Part 2: special populations. Can Fam Physician. 2011; 57(11):1269–76. e419–28.

36. Fiore MC, Bailey WC, Cohen SJ, Dorfman SF, Goldstein MG, Gritz ER, et al. Smoking cessation. Clinical practice guideline no. 18 (AHCPR Publication No. 96-0692). Rockville, MD: US Department of Health and Human Services. Public Health Serv Agency Health Care Policy Res; 1996.

37. Kahan M, Mailis-Gagnon A, Wilson L, Srivastava A. National Opioid Use Guideline Group. Canadian guideline for safe and effective use of opioids for chronic noncancer pain: clinical summary for family physicians. Part 1: general population. Can Fam Physician. 2011;57(11): 1257–66. e407–18.

38. Manchikanti L, Abdi S, Atluri S, Balog CC, Benyamin RM, Boswell MV, et al. American Society of Interventional Pain Physicians (ASIPP) guidelines for responsible opioid prescribing in chronic non-cancer pain: Part 2—guidance. Pain Physician. 2012;15(3 Suppl):S67–116.

39. Christo PJ, Manchikanti L, Ruan X, Bottros M, Hansen H, Solanki DR, et al. Urine drug testing in chronic pain. Pain Physician. 2011;14(2):123–43.

40. Helander A, Böttcher M, Fehr C, Dahmen N, Beck O. Detection times for urinary ethyl glucuronide and ethyl sulfate in heavy drinkers during alcohol detoxification. Alcohol Alcohol. 2009;44(1):55–61.

41. Manchikanti L, Abdi S, Atluri S, Balog CC, Benyamin RM, Boswell MV, et al. American Society of Interventional Pain Physicians (ASIPP) guidelines for responsible opioid prescribing in chronic non-cancer pain: Part I—evidence assessment. Pain Physician. 2012;15(3 Suppl): S1–65.

42. Sullivan MD, Edlund MJ, Steffick D, Unützer J. Regular use of prescribed opioids: association with common psychiatric disorders. Pain. 2005;119(1-3):95–103.

43. Cheatle MD, Gallagher RM. Chronic pain and comorbid mood and substance use disorders: a biopsychosocial treatment approach. Curr Psychiatry Rep. 2006;8(5):371–6.

44. Haibach JP, Beehler GP, Dollar KM, Finnell DS. Moving toward integrated behavioral intervention for treating multimorbidity among chronic pain, depression, and substance-use disorders in primary care. Med Care. 2014;52(4):322–7.

45. Petrakis IL, Carroll KM, Nich C, Gordon LT, McCance-Katz EF, Frankforter T, et al. Disulfiram treatment for cocaine dependence in methadone-maintained opioid addicts. Addiction. 2000; 95(2):219–28.

46. Campbell BK, Wander N, Stark MJ, Holbert T. Treating cigarette smoking in drug-abusing clients. J Subst Abuse Treat. 1995;12(1):89–94.

47. Lingford-Hughes AR, Welch S, Peters L, Nutt DJ, British Association for Psychopharmacology, Expert Reviewers Group. BAP updated guidelines: evidence-based guidelines for the pharmacological management of substance abuse, harmful use, addiction and comorbidity: recommendations from BAP. J Psychopharmacol. 2012;26(7):899–952.

48. Agerwala SM, McCance-Katz EF. Integrating screening, brief intervention, and referral to treatment (SBIRT) into clinical practice settings: a brief review. J Psychoactive Drugs. 2012; 44(4):307–17.

Index

© Springer International Publishing Switzerland 2016
A.M. Matthews, J.C. Fellers (eds.), *Treating Comorbid Opioid Use Disorder
in Chronic Pain*, DOI 10.1007/978-3-319-29863-4

N
Naloxone, 97
Naltrexone, 227
National All Schedules Prescription Electronic
    Reporting Act (NASPER), 144
National Center for Health Statistics, 166
National Center for Injury Prevention and
    Control, 166
National Comorbidity Survey (NCS), 199
National Comorbidity Survey Replication
    (NCS-R), 199
National Drug Control Strategy, 169
National Epidemiologic Survey on Alcohol
    and Related Conditions (NESARC),
    199, 201
National Institute of Neurological Disorders
    and Stroke (NINDS), 162
National Institute on Alcohol Abuse and
    Alcoholism (NIAAA), 158
National Institute on Drug Abuse (NIDA),
    133, 158, 164
National Institutes of Health (NIH), 162–165
National Pain Strategy Task Force, 163, 164
National Survey of Substance Abuse
    Treatment Services (N-SSATS), 161
National Survey on Drug Use and Health
    (NSDUH), 14, 160, 161
Nausea, 194
Neonatal abstinence syndrome (NAS), 95, 96
NESARC. See National Epidemiologic Survey
    on Alcohol and Related Conditions
    (NESARC)
Nicotine replacement therapy (NRT), 226
NIH Pain Consortium, 162
Nonmedical prescription opioid use (NMPOU)
    disorders, 91, 199, 201, 204
Non-opioid analgesia, 190–191
Non-opioid substance abuse, 215–217
Non-opioid substance use, 216
Nonpharmacologic approaches, 25
Non-steroidal anti-inflammatory drugs
    (NSAIDS), 109, 186, 190
Number needed to treat (NNT), 70
Numeric Rating Scale (NRS), 48

O
Obsessive-compulsive disorder (OCD), 205
Office of the National Drug Control Policy
    (ONDCP), 155, 169–170
Older adults, pain management
    assessment, 105–106
    chronic conditions, 105

    chronic pain assessment, 106
    complications, 104–105
    medication management, 110, 111
    neuropathic pain, 110–112
    non-opioid analgesics, 109
    nonpharmacological approaches, 108–109
    opioid pain management, 111–114
    pharmacokinetic changes, 104
    polypharmacy in, 104
    principles for, 106–108
Oligoanalgesia, 187
Opiates, 13
Opiate Treatment Programs, 143
Opioid abuse
    definition, 14
    epidemiology, 14, 15
    forensic studies, 16
    healthcare clinicians, 14
    incidence of prescription, 14
    and misuse, 19
    portenoy, 16
    potential study, 17
    prevalence rates, 19
    problematic use, 14, 19
    risk and rates, 16
    standardizing terminology, 17
    wide-ranging estimates, 17
Opioid Compliance Checklist (OCC), 54
Opioid maintenance therapies (OMT), 94
Opioid medications, 170
Opioid-related Behaviors in Treatment
    (ORBIT) scale, 217
Opioid risk tool (ORT), 105, 221, 222
Opioid rotation, 114
Opioids
    abuse (see Opioid abuse)
    drugs, 7
    immense medical utility, 13
    inhibition, 9
    medications, 170
    pain syndromes, 132
    prescription, 141, 142
    rotation, 114
    substitution therapy, 63
    tapering, 114
    therapy
        complex interventions, 133–135
        Multidisciplinary Pain Clinics, 177–179
        pill counts, 137
        primary care-based treatment, 134
        reimbursement system, 135
        substance use agreements, 137–138
        UDT, 135–136

Printed in the United States
By Bookmasters